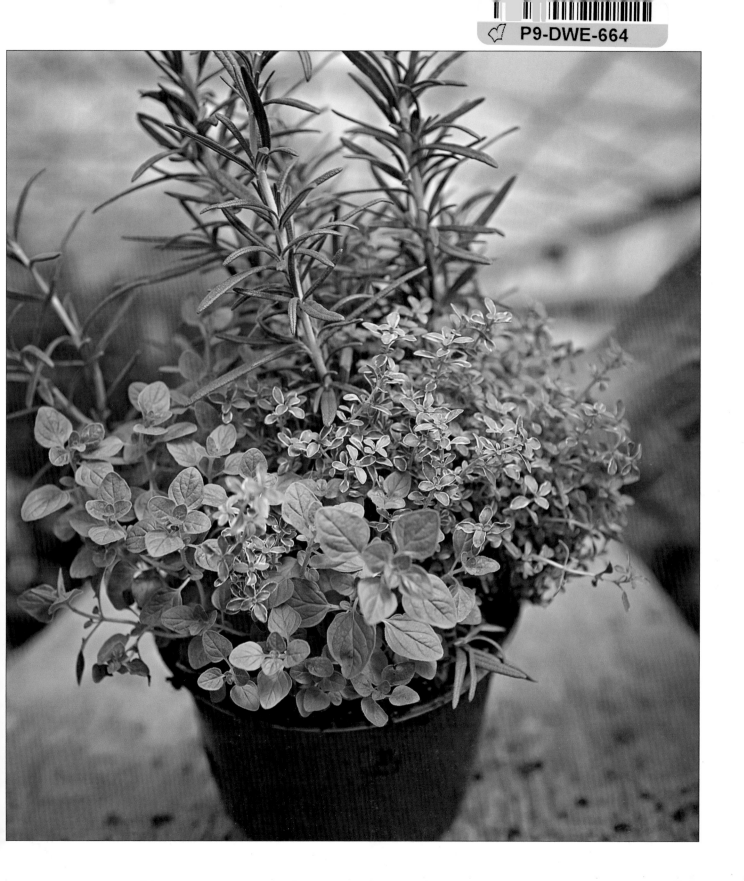

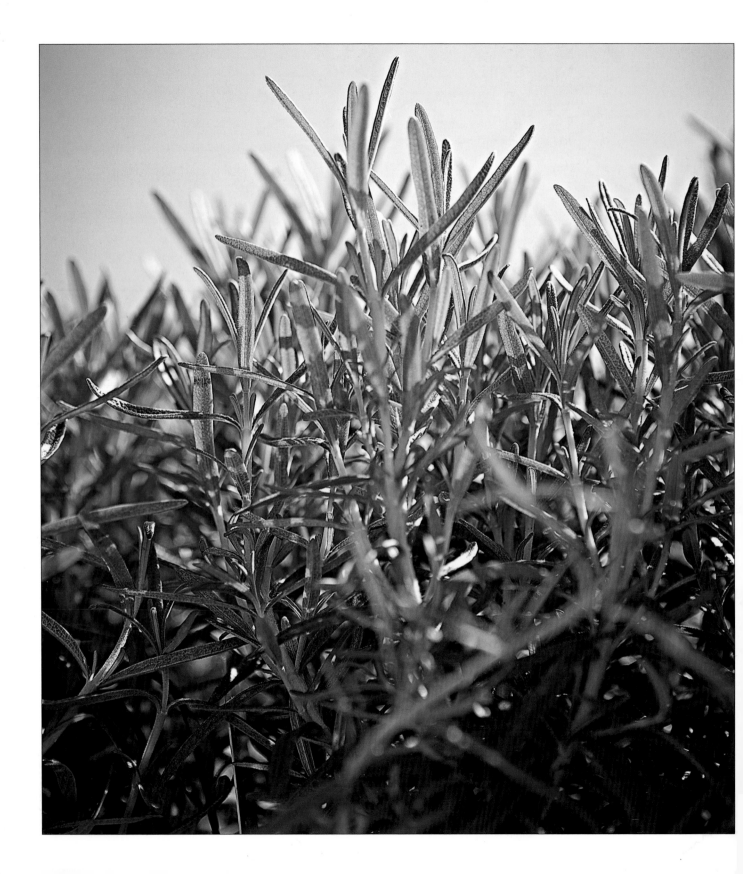

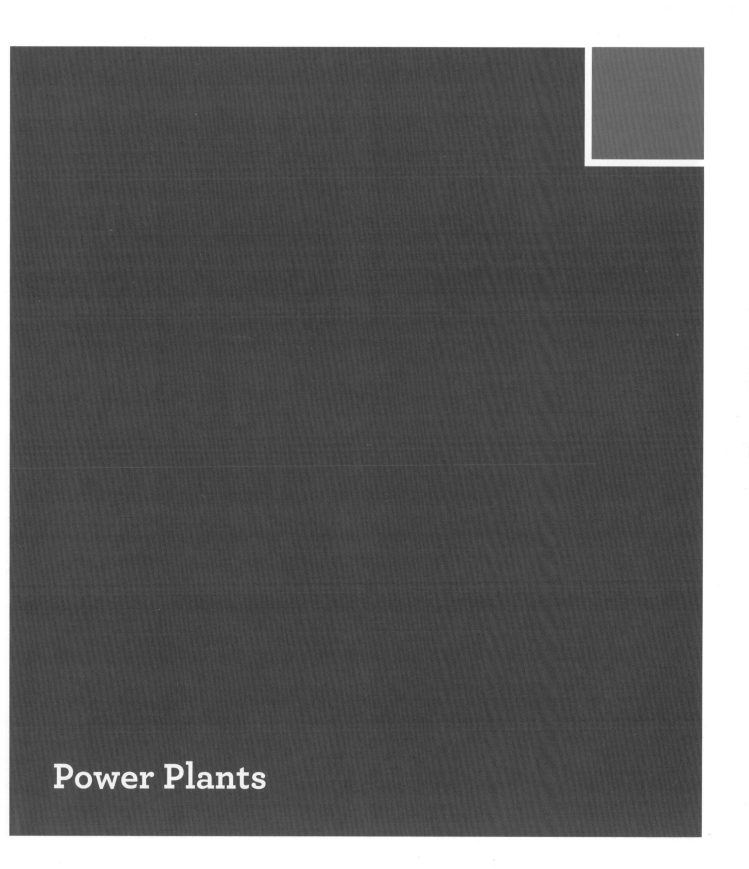

Power Plants

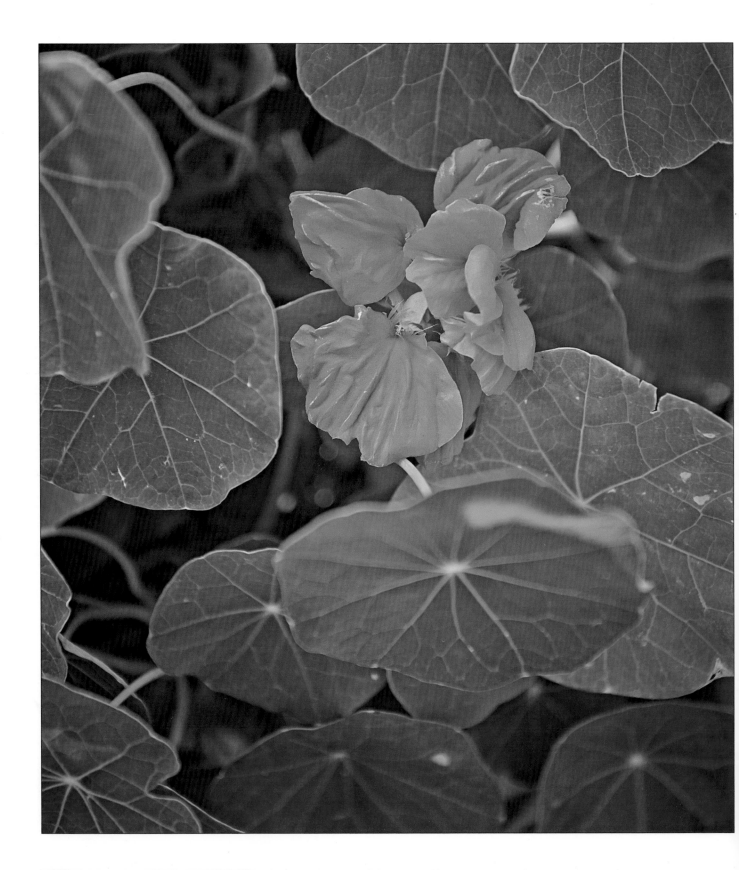

Collins

FRANKIE FLOWERS & BRYCE WYLDE

Photography by Shannon J. Ross

Power Plants

Simple Home Remedies You Can Grow

HarperCollins books may be purchased for educational,
business, or sales promotional use through our Special
Markets Department.

HarperCollins Publishers Ltd
2 Bloor Street East, 20th Floor
Toronto, Ontario, Canada
M4W 1A8

www.harpercollins.ca

Library and Archives Canada Cataloguing in Publication
data is available upon request

ISBN 978-1-44342-676-3

Printed and bound in Canada
DWF 9 8 7 6 5 4 3

Contents

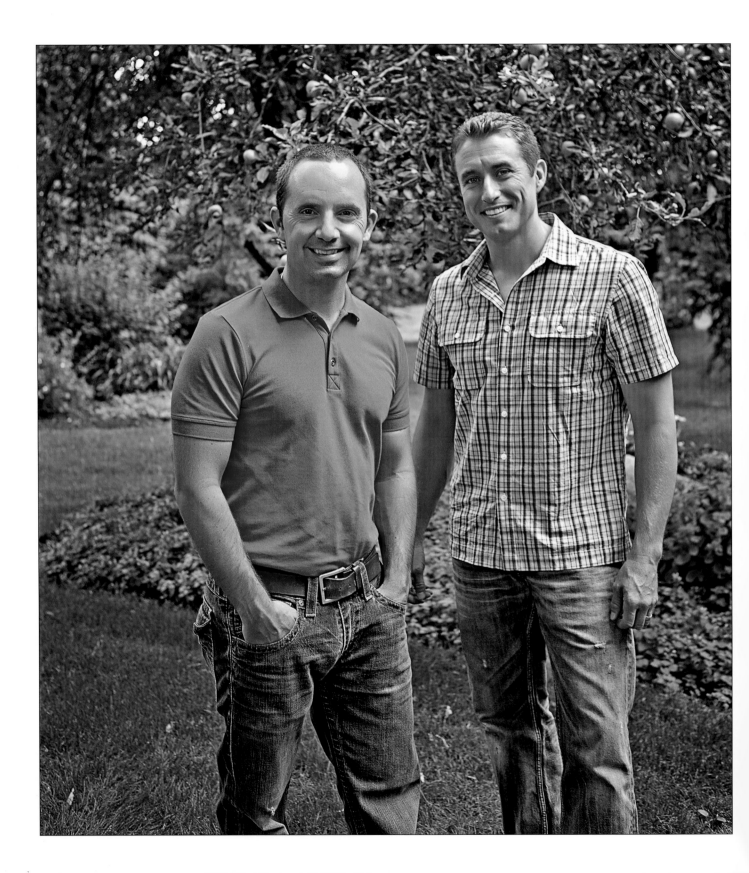

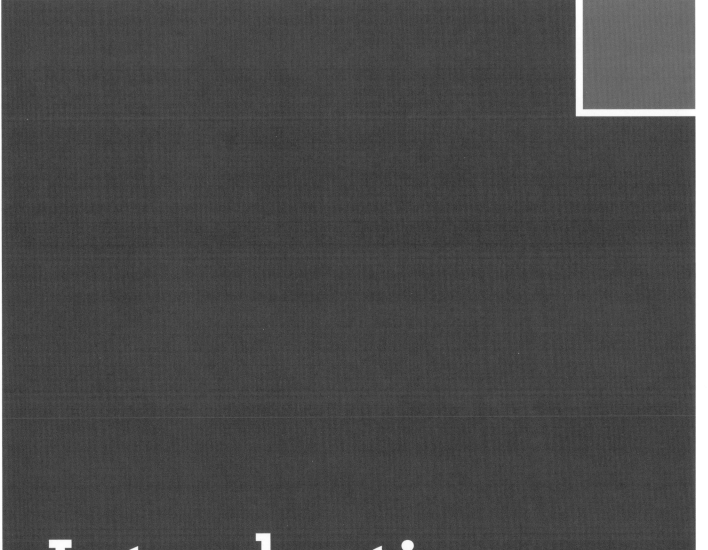

Introduction

What happens when an alternative health practitioner and a horticulturalist start talking? The conversation naturally turns to the relationship between plants and people—how working with plants is directly related to improved mood and overall health, and how so many ailments can be cured using plants. This conversation really did happen, and the result is the book you're holding now.

The two of us appear regularly on Breakfast Television and CityLine, where we share our passions with a large TV audience—Bryce as an alternative health practitioner and nutritionist, and "Frankie Flowers" as a popular and respected gardening expert. Eventually we decided to combine our talents and collaborate on a book that would help people improve their own health from the ground up.

In one of our early conversations, we considered the question "Does an apple a day really keep the doctor away?" Let's look at what science says an apple really is: It's made up of fibre, antioxidants, calcium, carotenoids, iron, lutein, magnesium, riboflavin, thiamine, tryptophan, and zinc, among many other things. All this "stuff" helps you lower cholesterol, reduce inflammation, lose weight and balance blood sugar, and feel better. The humble apple can even help manage our biggest modern health issues: heart disease, diabetes, and cancer.

But there are even more powerful allies in the garden: plants that don't just provide good nutrition over the long term, but also have healing abilities for acute ailments. That's what we wanted to focus on when we decided to team up for this book. We want to show you how to grow your own remedies—organic and local alternatives to overprescribed drugs and expensive health-store cures. It is a perfect partnership: Bryce explains how and why each plant is used in medicine, and Frankie shows readers how to grow it at home.

Bryce grew up in Canada, but in an English garden setting. His mother, born and raised on a farm in Colchester, England, had 10 green thumbs! Bryce and his two sisters were each responsible for their own plot in the back garden. Tending their plants was as common a chore as taking out the garbage.

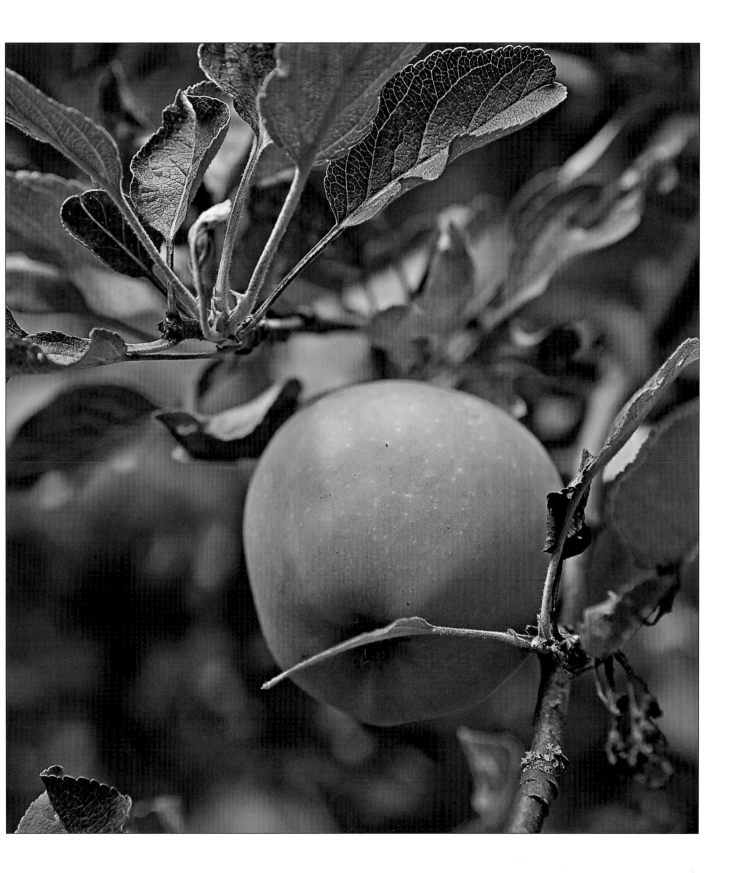

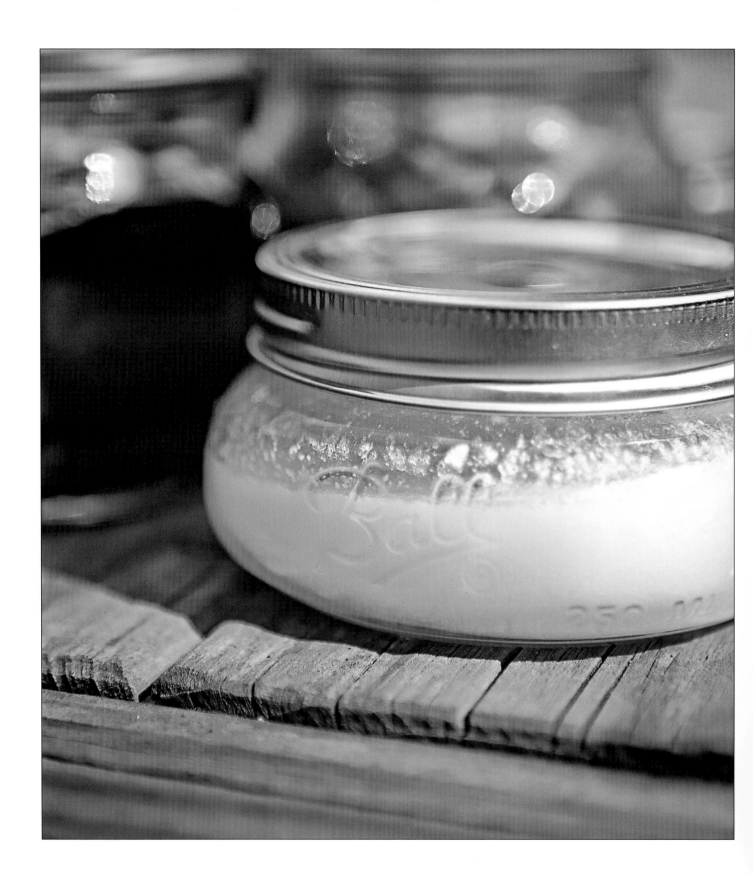

Frankie's first home was attached to a greenhouse. His grandfather, father, and uncles grew everything from pansies to produce on the rich soils of the Holland Marsh in southern Ontario. As immigrants from Italy, they built what is today Bradford Greenhouses, one of Canada's largest combined greenhouse and garden centre operations.

We don't see gardening as a chore or even a job—we never have. We find tilling, weeding, and growing to be relaxing, rewarding, and enjoyable. But don't just take our word for it: The latest research shows gardening really does help you ground yourself—excuse the pun—and manage the stress of day-to-day life.

This book combines our expertise and our passions to create an instructional guide—step by step, plant by plant, ailment by ailment, recipe by recipe—to help you achieve better health. *Power Plants* includes profiles of 49 different plants with medicinal value, all of which can be grown at home by anyone with modest gardening skills.

Each profile begins with an introduction to the plant and an overview of its health benefits, including a description of its active ingredients and how they work. Bryce explains how the plant can be used as a powerful alternative remedy, and how its medicinal uses have evolved over time.

Frankie then shows you how to grow these plants in your own garden. He tells you how to find the right location, when to plant, how to nurture your crop, and how to harvest. If you've got a little dirt under your fingernails you'll have no problem following these instructions. But if you're new to gardening, flip to "A Gardening Primer" on page 353 to learn some basic skills before you dig in.

We share several recipes and home remedies that harness the power of each plant. Before you use any of the preparations in these pages, understand that this book does not replace professional healthcare advice. It's intended as a reference volume only. We want to help you make informed decisions about what you might do to improve your health, but the remedies are not a substitute for any treatment that may have been prescribed by your family physician or any other licensed doctor. If you suspect you have a medical problem requiring professional care, we urge you to seek competent help.

We have listed a number of cautions you should observe when using each plant. However, these potential side effects and contraindications are not exhaustive. Before starting any new health program, or before you begin taking any medication or supplement—whether conventional, natural, or plant-based, and whether made on your own or bought from a store—always check with your primary health-care provider first.

Good things come to people who wait. But if you can't wait to grow your own—or you don't have the ability to do so—then look to the Fast Forward section we've included in each plant profile. Here we suggest a retail product with equal purity and efficacy. These can be found in health food stores or specialized pharmacies, or ordered online.

Having your own garden means you'll know exactly where your food and medicinal plants came from: they won't have travelled thousands of miles, and you can be certain that no chemicals, growth hormones, synthetic fertilizers, or preservatives have been used. And your garden won't just benefit your health; it will also give you the sense of ownership and pride that comes with being your own urban farmer. So let's get growing!

— *Bryce Wylde and Frank Ferragine*

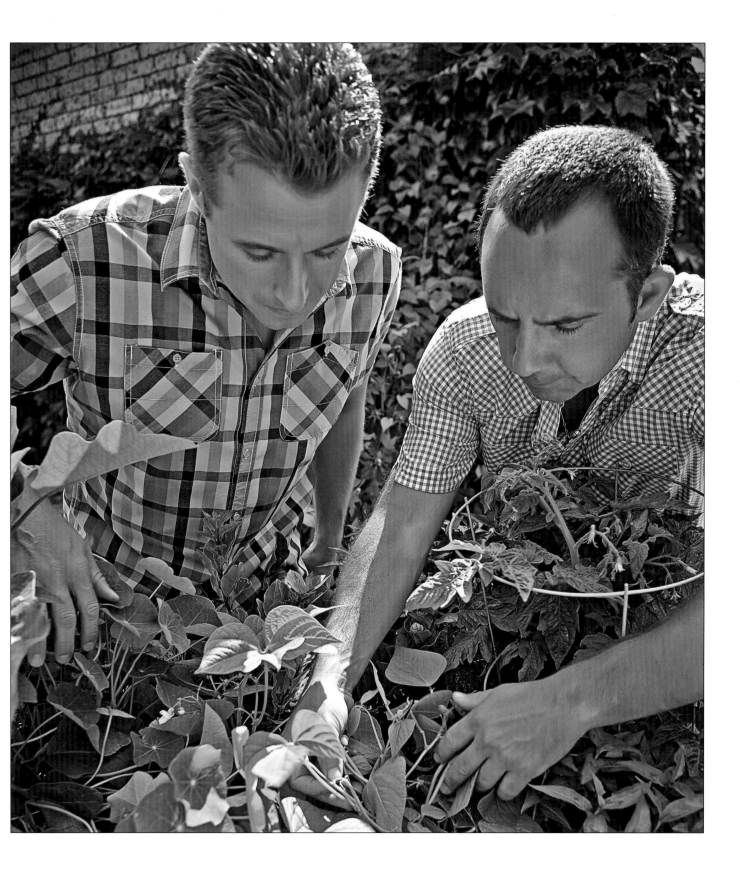

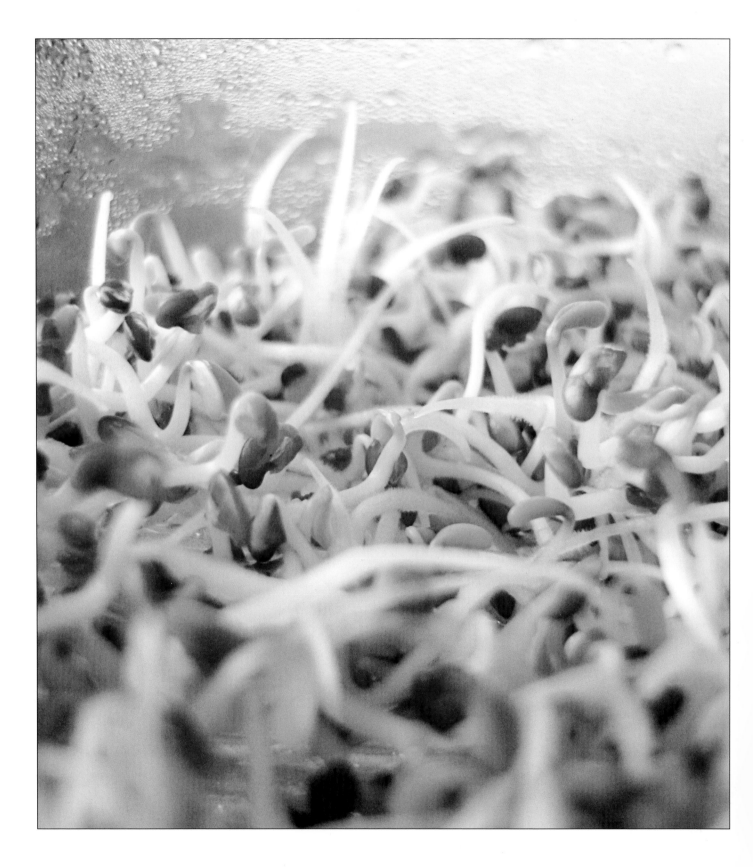

Alfalfa

When you think of legumes, peas and beans probably come to mind. You might not think of alfalfa: Like peanuts, it's a surprising addition to the legume family (*Fabaceae*). Also known as lucerne, alfalfa has a long history of dietary and medicinal uses. Native to western Asia and the eastern Mediterranean, alfalfa is common forage for cattle, and alfalfa sprouts are a popular food around the world.

Health Benefits

In traditional Chinese medicine, alfalfa has been used to treat gastrointestinal problems and coughs, while in India it has been used to support digestion and treat boils, water retention, and even arthritis. Native Americans used alfalfa to promote blood clotting and treat jaundice.

Preliminary research suggests alfalfa can reduce cholesterol and artery plaque formation. Alfalfa also seems to have some ability to lower blood sugar. Obesity is an epidemic in North America, and it contributes to diabetes and heart disease, so this humble little plant may have the potential to help with some of the most important health issues of our time.

Like all legumes, alfalfa contains some protein. It is packed with powerful antioxidants (vitamins A, C, E, and K) as well as vitamins B1 and B6. It also contains calcium, potassium, iron, and zinc.

As an herb, dried alfalfa leaf (as opposed to the more familiar sprouts) has a very mild grassy flavour and can be mixed in salads and soups without much change in taste. Alfalfa leaves contain saponins, compounds that block the absorption of cholesterol and prevent the formation of plaque. They also contain flavones and isoflavones, which are thought to be responsible for estrogen-like effects. Although it has not been confirmed in human trials, alfalfa is sometimes used to treat menopause symptoms.

Growing

Alfalfa sprouts are fast-germinating and easy to grow, and they require very little space: From sowing to serving can take as little as 5 days! That makes these instant gratifiers an excellent way to get kids into gardening. All you really need are some seeds,

DIFFICULTY
Easy

HARDINESS
Annual; best grown indoors

TIME TO PLANT
Can be grown indoors year-round

TIME TO HARVEST
5 to 7 days after sowing seeds or immediately after green tips emerge

SOIL TYPE
No soil required

water, a glass jar (like a Mason jar), a rubber band, and cheese-cloth. When growing alfalfa, healthy seeds are clean seeds—it's very important to rinse your seeds twice daily to reduce the risk of harmful bacteria growing in the jar.

Common Varieties: Purchase alfalfa seeds labelled "sprouting seeds" or "for sprouting." These will be pathogen-free.

PLANT

Measure a tablespoon of alfalfa seeds and place them in the bottom of a jar (1 tablespoon of seeds will yield about 1½ cups of sprouts). Cover the seeds with ½ cup of cool water. Cover the top of the jar with cheesecloth, secure it with a rubber band, and let the seeds soak overnight.

GROW

In the morning, without removing the cheesecloth, drain the water and thoroughly rinse the seeds by adding fresh water and swishing it around in the jar. Then completely drain the water and place the jar in indirect light at room temperature (about 20°C/68°F). Repeat this rinsing every 8 to 12 hours (once in the morning and again at night) for 3 to 5 days. After 3 days, white shoots will emerge. Within 4 or 5 days, the jar will fill with a tangle of growing sprouts.

The most common cause of failure when growing sprouts is inadequate drainage. You may want to place the jar sideways on a downward-sloping angle so any excess water drips through the cheesecloth and out of the jar.

This same process can be used for many types of sprouts: Consider bean, radish, beet, pea, and sunflower sprouts. As a general rule, any plant with edible stems is a good option for sprouting.

HARVEST

On approximately the sixth day or when leaves appear, the sprouts are fully grown. Taste them for crispness and flavour, and

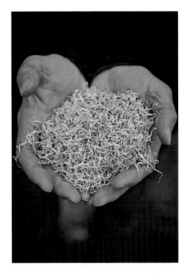

A fresh harvest of alfalfa sprouts.

if they're ready, rinse, drain, and enjoy. However, if your sprouts don't smell or taste right—for example, if they smell like rotten lettuce or a mouldy towel—don't eat them! Sprouts grown in dirty water or in a jar not properly drained can be contaminated with bacteria, including salmonella and *E. coli*.

STORE

Rinse the sprouts. Dry the sprouts on a clean paper towel or use a fine-mesh salad spinner to remove excess water. Use immediately or store in an airtight container in the refrigerator for up to 3 days.

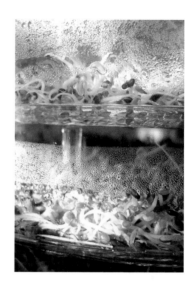

⚙ Put It to Work

Plugged arteries? Drink a degummer tea!

Alfalfa is sold in bulk as a dried herb or in tablets, capsules, and liquid extracts, but reaping its medicinal effects can be as easy as brewing your own alfalfa tea.

The active ingredient in alfalfa (saponins) can bind to cholesterol and prevent its absorption. Studies have reported reductions in total cholesterol and "bad cholesterol" (low-density lipoprotein or LDL) after taking 10 grams of dried alfalfa herb 3 times daily. This won't alter your "good cholesterol" (high-density lipoprotein or HDL) levels. Alfalfa also has been studied for its ability to reduce plaque buildup on the insides of artery walls.

If you're growing your own sprouts, buy extra seeds to make this potent artery degumming tea. Add 1 tablespoon of alfalfa seed to a clean coffee or spice grinder and pulverize. Tap the contents into a mug. Add boiling water and steep for 10 minutes. Strain the tea through a fine-mesh sieve lined with cheesecloth or a coffee filter. Drink 2 to 3 cups daily.

Blood sugar spiking? Help it take a dip!

Studies report that alfalfa can reduce blood sugar levels. Why not use your alfalfa sprouts to make a nutrient-dense chip dip to tide you over between lunch and dinner?

Enjoy this dip with black corn tortilla chips, which complement the flavour of the alfalfa and give you an extra dose of antioxidants. Portion control is key in the management of blood sugar, so allow yourself 10 chips per serving, which is equivalent to about 35 grams of carbohydrates and 140 calories. Use no more than ¼ teaspoon of dip per chip.

» Fast Forward

Fast forward to the health food store and purchase Solgar alfalfa leaf capsules or equivalent. Follow the instructions on the label.

! Cautions

With its ability to manage cholesterol, alfalfa can be heart-healthy but if you're also taking a blood-thinning medication, the high levels of vitamin K found in alfalfa can be a contraindication.

Some evidence suggests alfalfa might stimulate the immune system, so it might not be a good idea if you have an autoimmune disease such as multiple sclerosis, systemic lupus erythematosus, or rheumatoid arthritis.

Alfalfa might reduce blood sugar levels, so if you have diabetes you'll need to monitor your levels more closely when using it.

Since alfalfa may have mild estrogenic effects, women with hormone-sensitive conditions (including breast, uterine, and ovarian cancer, and endometriosis and uterine fibroids) should possibly avoid it.

Alfalfa Dip

1 cup alfalfa sprouts
1 yellow bell pepper, chopped
½ cucumber, peeled and chopped
¼ cup nutritional brewer's yeast
1 cup plain low-fat yogurt
1 tsp vegetable soup mix
¼ tsp paprika

Combine all of the ingredients except the paprika in a blender and blend on high speed until smooth. Transfer to a bowl and sprinkle with paprika. Garnish with a small bunch of alfalfa.

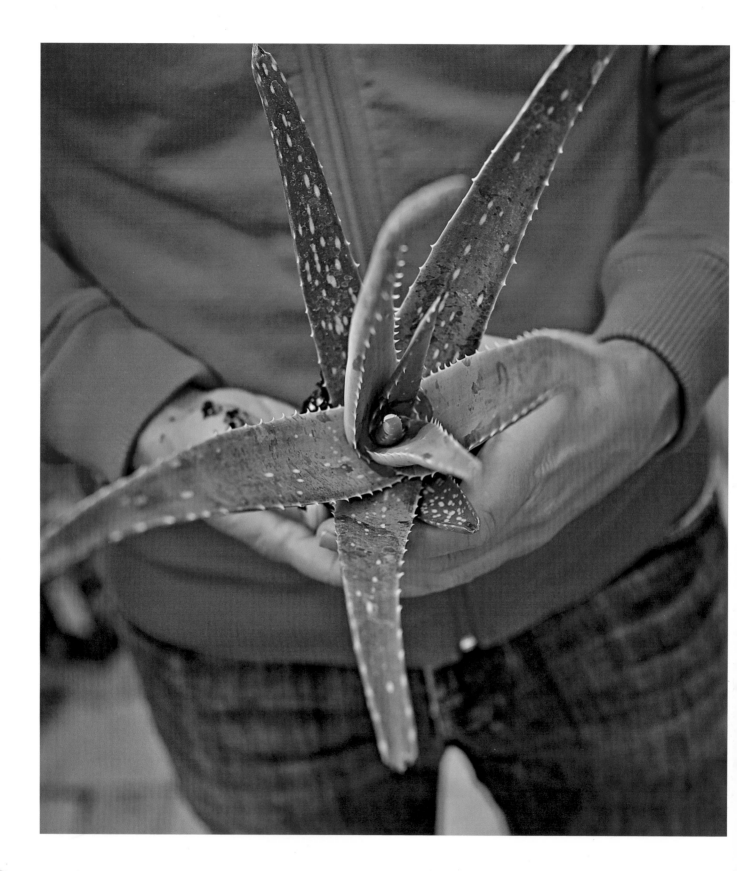

Aloe Vera

Aloe vera is a cactus-like succulent plant with thick, fleshy leaves. The aloe family probably originated in Africa, but it has been cultivated all over the world for centuries. The leaves contain two different substances that have long been used for medicinal purposes. The first is a transparent gel-like substance commonly used as an ointment. The second is the inner part of the leaf surrounding this gel, which contains a yellowish compound called aloe latex.

✚ Health Benefits

The gel from aloe vera leaves has been used for thousands of years to treat wounds, skin infections, burns, and numerous other skin conditions. More recently, promising research in both animal and human studies suggests that topical aloe gel has immune-balancing properties that improve skin inflammation.

It is thought that the moisturizing, emollient, and healing properties of aloe are due in part to its polysaccharides—long-chain carbohydrates such as aloeride and acemannan—as well as numerous powerful antioxidants. These work together to exhibit the immune-boosting, antiviral, and healing effects that become so evident when you apply aloe to your skin.

Aloe vera may also be the most important plant ever discovered for digestive health. Odds are high that you or a member of your family suffers from some sort of digestive disorder. More than 60 million North Americans suffer from frequent heartburn, 15 million experience it daily, 25 million have been treated for ulcers at some point in their life, and more than 30 million qualify for the diagnosis of irritable bowel syndrome.

The dried aloe latex has long been taken orally as a laxative. Aloe vera juice also contains a natural acid buffer called calcium malate (also known as malic acid). Drinking homegrown aloe juice will not only reduce the acid in your stomach immediately, but over time it will continue to buffer the hydrochloric acid your stomach produces and heal any tissue damaged by acid erosion due to heartburn and gastroesophageal reflux disease (GERD).

🌱 Growing

Aloe vera is inexpensive and easy to grow. It can be found almost any time of year at garden centres and big box stores. I think it's

Aloe vera was known to the Egyptians more than 6,000 years ago as the "plant of immortality," and Cleopatra reportedly used it to improve the beauty of her skin. The ancient Greeks thought of aloe as a "miracle health plant," and Alexander the Great is said to have conquered certain territories specifically to secure control of the plant.

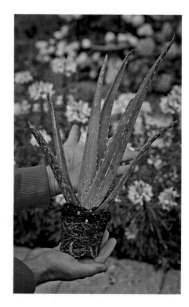

a must-have, whether you enjoy it as a houseplant or as a potted plant in your landscape. The key is to give it as much sun as possible and not to overwater. Aloe doesn't require fertilizer, and the more you leave it alone the better it grows!

Common Varieties: There are almost 500 varieties of *Aloe*, and several produce the latex used for medicinal purposes. But *Aloe vera* (which means "true aloe") is the only species that yields the iconic gel that is so wonderful for the skin.

PLANT

Aloe is so readily available and inexpensive that you may simply want to buy it. However, one of the reasons it is so inexpensive is that it's easy to grow! Take a cutting measuring 6 to 12 cm (2.5 to 5 inches) from a healthy leaf. Lay the cutting in a dry location for up to a week and allow the cut end to dry out or "scab." This reduces the risk of disease when rooting. Next, get a pot measuring 10 to 15 cm (4 to 6 inches) with good drainage (clay pots are ideal) and fill with store-bought cactus mix soil. Place the cutting into the soil with about a third of the leaf covered. Keep the soil moist for approximately 7 to 10 days, then reduce watering thereafter.

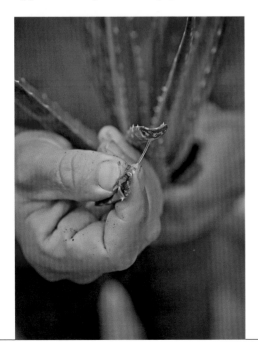

Here you can see both the aloe gel and the aloe latex—the yellowish inner edge of the plant.

DIFFICULTY
Easy

HARDINESS
Perennial in zones 9 to 11; can be grown indoors

TIME TO PLANT
Can be grown indoors year round; pots can be placed outdoors after all risk of frost has passed

TIME TO HARVEST
Harvest mature, rooted plants only: they should have 3 to 5 leaf stems

LOCATION
Full to part sun. Indoors: direct light in west- or south-facing window. Outdoors: indirect light at first to allow the plant time to adapt, then move into full sun

SOIL TYPE
Sandy; use potting soil formulated for cacti

GROW

Overwatering is the number 1 reason people fail at growing aloe vera. Remember, it's a drought-tolerant plant, and once rooted it prefers to be dry. Depending on the amount of light and humidity in your home or landscape, aloe vera may need as little as one watering per month. Test by placing your finger into the soil: only water if the soil feels completely dry to the touch. Another indicator of lack of water is leaves that become thin and curl.

Here's a good way to determine if your aloe is getting the right amount of light. Leaves turning brown? Your aloe is getting too much direct sun. Leaves lying flat? Your aloe is not getting enough sun.

HARVEST

Aloe vera can be harvested as soon as the plants are mature and healthy: The leaves should be fleshy and green and 20 to 25 cm (8 to 10 inches) long. Use the outermost leaves first, since these should be the oldest and largest.

Remove the leaf using a sharp, clean knife (1), slicing close to its base and away from the centre of the plant. A straight, clean cut is a must! Rinse the leaf and then soak it in a bowl with 3 cups of cold water mixed with 1 tablespoon of white vinegar for about an hour to allow the yellowish latex to release into the water.

Cut around the perimeter of the leaf to remove the serrated edges (2, 3), and then remove the skin by running the knife underneath it and peeling away (4). Presto, you're left with the pure gel!

STORE

Aloe vera is best used fresh, so I recommend harvesting it as needed. However, the leaves can be stored in an airtight container for up to a week. Some people place it in a resealable bag and freeze it, but I don't recommend this (it will lose potency). Fresh is always best.

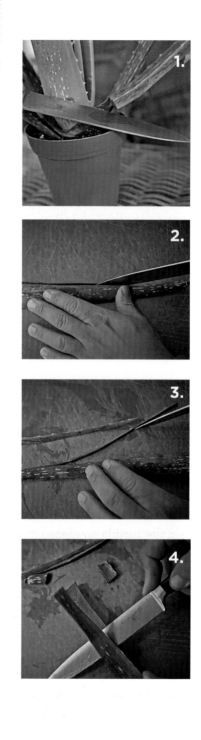

Put It to Work

Can't go? Drink some aloe!

A simple and effective formula to maintain soft stools and bowel regularity is to combine aloe gel with fibre and to drink this daily for 1 week.

Collect the aloe gel from 6 to 8 large leaves (about 6 ounces) as described on the opposite page, or simply peel away the rind from the leaves and squeeze out the gel. Transfer the gel to a blender, add 2 ounces of freshly squeezed citrus juice (orange, lemon, or grapefruit), and 1 teaspoon of psyllium powder or wheat bran. Blend on high speed until smooth. Drink immediately.

Heartburn? Drink up!

Here's how to make your own aloe juice. Using a very sharp knife, carefully peel away the rind from as many aloe leaves as necessary to extract 6 ounces of gel. Discard the rind. Peel away the top yellow layer (the aloe latex) and discard. Transfer the aloe gel to a blender and add the freshly squeezed juice of half a lemon and ½ cup of water. Blend on high speed until smooth (but not frothy). Drink immediately.

Sunburn or skin irritation? Aloe is soothing!

Evidence suggests aloe may aid healing of mild-to-moderate sunburn, eczema, dermatitis, and psoriasis. All you need to do is cut 3 medium-sized leaves from the aloe plant. Squeeze the gel out of the leaves into a sterile glass container. Add 2 ice cubes and stir gently to cool the aloe gel. Dip a clean paper towel or cotton swab into the liquid and apply liberally to affected areas. Repeat 3 to 5 times daily to speed healing, or as needed for relief.

⟫ Fast Forward

Fast forward to the health food store or the web to purchase AloeCure pure aloe juice or equivalent. Follow the instructions on the label.

! Cautions

There aren't many negative side effects from using aloe gel as a topical application; it is rare to have allergies to aloe. Recognize its limitations, however, and seek medical attention for severe burns.

Because aloe contains anthraquinones (compounds with laxative qualities), it should not be ingested by anyone with inflammatory intestinal diseases, including Crohn's disease or ulcerative colitis. It should also not be used by children or by women during pregnancy or breastfeeding. Aloe latex should not be used as a laxative for more than 10 consecutive days.

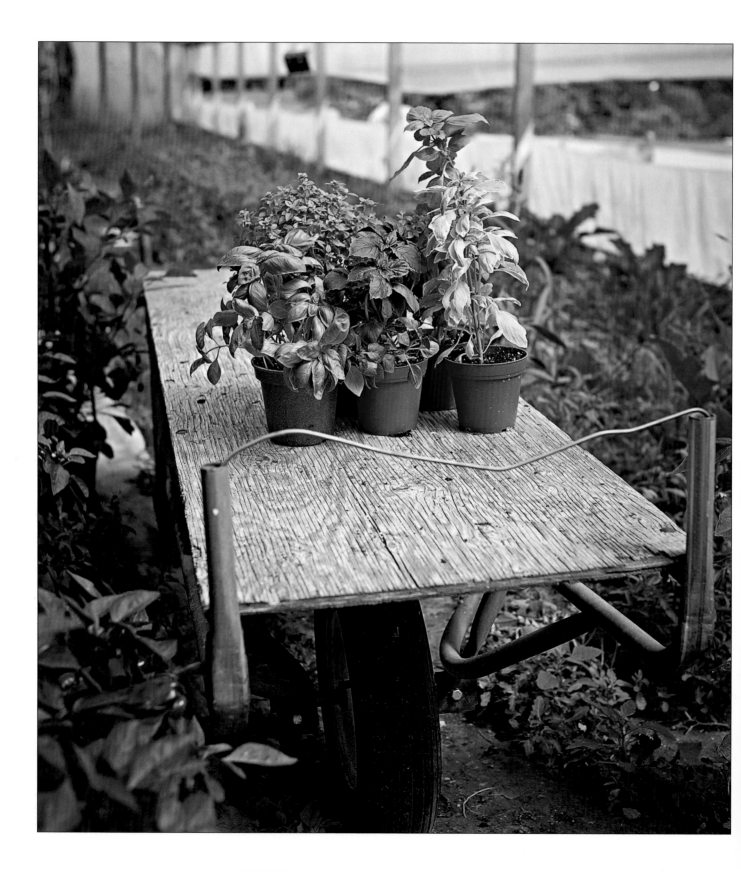

Basil

Basil is not only one of the tastiest herbs to use in the kitchen, but also one of the healthiest. Part of the mint family (*Lamiaceae*), basil likely originated in India, but today it is most commonly associated with Italian and Thai cuisine, and it grows in gardens all over the world. It is still used as a medicinal herb in India and elsewhere.

Health Benefits

Basil leaves have traditionally been used to provide relief from indigestion and as a remedy for irritation of the skin and digestive tract. In Thai herbalism, the plant is also used for coughs. It has a long list of other uses, including treatment for stomach spasms, kidney conditions, and insect bites. The plant has antiviral, antibacterial, and antiproliferative (inhibiting the growth of malignant cells) effects. It even has some insecticidal properties, possibly because it contains methyl cinnamate.

Basil has been used orally as an appetite stimulant, antiflatulent, diuretic, lactation stimulant, gargle, and mouth astringent. It's a rich source of vitamin C, calcium, magnesium, potassium, and iron.

The herb contains strong-smelling oils that are composed primarily of compounds called terpenoids, which give basil its unmistakable aroma. Essential oils such as these are used in perfume and aromatherapy. They are also the reason basil is such a health-promoting herb: some of these terpenoids—particularly eugenol, thymol, and estragole—play a role in the plant's antibacterial properties, for example. Thymol (which is found in even higher concentrations in thyme) is also a powerful antioxidant and anti-inflammatory.

Growing

Basil is one of the most popular and beloved of all herbs. Plucked fresh from the garden, it adds flavour to a simple caprese salad, pesto sauce, and countless other dishes in many cultures. Unfortunately, basil isn't the easiest plant to grow. Its delicate foliage can be fussy. High winds, hail, and frequent heavy rainfalls can all contribute to its demise.

DIFFICULTY
Medium

HARDINESS
Annual

TIME TO PLANT
Spring, after threat of killing frost has passed; can be sown indoors 6 to 8 weeks before last frost date

TIME TO HARVEST
Early summer through early fall

LOCATION
Full sun

SOIL TYPE
Well-drained

Common Varieties: Traditional sweet basil has many cultivars. My favourites include 'Genovese Gigante', 'Spicy Globe', 'Purple Ruffles', Thai basil (*O. basilicum* var. *thyrsiflora*) and Greek Columnar basil (*O. × citriodorum* 'Lesbos').

PLANT

Basil is cold-sensitive: if planted too early, when temperatures are cool and the threat of frost looms, it's doomed. So don't plant it outdoors until mid- to late spring, when both soil and air temperatures warm to approximately 20°C (68°F). Basil should be located in full sun and protected from high winds. Plant in well-drained soil and keep it evenly moist. Space the plants 25 to 50 cm (10 to 20 inches) apart, since most basils grow 45 to 60 cm (18 to 24 inches) tall and have a bushy appearance. If you plant it in containers, use a potting soil.

GROW

Basil will struggle with two things: lack of water and high humidity. During the growing season, water frequently and evenly, being careful to avoid watering the foliage. Basil doesn't enjoy overhead watering, and will benefit from mulching or use of a soaker hose. With the proper location and watering, basil can grow up to 2.5 cm (1 inch) per day. If it's planted in the ground and the soil is rich in organic matter, it will not require fertilizer. However, if you plant it in containers, it will benefit from an all-purpose fertilizer (20-20-20).

Diseases that attack basil include Pythium, verticillium wilt, stem canker, tomato spotted wilt virus, stem die-backs, leafspot diseases, and damping off. To keep your plants disease-free, use quality seed and seedlings, use disease-free soil, wash your hands and sterilize your tools after handling infected plants, and don't plant basil in the same spot two years in a row. If a basil plant becomes badly diseased, remove it to minimize the threat to others.

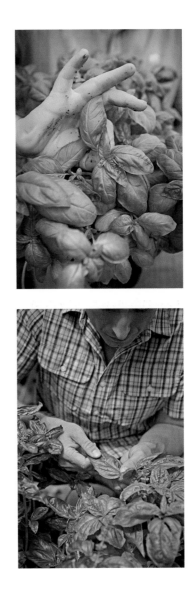

HARVEST

Basil benefits from frequent cutting and should be harvested often to maintain plant health, even if you don't require any leaves. It can be harvested immediately after it has rooted, or approximately 2 months after grown from seeds. Pick the leaves before the plant sets flower, and select leaves above the bottom 2 to 4 sets. Wash before using or storing.

STORE

Basil can be stored fresh or frozen. Gently wash it under cool running water and then hang it in a dark, dry place to air-dry. Roll it in damp paper towel and place it in a resealable bag in the refrigerator. To freeze basil, arrange washed leaves in a single layer on a baking sheet, freeze, then transfer the leaves to a resealable bag. You can also purée basil and freeze it in a BPA-free ice-cube tray. (Use basil purée in sauces, soups, marinades, or any recipe calling for the herb.) To garnish summer drinks, place a single basil leaf in each compartment of an ice-cube tray, cover with water, and freeze.

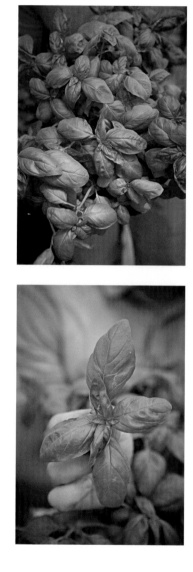

Put It to Work

Stomach upset? Sip basil tea!

If you're suffering from a stomach ache, basil tea is a natural way to ease the digestive system. It can calm your body, and the micronutrients (including potassium) can help rid you of feelings of nausea and cramping in the stomach.

Roughly chop 20 fresh basil leaves (to help release the oils) and place in a mug. Fill the mug with boiling water, cover with a saucer, and steep for 10 minutes. Strain before drinking, if desired.

Acne breakout? Make a blemish mask!

If you have acne, a basil blemish mask is your solution. In a blender, combine ¼ cup of plain yogurt with 25 fresh basil leaves and blend on high speed until smooth. Apply evenly to your face and leave on for up to 30 minutes. Rinse with cool water.

Aging skin? Tighten it with a basil toner!
Poor hygiene, oil, makeup, dead skin cells, and cumulative exposure to sunlight all contribute to enlarging your pores: the surrounding skin loses its firmness and the pore may appear larger because of the lack of support. Excessively clogged pores can lead to blackheads. Fortunately, basil can help.

In a blender, combine 30 fresh basil leaves with ½ cup of boiling water and blend on high speed until smooth. Let sit for 15 minutes to cool down, then strain through a fine-mesh sieve into a glass container with a tight-fitting lid. Use a cotton swab or ball to apply the toner to your face in the morning and evening. The toner will keep in the refrigerator for up to 7 days.

Love your pasta? Healthify it with basil!
Basil is a strong anti-inflammatory. But what causes inflammation in the first place is eating too many refined carbohydrates: cakes, cookies, breads, crackers, and—you've got it—pasta. There are a few things you can do to make your pasta healthier and taste better, too.

First, cook pasta until al dente or slightly firm to the bite. Mushy pasta makes it too easy for your digestive system to use the available carbohydrates. This means the energy extracted from the pasta enters the blood-

stream too quickly, causing a spike in blood sugar and a biological cascade that contributes to inflammation.

Second, make your pasta dish with a basil pesto instead of cream sauce. You'll save calories and garner the anti-inflammatory effects of the basil. You'll need the following ingredients:

3 cups fresh basil leaves
½ cup grated Parmesan cheese
½ cup pine nuts
Pinch sea salt and fresh ground black pepper
½ cup extra virgin olive oil
2 cloves garlic, chopped

In a food processor, finely chop the basil, Parmesan, pine nuts, and salt and pepper. Add the oil and garlic and pulse to combine. Be careful not to over-process—the pesto should be thick with some texture.

» Fast Forward

Fast forward to the health food store to purchase Simply Organic dried basil or equivalent.

! Cautions

People with serious kidney or liver damage should not consume basil essential oil, as they may have trouble eliminating it.

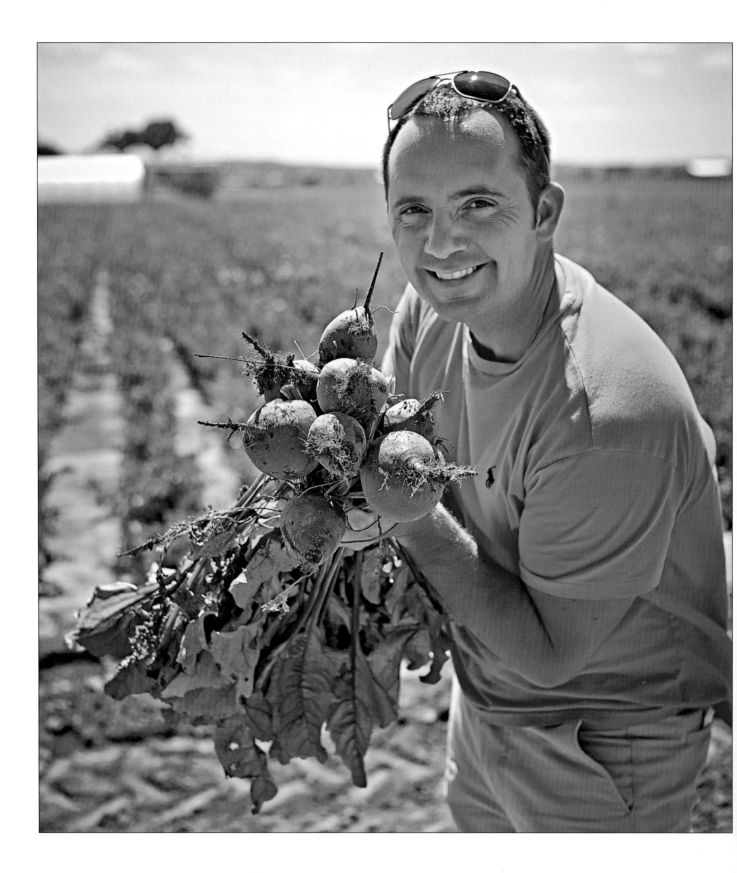

Beet

Beet (or beetroot) is a flowering biennial plant whose leaves and roots are edible sources of several vitamins and minerals, as well as fibre. Sugar has been extracted from certain varieties of *Beta vulgaris* since the 15th century. The plant contains natural pigments called betanins that account for the deep red colour of the root. The pigments are used as colourants in many foods. If you've eaten beets, you may have noticed how these pigments can produce red or pink urine (we call that beeturia).

✚ Health Benefits

Beets and their juices have been used since Roman times to treat various medical conditions. Some reports suggest beetroot was used to treat fever, constipation, digestive illnesses, blood conditions, and wounds. The plant is a great source of folate, potassium, vitamin C, fibre, and nitrates. The betanins that give beet juice its rich colour are also antioxidants.

Nitrates may be the hidden key to improving circulation throughout the body, including the brain, heart, and muscles. Current research demonstrates that beet juice is one of the richest dietary sources of nitrates. The body converts these nitrates into a powerful antioxidant called nitric oxide, a vasodilator (blood vessel enlarger) that increases blood flow and helps lower blood pressure, thus reducing the risk of heart disease.

A recent study showed that consuming beet juice daily for 6 days enhanced overall physical performance and heart functioning during exercise. A research team at the University of Exeter discovered that nitrates help people to exercise longer by reducing oxygen uptake, in essence making exercise less tiring.

🌱 Growing

I can grow beets, you can grow beets, my son can grow beets, and even my wife can grow beets (don't tell her I said that!). They're a very easy root vegetable, and they enjoy cooler climates like we experience in Canada. In fact, in places like Florida they're deemed a "cool crop" and are only attempted in early spring or late fall.

Common Varieties: My favourite red varieties include 'Ruby Queen', 'Early Wonder', 'Sweetheart', 'Pacemaker', and 'Warrior'. 'Little Ball' and 'Little Mini Ball' are great choices for smaller vari-

DIFFICULTY
Easy

HARDINESS
Biennial (will not grow well in hot areas or above zone 8)

TIME TO PLANT
Early spring, after ground frost and as soon as soil is workable

TIME TO HARVEST
Beet tops (leaves) can be harvested in late spring; harvest roots in midsummer to late fall

LOCATION
Prefers full sun, but can tolerate part sun

SOIL TYPE
Well-drained sandy loam free of stones

eties. There are also a number of specialty beets, including golden (yellow), 'Cylindra' (cylindrical shaped), and 'di Chioggia' (an Italian heirloom variety with a red-and-white striped interior).

PLANT

Beets can be grown in containers if you plan to harvest only the tops, but for best results plant them in the garden. I recommend using seed tape, but beets can also be sown by hand. Sow seeds 1.25 cm deep (½ inch), 5 to 10 cm apart (2 to 4 inches), in rows 30 to 75 cm apart (12 to 30 inches).

Due to their poor germination rate, beet seeds are compounded, which means what looks like an individual seed is actually a cluster of smaller seeds. Because of this, no matter how carefully you space them, you will always have to thin your crop by removing the weakest seedlings and giving the others room to thrive. Start thinning when the seedlings are 5 to 10 cm (2 to 4 inches) tall.

To avoid insects and disease, never plant beets in an area where their cousins spinach or Swiss chard were grown in the previous year.

GROW

Outside of the occasional weeding and watering, beets grow very easily. They rarely require fertilizer and often take care of themselves. Periods of intense heat and drought are their only nemesis: Water stress can cause them to become woody. Keep them well watered during heat waves and they will bounce back.

In my experience beets are fairly resistant to disease and insects, but leaf miners and flea beetles may offer challenges. If they attack, treat with insecticidal soap.

HARVEST

Beets mature within 55 to 75 days of being sown. The tops can be harvested as soon as they are large enough for use, but make

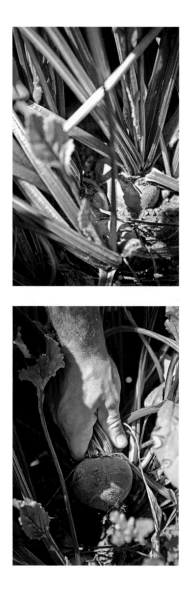

sure you take no more than a third of the greens at a time or you'll impede the growth of the root.

Roots are best harvested when they measure 2.5 cm (1 inch) or larger in diameter. The optimum size for flavour is 2.5 to 7.5 cm (1 to 3 inches). Use a garden fork to loosen soil and then just pull them up. Make sure you harvest them all before the first hard frost. When removing tops from the root, leave a section of the stem measuring 2.5 cm (1 inch) to prevent bleeding.

STORE

Beets can be stored in the refrigerator for several weeks. They will last 2 to 5 months if you layer them in boxes and fill with sand, sawdust, or peat and store in a dark, cool, frost-free place (like a cold cellar). Beets can be canned or pickled for lengthier storage.

Put It to Work

Working out? Get juiced!
Cooking depletes some of the nitrates in beets, so juicing them is a great way to reap their full benefit. Experiments suggest that dietary nitrate supplementation has the potential to improve athletic performance in events lasting 5 to 30 minutes (short bursts of activity). Eating raw beets or drinking beet juice may also have a positive impact on overall cardiovascular health. Try this natural energy drink.

1/2 cup fresh beet juice
1/2 cup pomegranate juice
1 tsp L-Glutamine powder

Combine all of the ingredients in a bottle and shake vigorously. Drink 20 to 30 minutes before working out.

High blood pressure? Beet it down!
Early evidence suggests beet fibre may modestly lower systolic blood pressure in patients with type 2 diabetes. This beet and spinach salad is a delicious way to get that effect!

3 cups baby spinach
2 beets, peeled
2 tsp mustard powder
¼ cup freshly squeezed lemon juice
2 tbsp cider vinegar
1 tbsp red fruit palm oil
2 tsp liquid honey
1 tbsp chopped fresh dill
Freshly ground black pepper

Place the spinach in a large bowl. Grate the beets overtop (wear gloves to avoid staining your hands). In a small bowl, whisk together the remaining ingredients until combined. Pour over the spinach and beets and toss to coat well. Season with pepper, if desired.

High cholesterol? Root out the problem!
Eating a diet rich in fibre can improve cholesterol levels and reduce the risk of heart dis-

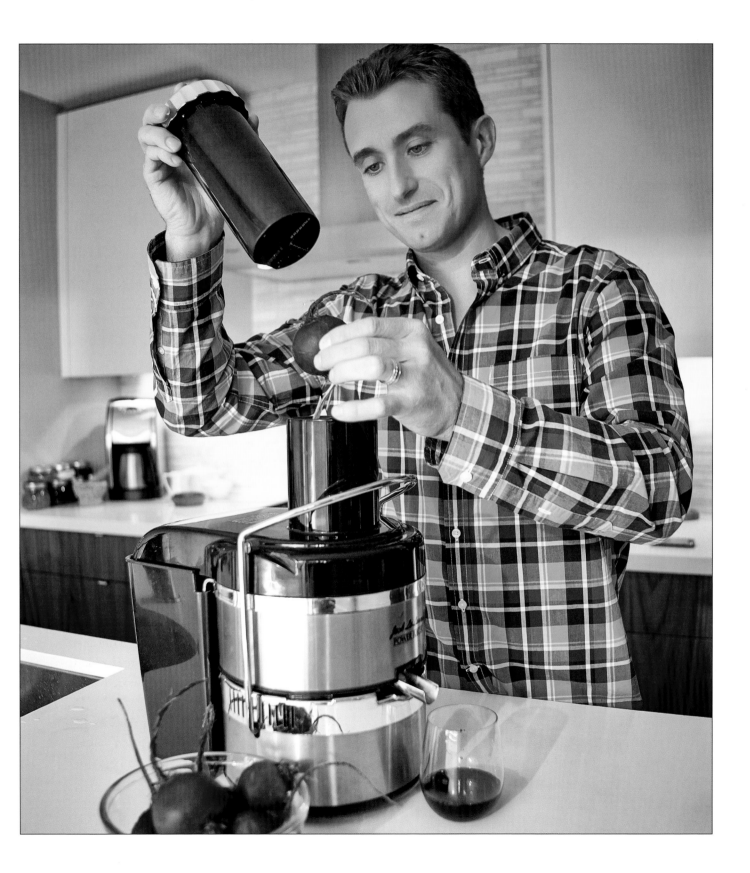

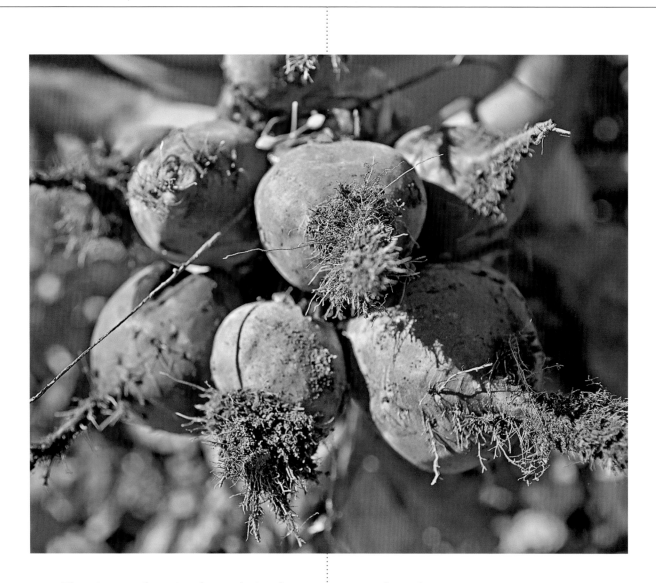

ease. The pigment that gives beets their colour is not only an antioxidant but may also reduce levels of LDL (bad) cholesterol, protect your artery walls, and help reduce the risk of heart disease and stroke. This beet salad is delicious and heart-healthy, too.

2 large beets
2 cloves garlic, minced
1 small Spanish onion, thinly sliced
2 tbsp red wine vinegar
3 tbsp finely chopped fresh dill
1 tbsp extra virgin olive oil
1 tsp brown sugar
¼ tsp pink Himalayan rock salt

In a small pot of boiling water, boil the whole beets until soft. Let cool and remove the skins (they should just slip off). Dice the beets and transfer them to a mixing bowl. Gently stir in the garlic, onion, vinegar, dill, oil, brown sugar, and salt. Chill in the refrigerator for 30 minutes before serving.

Forgetful? Boost brain power with a beet smoothie!

Research shows the high levels of nitrates in beets may help fight the progression of dementia by increasing blood flow to the brain. High concentrations of folic acid in beets may also play a part. Give your brain a boost with this delicious smoothie.

1 small beet, peeled and chopped
¼ cup blueberries (fresh or frozen)
¼ cup blackberries (fresh or frozen)
½ cup strawberries (fresh or frozen)
1 cup almond milk
1 tbsp cacao powder
1 tbsp pure maple syrup
Ice cubes

In a blender, combine all of the ingredients and blend on high speed until smooth. Serve immediately.

» Fast Forward

Fast forward to the health food store to purchase Genuine Health ActivFuel+ powder or equivalent, which features beetroot powder as a pre- and post-workout solution. Follow the instructions on the label.

! Cautions

Always drink beet juice when it's fresh: the nitrates present a potential risk if the juice is stored incorrectly. Bacteria can convert nitrate to nitrite, which contaminates the juice. If high levels of nitrite accumulate over time, it can be potentially harmful. Avoid giving beet juice to infants younger than 3 months to avoid the risk of nitrite poisoning.

Avoid beets if you have an allergy or hypersensitivity to any part of the beet plant or to plants in the Goosefoot family (*Chenopodiaceae*), including Swiss chard and spinach.

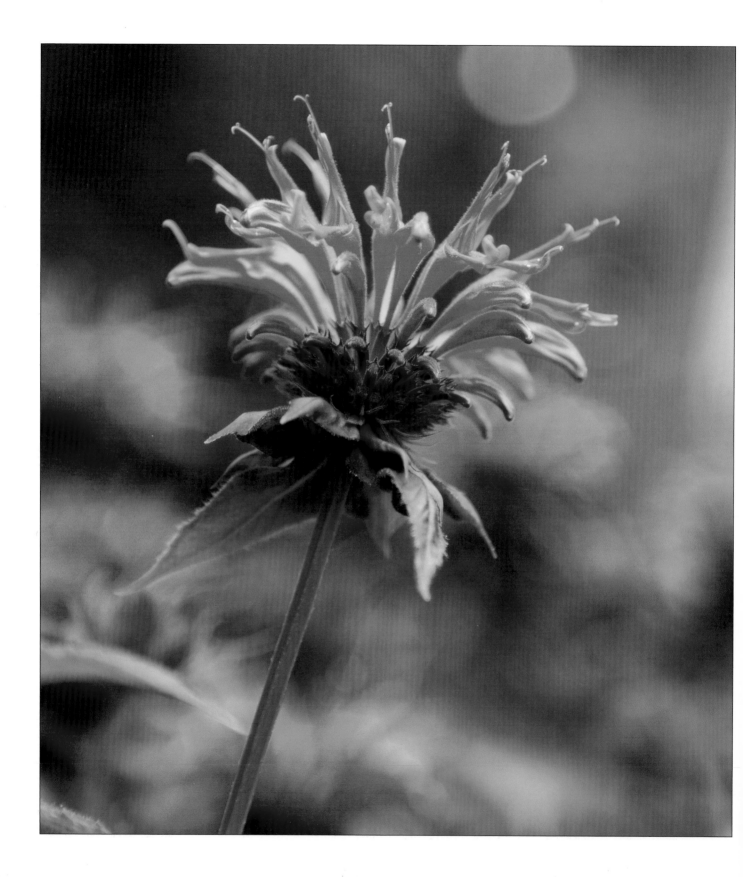

Bergamot

If you want hummingbirds and butterflies in your garden, this is the plant to grow! Its deep crimson colour attracts nearly everything in the business of dealing pollen. Bergamot—also called bee balm—is part of the mint family (*Lamiaceae*). It shouldn't be mistaken for the Bergamot orange used in Earl Grey tea, though it does smell very similar. It also shouldn't be confused with lemon balm (see page 187), which is also in the *Lamiaceae* family.

Health Benefits

If you rub the leaves of bergamot you'll smell the unmistakable aroma of lemon, a result of the high amount of medicinal oils (including thymol) found in this plant. Bergamot tea has been traditionally used to treat premenstrual syndrome, as it has anti-spasmodic (muscle relaxing) effects. It is now primarily used for digestive disorders and as an antiseptic. The tea has carminative properties, which means it can prevent the formation of gas in the gastrointestinal tract. It may also be a mild diuretic and has been used to decrease fever.

Growing

A traditional border plant in the perennial garden, bergamot offers aromatic blooms in several colours, including white, pink, and red. You can cut the blooms and enjoy them in a vase, but I prefer to leave them in the garden to attract bees, hummingbirds, and butterflies. The challenge with bergamot is its susceptibility to disease, especially powdery mildew, although resistant varieties are now available.

Common Varieties: Heirloom varieties include 'Cambridge Scarlet', 'Croftway Pink', 'Granite Pink', and 'Snow White', to name just a few. Look for mildew-resistant varieties, including 'Blaustrumpf' (Blue Stocking), 'Colrain Red', 'Gardenview Scarlet', 'Marshall's Delight', 'Sunset', and 'Violet Queen'.

PLANT

Bergamot can be planted in the garden almost any time during the growing season. It enjoys full sun and tolerates most soils: it will even thrive in clay soils. Bergamot is easily divided, and can even be propagated by taking a small section of stem and rooting

DIFFICULTY
Medium

HARDINESS
Perennial in zones 3 to 9

TIME TO PLANT
Spring through fall

TIME TO HARVEST
Summer

LOCATION
Full to part sun

SOIL TYPE
Any

it in soil. (Stem cuttings should be taken in mid-spring while foliage is young.) If you're growing it from seed, sow in early spring and space the seeds about 45 to 60 cm (18 to 24 inches) apart.

GROW

Bergamot enjoys damp soil and should be watered frequently. The key is to monitor it for disease and pests throughout the growing season. To prevent mildew, keep the soil evenly moist and provide good air circulation between plants by thinning stems early on. If mildew develops after flowering, cut the plant back to uninfected leaves at the base and discard the diseased foliage.

To improve its overall health and lengthen the bloom period, immediately deadhead spent flowers.

Bergamot is aggressive and may require frequent dividing and some removal to prevent it from taking over. Divide clumps every 2 to 3 years in early spring, just before vigorous growth begins. You should also divide any clump showing signs of dying out in the centre.

HARVEST

You can harvest leaves and flowers as needed during the growing season. The best time to harvest is mid-morning when the dew has dried and the plants are cool. Avoid harvesting during the peak heat of the day. If you plan to dry the leaves, harvest them just before flowering or while bergamot is in full bloom, and always discard any leaves affected by mildew.

To harvest bergamot seeds, wait until the flowers have dried on the stems. Remove the flowers and place them on a baking sheet in the sun to dry. Place the dried flower heads into a paper bag and shake to separate the seeds from the petals.

STORE

Bergamot can be used dried or frozen. Dry by hanging it in a cool, dark, dry place with good ventilation (see "Drying Herbs at

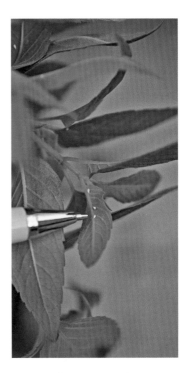

Whiteflies are pesky, invasive insects. While they will not immediately harm a plant, they are very unsightly and generally an indicator of poor plant health. For milder cases, treat with insecticidal soap (page 362). If the infestation is severe, though, discard the entire plant to prevent the spread of whiteflies to other plants.

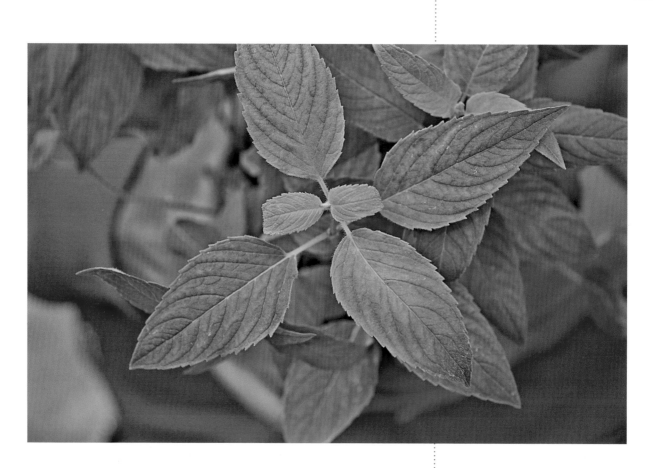

Home" on page 365). Or you can chop fresh bergamot and place it in resealable bags in the freezer. The seeds can be stored for up to 3 months in a paper bag or envelope; keep them at room temperature out of direct light.

Put It to Work

Bad gas? Steep this!

Bergamot is delicious as a hot or iced tea, by itself or in combination with citrus peel and other mints. Pick about 20 fresh bergamot leaves. Place them in a mug and pour 1 cup of boiling water over the leaves. Cover with a saucer and steep for 10 to 15 minutes, then strain. Add 1 teaspoon of manuka honey or blue agave nectar. Garnish with a fresh edible bergamot flower for a splash of colour and for extra bioflavonoids.

Stinky breath? Make your own mouthwash!
World-renowned pharmacognosist Dr. James Duke recommends bergamot for treating halitosis (bad breath) and tooth decay. The plant contains thymol, a potent antiseptic and an active ingredient in Listerine mouthwash. If you have bad breath, wash 5 leaves and chew them. One minute is all it takes. (Spit or swallow as you chew.) The leaves are also very high in the powerful cavity-preventing compound geraniol.

Stomach upset? Settle it with a salad!
If you have an upset stomach, or if you're bloated and constipated, this could be your cure. In addition to the bergamot, the other ingredients in this light salad are also healing to your digestive system.

Salad:
1 cup bergamot leaves
2 cups spinach
½ green apple, cored and sliced
2 Belgian endives, chopped
¼ cup chopped walnuts
½ red onion, sliced

Dressing:
½ cup plain Greek-style yogurt
2 tbsp apple cider vinegar

1 tbsp liquid honey
1 tbsp freshly squeezed lemon juice
½ tsp mustard powder
1 clove garlic, finely chopped
½ tsp ground turmeric
Sea salt and freshly ground pepper

Place the spinach and bergamot leaves in a large salad bowl. In a separate bowl, whisk together the yogurt, vinegar, honey, and lemon juice. Add the mustard powder, garlic, and turmeric. Season with salt and pepper to taste and mix well. Drizzle the dressing over the greens and toss to coat well. Top the salad with the apple, endives, walnuts, and red onion.

To make this salad a complete meal, add cubed tofu, salmon, or grilled chicken—once your tummy is better!

Home odours? Freshen up with bergamot spray!
Bergamot is an antiseptic and has a clean, refreshing citrus-mint aroma. It might be the perfect one-two punch to clean and deodorize the air in your home naturally.

You can make your own hydrosol using a simple process called steam distillation. Collect 2 cups of fresh bergamot leaves. Place a heavy bowl upside down on the bottom of a large pot. Fill the pot with water until it almost covers the bowl and place on the stove. Add the leaves to the water. Place another bowl on top of the upside-down bowl.

Cover the pot with an upside-down lid (the idea is to allow the evaporating water to collect on the lid and then run into the bowl that's sitting right-side-up). On top of the lid, place yet another bowl and fill it with ice. The ice will keep the lid cool and create condensation.

Turn on the burner to medium-low heat and simmer for an hour or two, until the bowl is full of "distillate." Pour this liquid into a spray bottle. Use it anytime you want to aromatize a room in the house. The hydrosol will keep in the refrigerator for up to 4 weeks.

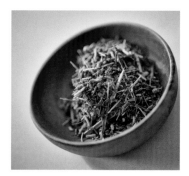

Fresh is best, but dried bergamot can make a delicious tea.

» Fast Forward

Fast forward to the health food store to purchase Oswego tea, which is made from bergamot. Follow the instructions on the label.

! Cautions

Bergamot is safe: There are no known interactions or harmful side effects. If you are harvesting leaves from your own garden, just be sure they are thoroughly washed and free of mildew.

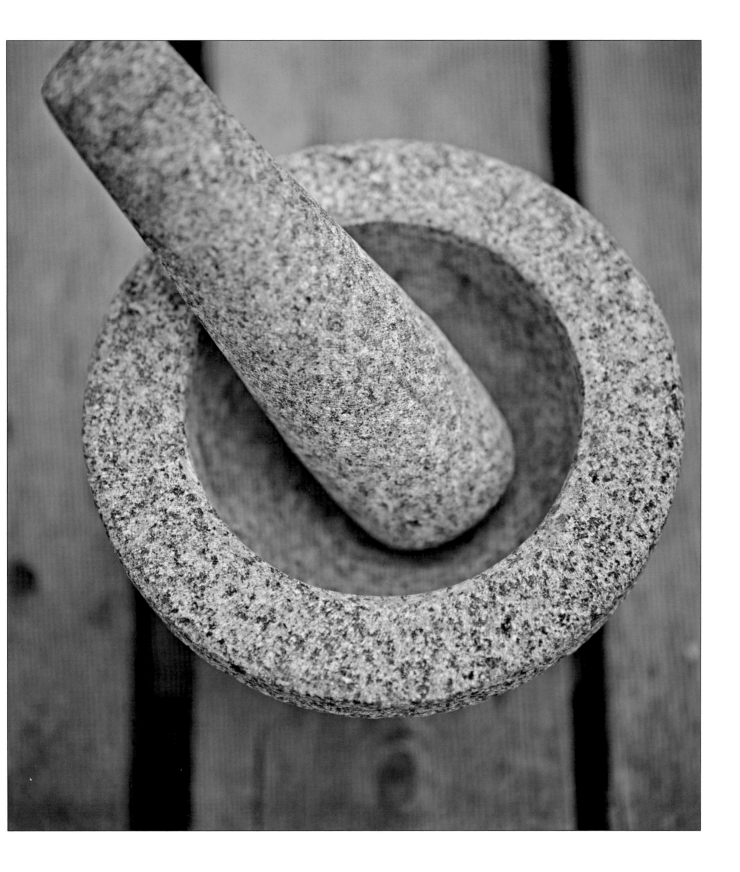

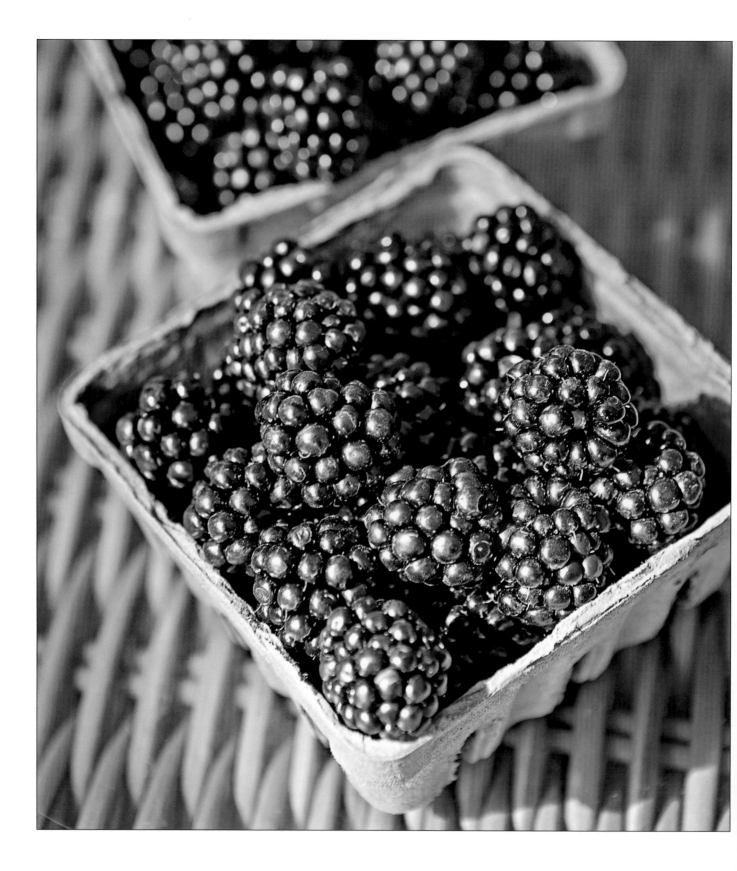

Blackberry

Blackberries are the dark purple-black fruits of several species of *Rubus*. They grow on prickly canes and are often found in the wild. The fruit is not a true berry. It's more accurately called an "aggregate fruit," because it is a cluster of many small fleshy fruits (called drupelets) that each develop from separate ovaries. Blackberries can be easily confused with raspberries, but the latter (including black raspberries) have a hollow centre, while blackberries have a greenish-white core. The other way to tell them apart is by looking at the leaves: raspberry leaves are silvery on their undersides, whereas blackberry leaves are light green. Both plants are members of the same genus (in the rose family), and related species are known by a variety of other names, including bramble, dewberry, and thimbleberry.

✚ Health Benefits

Blackberries have one of the highest antioxidant levels of all fruits, based on their ORAC value. (ORAC stands for "oxygen radical absorbance capacity," which measures the ability of a food to clean up the mess left behind by free radical damage—oxidative stress—in the body.)

If you want to slow down the aging process, blackberries can help promote the healthy tightening of tissue, a non-surgical procedure that can make skin look younger. Prolonged consumption also improves clarity of thought and memory. The fruit contains anthocyanins, salicylic acid, and ellagic acid, which are all heart- and brain-healthy.

The plant's root, bark, and leaves are also packed with tannins, which have historically been used as an astringent, a tonic for diarrhea, and a treatment for whooping cough.

Blackberries are rich in bioflavonoids and contain soluble and insoluble fibre. One cup of blackberries has nearly 8 grams of fibre and contains half the daily recommended dose of vitamin C, which protects the immune system and can lower the risk of developing certain cancers.

🌱 Growing

Blackberries are easy to grow, but they are not maintenance-free and they require space. Like raspberries, the canes are not only vigorous, but may be invasive. You need to be willing to spend time pruning them to prevent them from spreading to other areas in the garden.

Common Varieties: Varieties abound, but they can be broken down into three types: training, erect, and semi-erect. Training blackberries are not hardy in cooler climates. Erect varieties ('Darrow', 'Cheyenne', and 'Illini Hardy') produce fruit with larger

DIFFICULTY
Easy to medium

HARDINESS
Perennial in zones 5 to 8

TIME TO PLANT
Spring or early fall

TIME TO HARVEST
Late spring to early fall
(depends on variety)

LOCATION
Full sun

SOIL TYPE
Moist, well-drained

seeds on old wood, and the canes are self-supporting. Semi-erect varieties ('Chester', 'Triple Crown') require staking and produce higher yields on thornless canes.

PLANT

Plant in early spring or as soon as soil can be worked. Blackberries can be planted in most soil types, including clay, but they enjoy well-drained soils rich in organic matter. Canes can last up to 15 years if you regularly amend the soil to replace much-needed nutrients (my favourite addition is sheep manure).

Plant blackberries in full sun and leave lots of space between them; depending on the variety that can mean 0.5 to 2 metres (2 to 6 feet). Plant at the same depth as the pot they came in. Blackberries are not the most attractive plant, so they should probably go at the back of the landscape. Plant in groupings or rows, and avoid planting them next to raspberries to minimize the spread of viruses.

Aphids are a threat to blackberries, but never fear, Mother Nature is here! To minimize the threat of these pests, improve the environment for ladybugs, which eat aphids. You can purchase ladybug lures to encourage them to visit your garden, or even buy the ladybugs themselves.

GROW

Growing blackberries isn't rocket science. It takes regular weeding, occasional watering, annual soil amendment, and early-spring pruning. Most blackberries produce fruit on last year's growth (old wood), so the only canes that should be removed in early spring are those that produced fruit last season (as well as any dead canes). You'll be able to see where you picked last year's fruit: these canes will probably be thicker than the new growth. Canes that emerge this year will produce next season.

As a general rule, remove the canes of erect blackberries immediately after harvest. In spring, remove any dead or weak canes, selecting the healthiest 8 to 16 canes for staking.

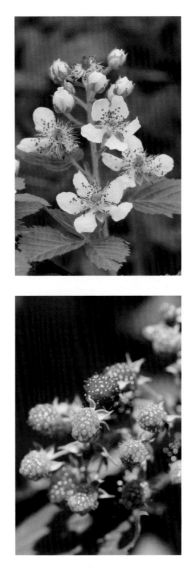

Blackberry blossoms and then unripe fruit. Blackberries look nearly identical to black raspberries but are often slightly rounder in their shape.

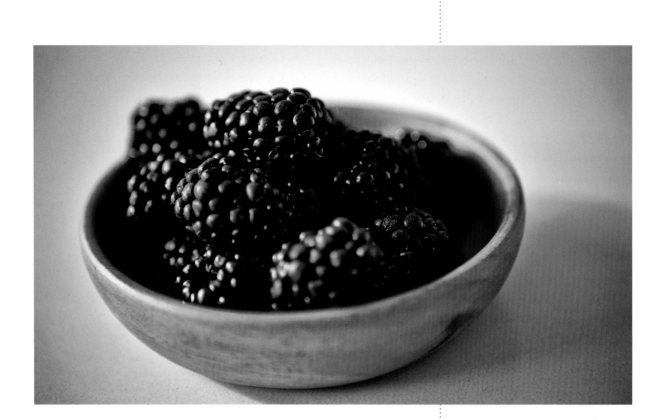

Monitor blackberries for signs of insects or disease, including spider mites, aphids, beetles, rusts, or blights. Identify the specific problem and treat as necessary, but be aware there are few organic controls for disease.

HARVEST

Depending on the variety, blackberries can be harvested from late spring all the way into early fall. Harvest them when the colour appears deep black; if the fruit is red or purple, it's not ripe. Don't forget to reach between the canes to locate ripe fruit hidden by foliage. Pick late morning and avoid harvesting midday.

STORE

Don't wash the fruit until you are ready to use it. Store blackberries uncovered in the refrigerator for up to a week, depending on the initial quality. After a few days in storage, however, the fruit loses its bright colour and fresh flavour and tends to shrivel. To freeze blackberries, wash, drain, and freeze on a baking sheet before transferring to resealable bags. Blackberries can also be preserved in jams and jellies.

Put It to Work

Canker sores? Chew blackberry leaves!

Chewing fresh blackberry leaves can help canker sores and inflamed gums. Chewing releases the astringent tannins, which heal and soothe the mucous membranes of the mouth. It also releases vitamin C, which is essential for gum health. Just pop a carefully washed handful into your mouth and chew for a couple of minutes. Spit out the leaves when you're done.

Inflamed gums? Gargle with blackberry!

If you're not a fan of chewing leaves (see above), they can also be brewed to make a refreshing cup of tea. They carry a slight bitter taste, so you'll want to add manuka honey, which also improves oral health. Place about 10 leaves in a mug, pour boiling water over them, cover, and steep for 10 to 15 minutes. Swish the tea around your mouth a few seconds before swallowing—the astringent tannins are also effective as a gargle or mouthwash.

High blood sugar? Make blackberry jam!

If you're watching your sugar levels, jam may not be your best choice. But if you can't give up a smear of fruity goodness on your toast in the morning, replace your super-sweet strawberry jam with this low-sugar blackberry jam.

2 cups blackberries (fresh or frozen)
2 cups granulated sugar
Freshly squeezed juice of 1 small lemon

Using the back of a spoon, press the blackberries through a fine-mesh sieve (to remove the seeds), letting the juice and pulp drain into a pot. Stir in the sugar and lemon juice. Cook over high heat for 5 minutes, then reduce the heat to medium and cook, stirring occasionally, for an additional 15 minutes. Skim off the foam with a slotted spoon and discard. The jam will thicken as it cools. Store in a resealable glass jar (like a Mason jar) in the refrigerator for up to 3 weeks.

Fast Forward

Fast forward to the health food store to purchase Celebration Herbals blackberry leaf tea or equivalent. Follow the instructions on the label.

Cautions

Blackberries have no known interactions or harmful side effects.

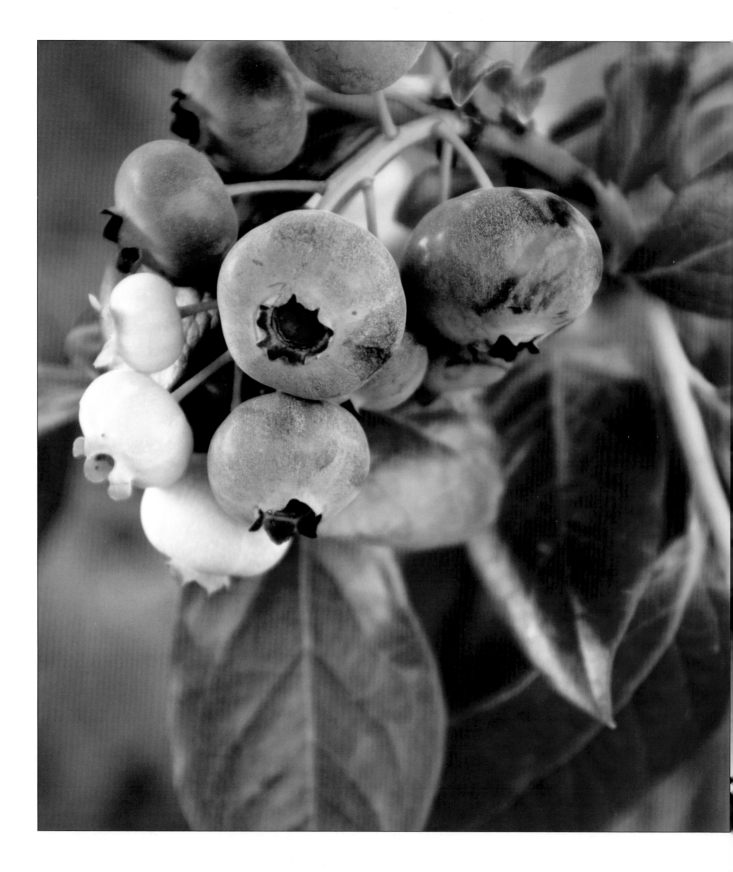

Blueberry

Blueberry is a shrub in the heather family (*Ericaceae*), which also includes cranberries, azaleas, and rhododendrons. Blueberries grow all over the world, but they are native to North America. Aboriginal peoples dried them in the sun and stored them for use year-round. Blueberries are big business in North America, with major growing regions in Maine, Michigan, New Jersey, Nova Scotia, Quebec, and British Columbia.

Health Benefits

The health benefits of blueberries come from a class of antioxidants called anthocyanins; these are the deep blue-purple pigments the plant produces to attract birds and insects. The anthocyanins are thought to pass through the blood-brain barrier to improve the health of the brain—memory in particular.

The antioxidant benefit from blueberries seems to be DNA-dependent. Research has shown the effectiveness of these berries (how well they protect the heart and brain) is much greater in some people than in others.

Blueberries have also been shown to have anti-inflammatory effects and the potential to lower blood sugar levels.

Growing

Blueberries can be grown anywhere, from pots to formal gardens; they're typically used as hedges or grown in clusters. They offer three seasons of interest in the garden: In early spring, the shrubs produce delicate white or pink flowers. In summer, the fruit has an attractive sky-blue colour. In fall, the foliage adds explosions of red and yellow to end the garden season.

Common Varieties: There are three basic classifications: highbush, lowbush, and hybrid half-high. Highbush varieties ('Blue Crop', 'Blue Ray', 'Jersey', 'Pioneer') are the most common and are typically hardy to zone 4. Lowbush varieties are best for colder climates (up to zone 3). Hybrid half-high varieties ('Northcountry', 'Northland', 'Northblue') combine properties from the other two.

PLANT

Plant blueberries in early spring or as soon as your soil is frost-free and workable. Locate them in full sun, and space them 1 to

DIFFICULTY
Easy to medium

HARDINESS
Perennial in zones 3 to 4 or above, depending on variety

TIME TO PLANT
Early spring, as soon as soil is workable

TIME TO HARVEST
Mid- to late summer

LOCATION
Full sun

SOIL TYPE
Moist, slightly acidic (see opposite)

2 metres (3 to 6 feet) apart. Plant more than one to ensure ample pollination.

It's difficult to find the ideal soil for blueberries. This plant likes soil that is both well-drained and acidic. Unfortunately, clay soils are naturally acidic but poorly drained, while sandy soils are well-drained but lack acidity. You can amend clay soils with a peat/sand mixture, or amend sandy soils with peat to improve absorption and acidity. But in most cases you'll need to apply sulphur to lower the pH.

The pH level in the soil affects a plant's ability to absorb nutrients and minerals. The lower the number, the higher the acidity. Most plants like soils with neutral pH (6.0 to 7.0). But some, including clematis, enjoy alkaline soils (pH 7.1 to 8.0), while many fruiting plants enjoy acidic soils. Blueberries are in that latter category: it's essential to grow them in soil with a pH of 4.5 to 5.2. Before planting, pick up a soil tester at your garden centre.

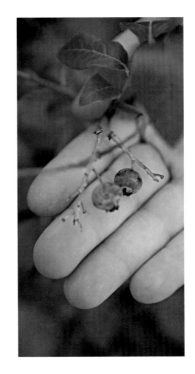

GROW

Blueberries require ample water to improve fruit size and yields. Water deeply, ensuring the water penetrates into the soil, as often as 3 times per week. Use a soaker hose to avoid watering the foliage. Mulch is also a big help: It not only helps maintain moisture, but mulch of pine or spruce needles will naturally improve soil acidity.

Prune any dead or weak stems early in spring. Prune to shape in fall or after harvest.

Blueberries are resistant to most diseases and insects, so they can easily be grown organically. The challenge will be battling the birds and bears for the fruit! Garden mesh or owl statues will discourage birds and smaller rodents. Larger furry friends pose greater challenges: call your local Ministry of Natural Resources!

HARVEST

Yields in the first couple of seasons will be modest, but when the bushes mature they can produce up to 6.75 kg (15 lb) of fruit annually. To see if the blueberries are ready to pick, place a bucket under the bush and gently move the foliage around with your hand: ripe blueberries will fall into the bucket. Many varieties will produce berries continuously and can be picked every 5 to 10 days.

STORE

Do not wash blueberries until you need them. Store blueberries in an airtight container in the refrigerator for up to 2 weeks. To freeze, wash, drain, and arrange in a single layer on a baking sheet. Once frozen, transfer to resealable bags. You can also preserve blueberries in jams and spreads.

Put It to Work

Need a breakfast makeover? Have a blueberry smoothie!

If you want to remain in good health, breakfast is the most important meal of the day. "Breaking your fast" is important for your brain and blood nutrient levels, and for increasing your energy. Smoothies have become a popular breakfast because they are fast, simple, easy to digest, and super-healthy. Toss these ingredients in a blender to kick-start your morning:

1 cup blueberries (fresh or frozen)
1 red pear, peeled and cored
½ apple, peeled and cored
1 cup plain low-fat yogurt
1 tsp vanilla whey, soy, or rice protein powder

Coping with stress? Don some antioxidant armour!

Stress is North America's number 1 silent killer, because it contributes to the development of free radicals. These aren't right-wing political activists: they're atoms with unpaired electrons that cause cell-damaging chemical reactions in the body, leading to heart disease, diabetes, and even cancer. Blueberries can help! They contain a wallop of antioxidants that help protect the body's cells.

You can arm yourself with antioxidants by drinking a shot of blueberry juice every morning. Toss 1 cup of blueberries into a blender and purée. Strain through a fine-mesh sieve (discard solids).

Drink 1 ounce every morning. Store the juice in an airtight container in the refrigerator. (Don't make more than 5 ounces at a time. It will oxidize quickly in the refrigerator.)

Diabetic? Snack on these!

Whether you're looking to prevent type 2 diabetes (one of the most epidemic health problems of our time) or manage it better, your fruit of choice should be the blueberry. Eat them straight-up as a snack between meals—right

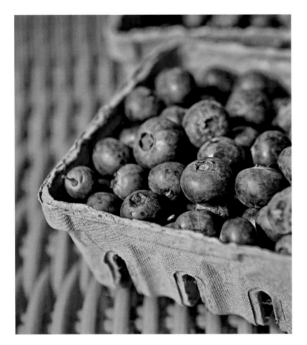

off the bush and into a Tupperware they go. Use an ice pack if you're on the road.

Research has found that higher consumption of anthocyanin-rich fruit like blueberries is associated with a lower risk of type 2 diabetes (but not the juice: that's too high in sugar). If you are trying to better manage your blood sugar, consider eating ½ cup of blueberries with 10 almonds between meals.

As always, keep your overall diet in mind. There may be an interaction in individuals with diabetes or who use blood-glucose-lowering agents. Blueberries have been found to lower blood glucose levels if consumed too frequently.

» Fast Forward

Fast forward to the health food store to purchase Douglas Laboratories pTeroPure capsules or equivalent. Follow the instructions on the label.

! Cautions

Avoid if you have a known allergy or hypersensitivity to blueberries or other members of the *Ericaceae* family.

Use cautiously with certain lipid-lowering drugs such as fibrates, as research has indicated an ingredient in blueberries called pterostilbenecan can reduce cholesterol and other lipids.

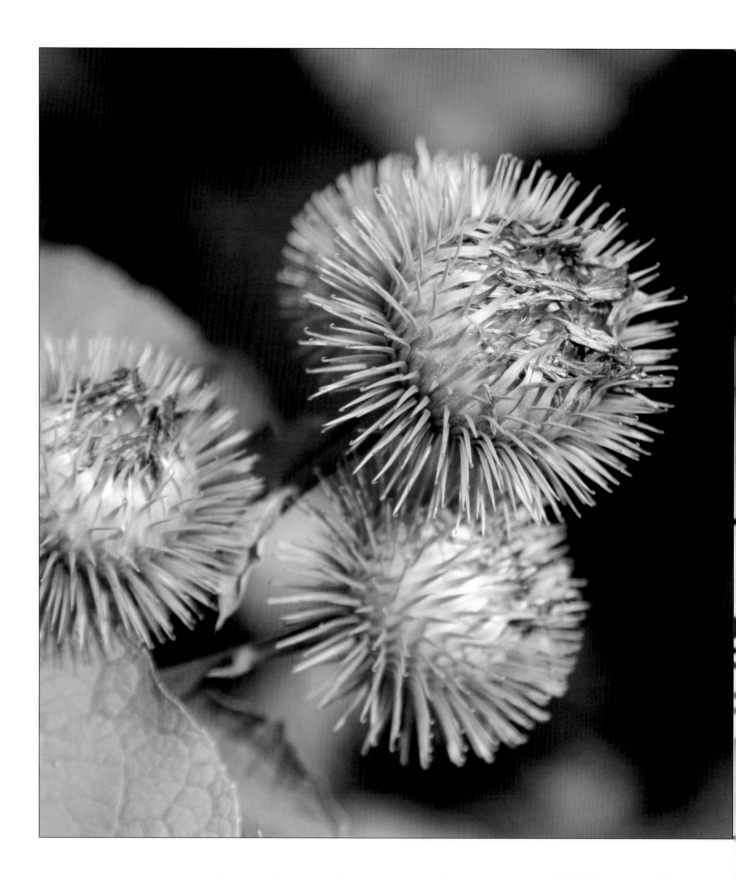

Burdock

If you've ever picked a sticky round burr from your clothes after walking in the countryside, there's a good chance you've encountered burdock. This plant's ingenious mechanism for seed dispersal was the inspiration for Velcro! Burdock is in the *Asteraceae* family, which makes it a relative of daisies and coneflowers (see Echinacea, page 105). It is native to Europe and Northern Asia, but it now grows as a weed throughout North America. In Japan, burdock is cultivated for its root and eaten as a vegetable called *gobo*. The root is crispy, with a sweet, earthy flavour that resembles celery and is jam-packed with micronutrients.

Health Benefits

Historically burdock was used to treat a wide variety of inflammatory ailments such as arthritis. In 14th-century Europe, burdock and wine were supposedly used to treat leprosy. Later European herbalists tested it on a variety of skin-related conditions (baldness, scrapes, and burns), syphilis, and even gonorrhea. However, no evidence currently supports using it for any of these cases.

Beginning in the 1920s, burdock gained popularity as part of an herbal remedy intended to treat cancer. The formula—which also contains rhubarb, sorrel, and slippery elm—was created by a Canadian nurse named Rene Caisse, who claimed she learned about it from an Ojibway healer. She reversed the letters of her surname and called the concoction "Essiac." It is still available today in various forms, including the brand Flor Essence, though it is not an approved cancer treatment in either Canada or the United States.

Research suggests burdock root may have blood-sugar-lowering effects. The root contains inulin (not to be confused with insulin), a type of fibre that is not digested or absorbed in the stomach. It moves through the intestines, where probiotics (friendly bacteria) use it to flourish. Inulin also decreases the body's ability to make certain kinds of fats. Research has also looked at burdock root as a way to help manage diabetes.

Other studies have explored the use of burdock for bacterial infections, HIV, and kidney stones. Although it is believed to exhibit a range of healing properties when used orally or topically, there is no consensus on the most important active constituents.

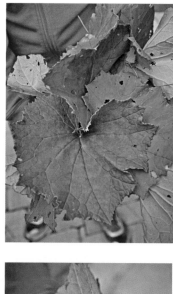

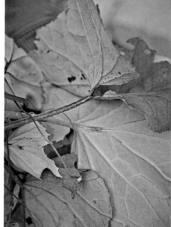

Freshly harvested burdock leaves and stems. Notice the white undersides of the leaves.

Growing

Burdock is a weed and can easily be found growing along just about any country road. It's a stout plant that demands space: it will grow up to 2 metres (6 feet) high, with a similar width. Burdock is best identified by its heart-shaped leaves, which are green on the top and whitish on the bottom. Purple flowers bloom between June and October. The spent flowers produce seed burrs that stick to clothing and pets.

PLANT

You can probably find all the burdock you need by taking a walk in the country, but if you want to grow your own, I recommend sowing seed in pots. That way there's less danger of them spreading out of control in your garden. You can harvest the seed from burrs you find in the wild and plant them the following season. The seeds only need to be lightly covered in soil and will germinate in 4 to 7 days.

GROW

Burdock is a maintenance-free plant—in other words, it's a weed! However, if you water and fertilize it you'll get bigger leaves and healthier roots. Remove flowers and burrs during the growing season to improve growth of roots and foliage.

HARVEST

You can eat burdock foliage, but its main appeal is the root. Harvest only mature burdock, typically in late summer. Roots can penetrate up to 2 metres (6 feet) in depth, so they should be removed only after loosening the soil with a garden fork.

DIFFICULTY
Easy (it's a weed!)

HARDINESS
Biennial in zones 3a and above

TIME TO PLANT
Sow seeds in spring

TIME TO HARVEST
Roots can he harvested from mature plants any time

LOCATION
Full to part sun

SOIL TYPE
Will grow in most soils but prefers good drainage

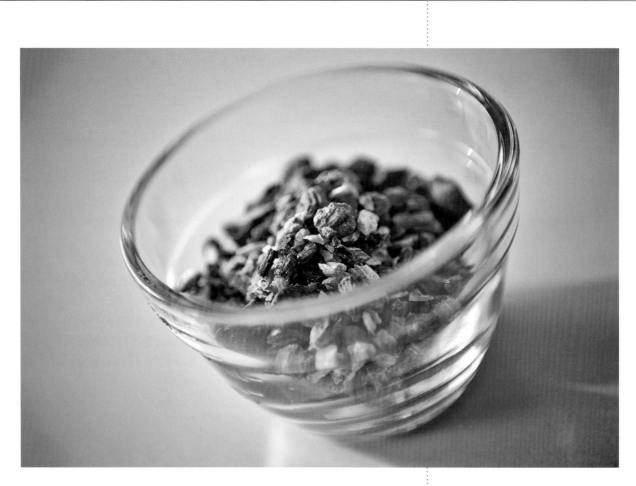

Chopped and dried burdock root.

STORE

Burdock foliage should be treated like spinach and harvested only as needed. The roots can be eaten raw or cooked in stir-fries, but it is best to dry them. After excavating the roots, cut them from the plant and wash well with a vegetable scrubber. Cut the roots into small pieces and arrange them in a single layer on a baking sheet to dry in the hot sun for 3 or 4 days or bake them at 120°C (250°F) for 4 hours. To air-dry indoors, cut clean roots into small pieces and place on a drying screen in indirect light for up to 2 weeks or until brittle. Dried roots will keep in an airtight container for up to a year.

Put It to Work

Blood sugar blues? Take this tincture!

Less than 20% of dieters can keep the weight off for more than 2 years. It's time to shift your mindset when it comes to dieting, focusing less on fads and more on maintaining a healthy balance and stabilizing your blood sugar. Imbalanced blood sugar (not to be mistaken for undiagnosed hypoglycemia or diabetes) can cause mood swings and lack of energy as well as weight gain, and burdock root might help.

To make your own tincture, using a clean coffee or spice grinder, grind ½ cup of chopped dried burdock root to a powder. Transfer the powder to a resealable glass jar (like a Mason jar). Add enough vodka (at least 80 proof) to cover the powder by 6 mm (¼ inch). Place wax paper over the jar and then screw the lid on tightly to seal it. Set it aside in a cool, dark place for 12 hours.

Check the jar after 12 hours. If the powder has absorbed the vodka, top it up until it is once again covered by 6 mm (¼ inch) of vodka. Set aside in a cool, dark place for 14 days, shaking the jar once daily.

After 2 weeks, cover the mouth of the jar with a coffee filter and strain the liquid into a glass bowl (discard solids). Extract as much liquid as you can by carefully squeezing the coffee filter. Store the tincture in a glass container, ideally equipped with a glass dropper.

Take 1 teaspoon in water 3 times daily with meals. The tincture will keep in a cool, dark place for at least a year.

Suffer from eczema? Here's your salve-ation!

Eczema is usually a signal that a deeper issue is brewing, such as lack of omega-3 fatty acids, food intolerances, or stress. A burdock root salve can be a godsend to manage the itchy, sore, and often raw and aggravated skin symptomatic of eczema. A salve is a semi-solid herbal mixture applied to the skin for its healing, protective, and nourishing effects. The base for most salves is a mix of wax and oil: the wax firms the texture to make it easier to apply, and the oil enhances the absorption of the medicinal plant into the skin.

You can make your own burdock root salve with a base of beeswax and olive oil. Start by grinding ¼ cup of chopped dried burdock root in a clean coffee or spice grinder until it becomes a powder. Stir the powder into 1 cup of extra virgin olive oil and transfer the mixture into an uncovered heatproof container. Heat in the oven at (50°C/120°F) for 3 hours, stirring periodically.

Line a large strainer with cheesecloth or a coffee filter. Pour the oil infusion through the strainer into a saucepan over low heat (discard solids).

Add about 1 ounce of shaved beeswax to the pan and stir until completely melted. Now comes the tricky part: determining how much beeswax to add to get the right consistency after the salve has cooled. To test the firmness, dip a spoon into the warm mixture and place in the freezer. After 10 to 15 minutes, the mixture should be hardened on the spoon. Try it: If it's too soft, add a little more beeswax. Repeat this process until you reach the desired consistency. Pour the salve into small glass jars with tight-fitting lids and set aside at room temperature to cool and harden.

» Fast Forward

Fast forward to the health food store to purchase Clef des Champs burdock root tincture or equivalent. Follow the instructions on the label.

! Cautions

Both oral consumption and topical use of burdock may cause severe allergic reactions. Avoid this plant if you have any allergy or sensitivity to members of the *Asteraceae* plant family (including ragweed, chrysanthemums, marigolds, and daisies). Caution should also be used if you have an allergy or an intolerance to pectin.

Although its primary indication is to help control blood sugar, caution is advised in people with diabetes (or low blood sugar) and especially in those taking drugs, herbs, or supplements that affect blood sugar. If you have diagnosed diabetes, always speak to a qualified healthcare practitioner before using anything that may adjust your blood sugar.

Taking burdock with anticoagulant or antiplatelet drugs (including aspirin) might increase the risk of bleeding.

Burdock may also cause oxytocin-like effects and stimulate the uterus. Because it has not been thoroughly studied, burdock is not considered safe during pregnancy or breastfeeding.

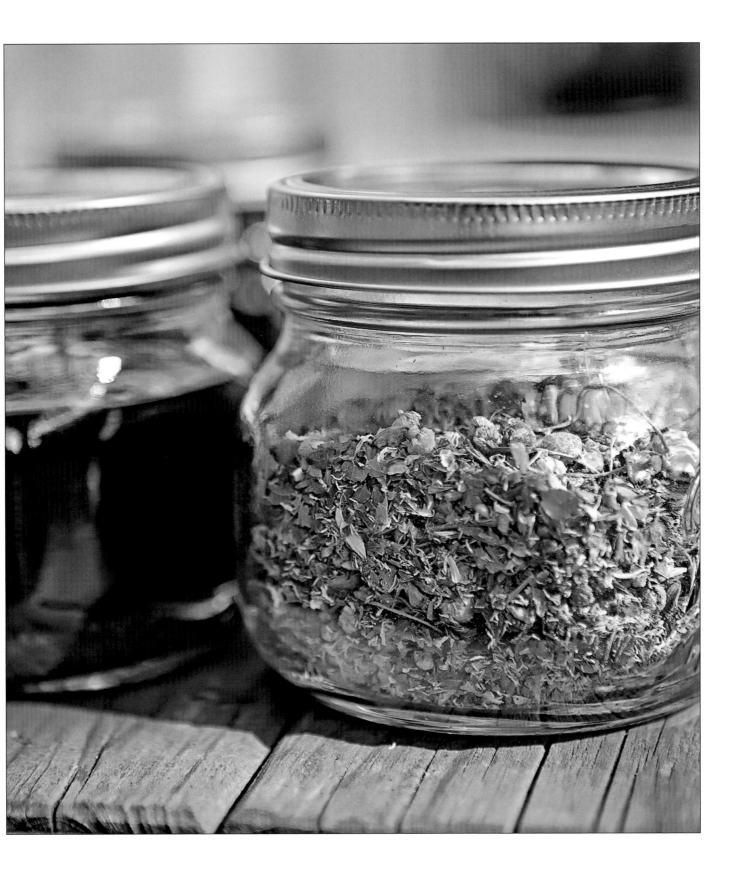

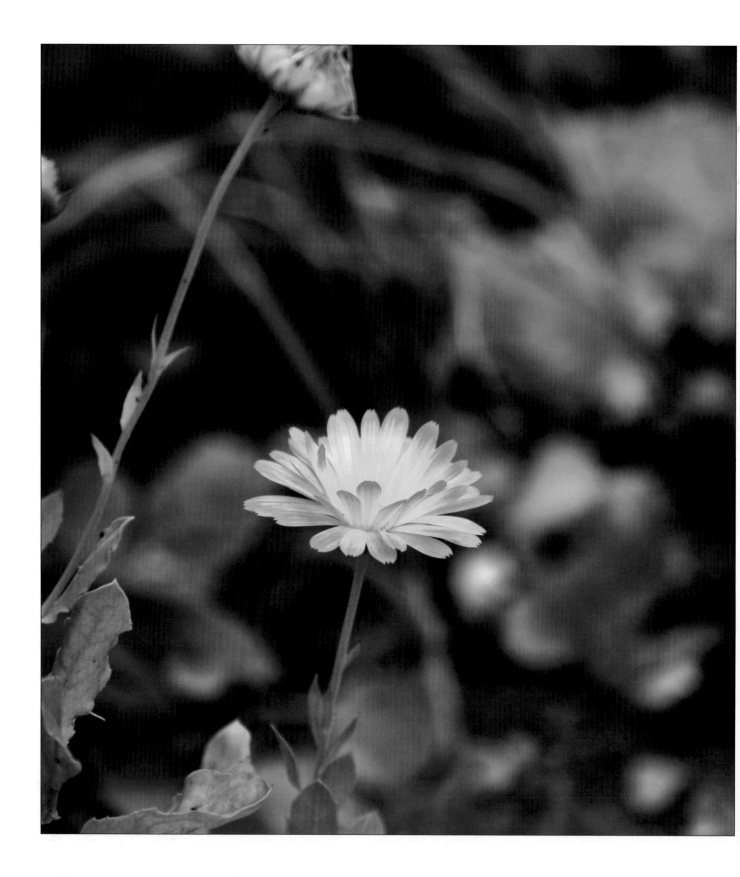

Calendula

This sunny yellow-orange flower—also called pot marigold or English marigold—is found in gardens all over the world. Calendula should not be confused with other marigolds of the *Tagetes* genus: these ornamental varieties have no medicinal value and won't do anything for you but look good. Calendula belongs to the same family (*Asteraceae*) as daisies, chrysanthemums, and ragweed. The plant's name is related to the Latin word *calens*, meaning the first day of the month. The flower has been known since Roman times and was rumoured to bloom on the first of each month. Christians called it "marygold" or "marybud" because it bloomed at festivals celebrating the Virgin Mary.

Health Benefits

Calendula officinalis is one of the most important plants in your medicinal garden. The dried petals make a miracle anti-inflammatory agent and wound healer. It can be used for leg ulcers and has been shown to help wounds heal faster and suppress minor infections.

It is speculated that calendula works by increasing blood flow to the affected area, which helps new tissue grow faster. In fact, it is such a powerful healing agent that you should avoid putting calendula cream on a deep wound, since it may induce the top skin layer to heal before the deeper layer has a chance to close, causing a pocket to form.

Some evidence suggests that calendula can reduce or prevent dermatitis and skin inflammation in breast cancer patients while they undergo radiation therapy. It is also effectively used for chronic nosebleeds, varicose veins, hemorrhoids, and even in dilute solution for conjunctivitis (inflammation of the white of the eye).

One of the many important ingredients in calendula may be its high concentration of flavonoids, a class of antioxidants. Calendula is also a natural weapon against harmful bacteria, fungi, and viruses.

Growing

Pot marigold is a tried-and-true annual that has been grown for centuries in both herb and flower gardens. With bright yellow or orange blooms, this plant is as colourful as it is easy to grow! It's so easy, in fact, that even beginners can grow it from seed. Calendula can be enjoyed as an ornamental and harvested as a cut flower, and its blooms can be used in salads or medicinally.

DIFFICULTY
Easy

HARDINESS
Annual

TIME TO PLANT
Mid-spring after risk of frost

TIME TO HARVEST
Summer (in bloom)

LOCATION
Full sun

SOIL TYPE
Well-drained, rich in organic matter

Common Varieties: Be sure you look for *Calendula officinalis*—other types of marigold do not have medicinal value. There are many varieties, but for best performance I recommend 'Calypso Orange'.

PLANT

Calendula can be grown from seed or purchased as a transplant. Fast to germinate, the seeds can be sown directly in the garden in mid-spring after the risk of hard frost. For best results plant in full sun. Calendula will grow in almost any soil type, but it will be most vigorous in soils that are well-drained and rich in organic matter. For small spaces, calendula does beautifully in containers.

In addition to their medicinal properties, calendula flowers are edible and will brighten any salad!

GROW

Calendula enjoys warm days, cooler nights, and adequate moisture. During the growing season it may lag during lengthy periods of hot weather, but it will rebound in late summer and fall when evening temperatures cool. Keep calendula free of weeds and water regularly—do not allow the plants to dry out.

The leaves may be vulnerable to white powdery mildew. Improve the air circulation by allowing adequate space between plants. If you spot any badly infected plants, remove them immediately to prevent spread. Pick flowers early and often, removing any spent flowers, as this too will reduce the risk of powdery mildew.

HARVEST

Calendula is a repeat bloomer, so you can harvest often, picking the flowers in the morning. The flowers are so easy to remove that some commercial varieties of calendula are harvested with combs! For optimum plant health, remove both the flower and stem.

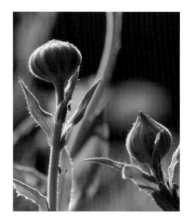

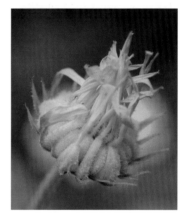

Calendula buds about to bloom.

Use the flowers when they're fresh. Although calendula flowers can be dried, this is difficult to do without artificial heat, as the flowers have many folds where moisture can hide and cause rotting.

Put It to Work

Eye problems? Serve them tea!

If you have conjunctivitis or dry, irritated, red eyes you can make a simple calendula infusion eye bath to help. Don't be scared off—it's just like making tea! It is highly recommended that you invest in a glass eye bath (it is inexpensive and can be found at your local pharmacy). Note that absolute sterility must be maintained in this practice.

Put 2 tablespoons of fresh whole flower tops in a small bowl. Boil 1 cup of water and pour over the flowers. Cover with a saucer and steep for 30 minutes. Strain through a coffee filter. Pour the calendula infusion into a sterile eye bath and use only when the liquid is cool enough. If you intend to treat both eyes, before repeating with the opposite eye, discard the used infusion, sterilize the eye bath by boiling in fresh water for 5 minutes, and then fill with new infusion. Discard any remaining infusion. Do not store.

Boo-boo or ouchie? Petal plasters to the rescue!

The painful wail of a hurt child is heartbreak-ing. Once you've hugged your child and assessed the scratch, scrape, or abrasion, it's time to offer a novel type of Band-Aid. Distraction is half of this successful treatment; the other half comes from the true healing power of calendula's petals.

Pick 4 or 5 petals from your calendula flower and have your child help apply them over the affected area, keeping the petals in place using a conventional bandage. Change the petals every 3 to 4 hours. If any small pieces stick to the wound, don't worry; they will easily come off with a water rinse or with the scab.

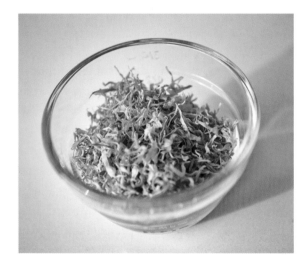

Commercially dried calendula is widely available if you want to try any of these fixes in the depths of winter! You can even just open up a calendula tea bag.

Stinky feet? Soak them in a calendula foot bath!

Funky feet are usually signs of a fungal infection (whether you see one or not). Calendula flowers have antifungal properties that make them good for a foot soak. Fungus is relentless and difficult to eradicate, so you will need to soak your feet daily for at least 6 weeks to make sure the fungal infection is fully healed.

Start by making a calendula infusion. Put ¾ cup of fresh calendula flowers in a jar that will hold about 4 cups of water. Fill the jar with boiling water and let it sit for about an hour. Strain it through a fine-mesh sieve directly into a foot bath container. Add enough hot water to the infusion to make the foot bath deep enough to cover your feet. Soak feet for about 20 minutes.

Here's a tip: Line the bottom of your child's gym, soccer, or hockey bag with dried calendula petals, or throw a handful into a sock. Not only will they impart a mild and pleasant scent, they can help to ward off the looming fungus that causes a stench.

Got a dash of a rash? Apply this!
This simple calendula ointment can be used topically to provide relief from eczema or psoriasis, and to heal abrasions, bedsores, cracked heels, chapped hands, and superficial cuts and other surface wounds.

Pick about 20 fresh calendula flowers and roughly chop them into 1 cm (½ inch) pieces. In a heatproof bowl over a pot of boiling water (acting as a double boiler), combine the flowers with about 10 teaspoons of petroleum jelly or shea butter, stirring occasionally until completely melted. Reduce the heat, cover, and simmer very gently for up to 3 hours (check

occasionally to ensure there is enough water in the pot and the mixture isn't burning). After 3 hours, the petroleum jelly will have turned the yellow-orange colour of the flowers.

Strain the mixture through a fine-mesh sieve into a sterilized, dark-coloured glass jar with a lid. (The dark glass will prevent the damaging effects of light.) Cover loosely with the lid and allow the ointment to cool. Apply sparingly to affected areas 2 to 3 times a day until healed. Store the ointment in a cool, dark place. Discard after 3 months.

» Fast Forward

Fast forward to the health food store to purchase St. Francis Calendula Vitamin E Cream or equivalent. Follow the instructions on the label.

! Cautions

Avoid using calendula if you have an allergy to plants in the *Asteraceae* family, including ragweed, chrysanthemums, marigolds, and daisies. Allergic reactions to calendula creams are rare.

As with most herbs or supplements, it is not clear whether calendula is entirely safe for use during pregnancy or breastfeeding, so it is best to avoid it during those times.

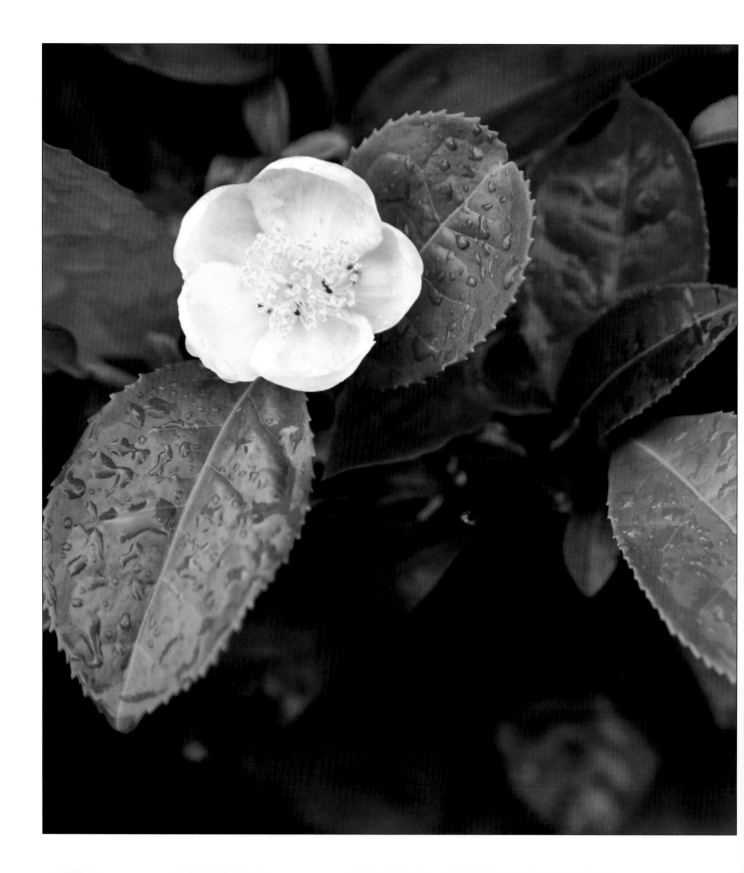

Camellia

Most people have never heard the scientific name *Camellia sinensis*, even if they encounter this plant every day. You know it by its more familiar name: tea. All non-herbal tea originates from the same plant! Whether you prefer black tea, white tea, green tea, oolong tea, or pu-erh tea, you've enjoyed *C. sinensis*, which is native to Asia but is now grown around the world. The various types of tea differ in the way the leaves and leaf buds are processed after harvesting. Black tea is made by cleaning, withering, cutting, and then fermenting the leaves. To make white tea, the very young leaves and buds are harvested, cleaned, and dried. Green tea is generally the least-processed variety, and it's the one most likely to be used for medicinal purposes.

Health Benefits

The main types of tea have nearly equal health benefits, but green tea is by far the most researched, as well as the easiest to harvest and prepare.

The *C. sinensis* plant is a superhero, with tremendous health benefits and a remarkable amount of research behind it. Studies have shown green tea is heart-healthy because it contains catechins—a class of antioxidants—that help reduce LDL (bad) cholesterol. Catechins are also believed to play a key role in reducing the risk of diseases like breast, colon, prostate, and esophageal cancers.

The most powerful catechin in tea is called EGCG (epigallocatechin gallate). Along with other antioxidants, EGCG is believed to help fight off the flu, improve symptoms of depression, and make skin appear younger by protecting against sun damage and reducing wrinkles. EGCG has also been proven to aid in weight loss, possibly by blocking fat tissue expression: In other words, tea burns fat cells! It may also benefit diabetics because of its ability to regulate blood sugar levels after eating.

The antioxidant effects of green tea appear to be boosted when it's taken with a twist of lemon. A recent study discovered citrus juices significantly increased catechin levels in lab tests, as did ascorbic acid, soy milk, rice milk, and cow's milk. The researchers found that beverages prepared with ascorbic acid increased the available catechin levels from less than 20% to as much as 69%, and citrus juices had the strongest benefit.

Growing

C. sinensis is an acid-loving broadleaf evergreen that has been grown and loved in Chinese gardens for some 3,000 years. It's

DIFFICULTY
Medium to hard

HARDINESS
Perennial in zones 7 to 9 (grow indoors in lower zones)

TIME TO PLANT
Year-round indoors; outdoors in pots after risk of frost

TIME TO HARVEST
Mid-spring to summer (tender shoots)

LOCATION
Indirect light

SOIL TYPE
Acidic potting soil

hardy to more southern climates (zone 7 to 9), but it still enjoys cooler temperatures, and when grown indoors it requires a period of dormancy. In nature, tea plants can grow over 4 metres (15 feet), but in a pot they will grow no more than 1 to 2 metres (3 to 6 feet). Enjoyed as an indoor plant for its foliage, *C. sinensis* will flower in late fall with white blooms and yellow stamens.

Common Varieties: *C. sinensis* isn't readily available. You will likely have to request it from your garden centre or source it online. There are many cultivars, and whatever is available locally should be suitable. Just be sure not to confuse this plant with its more popular cousins *C. japonica* and *C. sasanqua*, which have no medicinal value.

PLANT

Transplant your tea plant into a container at least twice as large as its root ball. Ensure the container has adequate drainage holes, or improve drainage by drilling additional holes or adding a coarse material like broken clay pots to the bottom. Use potting soil only and improve acidity by amending with garden sulphur or increasing the percentage of peat moss.

When repotting, score the roots and firmly pack soil around the side, making sure you don't plant the root ball deeper than the previous soil line. *C. sinensis* will require repotting every 2 to 4 years.

GROW

Place the plant in a room with bright indirect light. West- or south-facing rooms are best; don't place the plant directly in front of a window. Ideal room temperature is 20°C (68°F), with cooler evening temperatures desired.

Keep the soil evenly moist but allow the top 5 cm (2 inches) to dry between waterings. Watering frequency depends on the light and humidity in your home. Use the finger-touch method to monitor soil moisture. Use 10-10-10 fertilizer once a

Even indoor plants may require a period of dormancy. This is a period of rest when plants are exposed to reduced light levels and temperature, as they are in winter. Allow your tea plant to rest from late fall into late winter by reducing watering, eliminating fertilizer, and placing it in a cooler room with reduced temperatures (about 10° to 15°C/50° to 59°F) for 1 to 3 months. This dormancy period will help aid flower production.

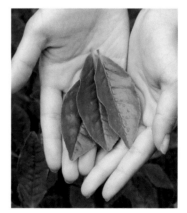

month while the plant is actively growing, from spring to fall. Prune after the plant blooms, removing spent flowers and dead and/or diseased wood.

In late spring, once the risk of frost has passed, you can move *C. sinensis* to a shady spot outdoors; bring it indoors again in late summer, before the risk of frost. Spray with insecticidal soap before returning indoors. Let the plant go dormant in winter (see page 71).

HARVEST

It's very important to harvest the tea leaves only while the tea plant is actively growing. Pluck only the 2 or 3 tender new leaves on the end of each stem, not the old growth. If the plant is outdoors, the leaves should be harvested mid-morning after the morning dew has evaporated.

STORE

Allow the leaves to dry for 2 hours out of direct light, then steam them like you would spinach. Rinse the leaves thoroughly under cold running water and shake, leaving some water clinging to them. Place the leaves in a large saucepan over high heat. Cover and cook for 1 minute. Arrange the steamed leaves in a single layer on a baking sheet and bake in a preheated 120°C (250°F) oven for 25 minutes. Store the dried leaves in an airtight container in a cool, dark place for up to a year.

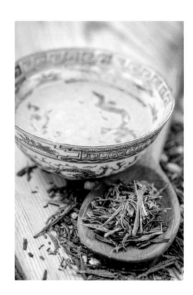

Whether you like green tea, white tea, or black tea, you're drinking the bounty of *Camellia sinensis*.

🔧 Put It to Work

Weight gain? Cravings? Three cheers for tea!
You don't need to avoid chocolate altogether if you're trying to lose weight. Whenever you have a craving, make a cup of tea and stir in ¼ teaspoon of grated chocolate. This will sweeten the tea, but more importantly, your taste buds will tell your brain that you are satisfying that craving.

To effectively cut down your food cravings and boost your metabolism, keep hot or cold tea close at hand in your house, workplace, and car. Carry a Thermos of hot tea with you or add cold tea to your water bottle. Keep your home-made loose-leaf green tea in resealable bags or small tins and pack a tea strainer in your brief-case or purse, or leave one in your desk drawer at work. When you're at a restaurant, order hot water and add your tea to it (don't forget to ask for a slice of lemon!). Drinking tea during and between meals can reduce the amount of food you eat.

Blackheads? Green solution!

Most blackheads are caused by skin debris and oil that block pores. Don't pick them! A green tea poultice, which contains tannins and anti-oxidants, can help flush out the pore, reduce inflammation, and detoxify and tighten the skin to prevent reoccurrence. This treatment is also useful for non-serious infections in the hair follicles.

Place about 4 tablespoons of dried green tea in a bowl. Pour boiling water over the tea until it just covers the leaves. Steep for 10 minutes. Wet a dark-coloured wash cloth (or face towel you don't mind staining!) with hot water. Lay it over a clean countertop or plate and spread the mixture evenly onto half of the cloth. Fold the cloth over quickly so as not to lose too much heat. Lie down on your back and place the poultice over your face, being careful not to burn yourself. Leave the cloth in place

for 10 minutes. Repeat this every night before bed for 1 to 2 weeks and enjoy the difference!

» Fast Forward

Fast forward to the health food store to purchase AOR Active Green Tea capsules or equivalent. Follow the instructions on the label.

! Cautions

Green tea is generally free of side effects, although people who consume several cups per day have reported insomnia, anxiety, and other symptoms from the caffeine. If you are sensitive to caffeine, limit yourself to one cup daily.

Green tea also contains tannins, which can decrease the absorption of iron and folic acid, so if you are pregnant or trying to conceive, then green tea may not be for you.

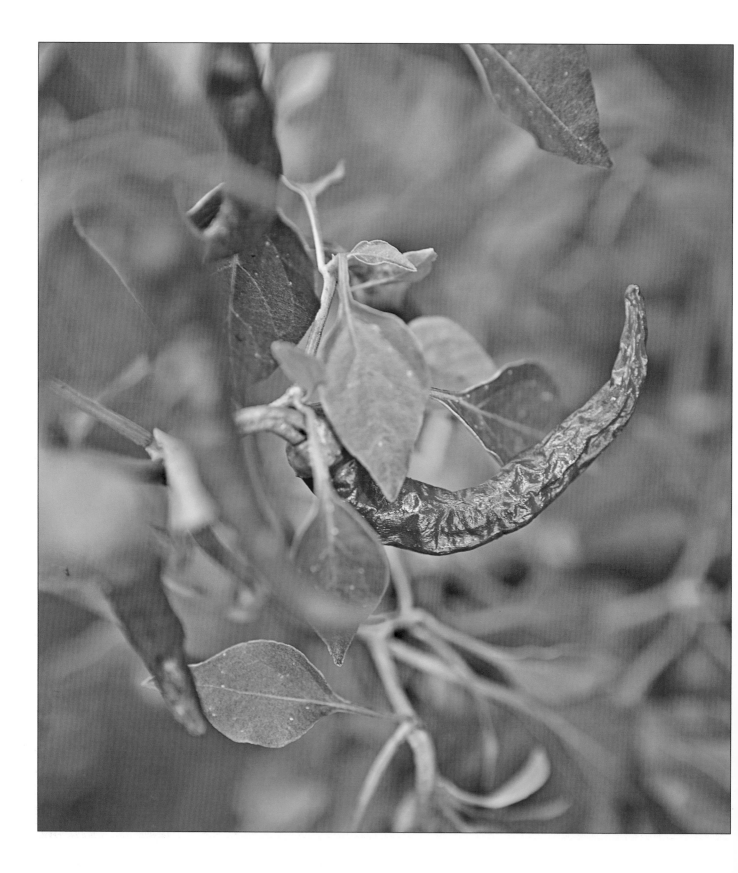

Capsicum

Capsicums—more commonly known as peppers—add brilliant colour, robust flavour, and often tremendous heat to dishes around the world. The most common varieties come from two closely related species: *Capsicum annuum* and *C. frutescens*. These include mild types such as bell peppers as well as hotter varieties used to make Tabasco sauce, chili powder, and paprika. A pepper's heat depends on the concentration of a phytochemical called capsaicin. This compound causes a burning sensation on the tongue, mucous membranes, and skin. In reasonable quantities it gives foods a pleasant, spicy taste. In high concentrations it is so powerful it can be used as a weapon: It's the active ingredient in pepper spray.

Health Benefits

Capsaicin has a numbing effect: It interferes with a neurotransmitter called "substance P," which sends pain signals from nerves to the brain. Capsaicin creams can alleviate pain when rubbed on the affected area, though the effect is temporary. Research proves capsaicin creams are effective for a wide range of problems including neuropathy (painful nerve endings common in diabetics), post-surgical pain, psoriasis, shingles, arthritis, and fibromyalgia.

Low back pain is one of the most common reasons people see their family doctor, and the evidence is very good that topical capsaicin cream helps. It is approved by Germany's Commission E (a board of scientific advisors who investigate traditional medicines) as an ointment for the relief of painful muscle spasms.

Capsicum isn't just helpful for pain: It could also be a key weapon in the battle of the bulge. If you already "like it hot," you may have an advantage when it comes to keeping off the pounds. Research shows capsicum can help you lose weight in three ways: by increasing your metabolism (you can burn an extra 50 or more calories per day), improving your energy expenditure, and reducing your appetite.

Growing

Peppers have been spicing up gardens around the world for centuries. They can be a challenge to grow in cooler climates, however, as they require a lot of heat and a long time to mature. When choosing among the many varieties of capsicums at your garden centre, check the tags for maturity dates (see page 77).

Common Varieties: There are many cultivars of *Capsicum annuum* and the closely related *C. frutescens*, in a range

DIFFICULTY
Medium

HARDINESS
Annual

TIME TO PLANT
Late spring

TIME TO HARVEST
Summer

LOCATION
Full sun

SOIL TYPE
Rich, well-drained

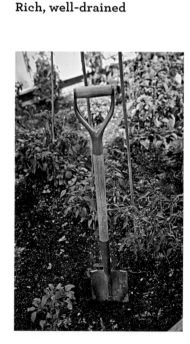

of colours, shapes, sizes, and heat intensity. For medicinal use, look for varieties that fall between 30,000 to 50,000 units on the Scoville heat scale. This includes cayenne and Tabasco peppers. (Hotter varieties typically belong to different species.)

PLANT

Growing peppers from seed isn't for the novice. Even for experienced gardeners I recommend purchasing transplants, and for those in cooler climates I recommend purchasing slightly mature plants.

Peppers can be grown both in the garden and in pots. Plant them in late spring once soil temperatures have warmed to 20°C (68°F). Planting them in cooler soils will stunt plants. Make sure they're located in full sun and in rich, well-drained soil.

Peppers are heat lovers: The more sun and the more heat you can give them, the better they do. I often plant peppers in black pots, since black absorbs heat and helps them grow!

GROW

Peppers are tender plants that will suffer from cold wind, frosty nights, and thunderstorms. Plant them in a wind-sheltered location and cover them on spring evenings when frost looms.

Water deeply and infrequently, maintaining adequate moisture and never allowing the plants to completely dry out. Water the roots only, not the foliage. Peppers benefit from mulching in the garden: Mulch helps retain moisture and prevents splashing on the foliage during intense rains, reducing the risk of disease. In containers and areas with poor soil, use a general-purpose fertilizer (20-20-20) or organic fish emulsion twice monthly after watering.

Inspect the plants regularly for insects and disease. Peppers will benefit from preventive sprayings of insecticidal soap to reduce aphid and whitefly populations. If plants appear to be wilting and losing bottom leaves, or if they have black marks on

A plant's maturity date is the number of days it requires to produce fruit. To make sure your growing season is long enough, count the number of days between average last frost date and average first frost date in your area. Some varieties of capsicum need 80 days or more to produce fruit, which is a challenge in some regions of Canada.

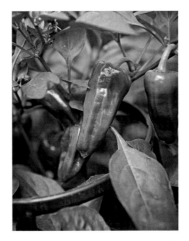

Don't panic if your hot pepper plant starts growing green peppers like these—with enough time and hot sun they'll turn fiery red.

lower foliage, remove and discard the entire plant, as they are most likely suffering from disease.

HARVEST

Harvest peppers in summer, allowing the fruit to reach their full size and colour on the vine. Remove by twisting and plucking or cutting them from the stem.

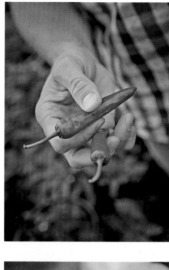

STORE

Fresh peppers can last for weeks in the refrigerator, and will even keep for 5 to 7 days at room temperature when left out of direct light and kept dry. Peppers can be sun-dried, air-dried, baked, or dehydrated and stored in airtight containers for months. They can also be pickled or packed in oil. Peppers lose flavour when frozen, but roasting them prior to freezing will help.

To sun-dry hot peppers, wash and then dry them with a paper towel. Using a sewing needle and thread, string 20 to 30 of them together by pushing the needle through their stems and then tying the ends together. Hang indoors in direct sunlight until dry. Monitor and remove any peppers that spoil (blacken).

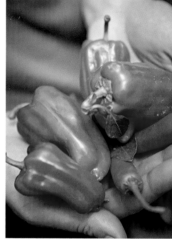

⚒ Put It to Work

Fibromyalgia or arthritis? Set fire to the pain!
Topical creams containing 0.025% to 0.075% capsaicin are generally used for pain relief. People often apply the cream to the affected area 3 or 4 times per day. A burning sensation may occur the first few times the cream is applied, but this should gradually decrease—that's "substance P," the cause of your pain, going to sleep.

You can make your own capsaicin cream with homegrown peppers, but be careful! Wash your hands thoroughly after handling the peppers. If you get capsaicin in your eyes or on mucous membranes it can cause a terribly intense burning.

Measure enough dried cayenne peppers to fill a large resealable glass jar (like a Mason jar). In a blender, pulse the peppers for about 1 minute or until coarsely ground. Do not overgrind—this will make the mixture difficult to strain later. Empty the ground peppers into a clean jar and pour in enough vodka (at least 80 proof) to cover the peppers by 6 mm (¼ inch). Place wax paper over the jar and then screw the lid on tightly to seal it. Set aside in a cool, dark place for 3 days, shaking the jar vigorously for 1 minute every day. Once the peppers have been soaking for 72 hours, you'll see the vodka has turned a pretty red.

After 3 days, cover the mouth of the jar with a coffee filter and strain the mixture into a bowl. Carefully discard the pepper pieces. You will be left with a mixture of alcohol and capsaicin oil. Pour the liquid back into the jar, but do not cover it. Leave the jar in a dry, warm place (out of the reach of children!) until the alcohol completely evaporates.

After a day or two, the bottom of the jar will be full of bright red capsaicin oil. Do not touch this directly with your hands—it is incredibly potent! Pour the oil into at least twice as much shea butter and mix well using a small spoon (if you have sensitive skin, add three times as much shea butter). Transfer this mixture to an airtight container and store it in a cool, dry place. The cream will keep for up to a year.

Whenever you experience pain from fibromyalgia or arthritis, use a cotton swab or ball to apply a small amount of the cream to the affected area. At first, you will feel a tingling, hot sensation, but this will fade, taking the pain with it. Continue to rub it in until the area feels slightly numb. Avoid using capsaicin cream on particularly sensitive areas or anywhere near your eyes.

Monitor how your skin and the deeper muscles react. If a small rash develops, it may mean you need to add more shea butter to the mix to dilute it further. If the rash persists, stop using the cream.

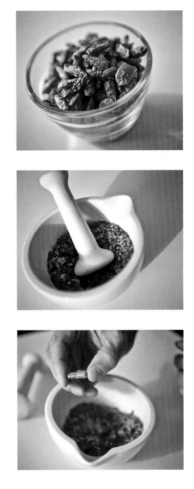

Grinding cayenne peppers for capsules can also be done with a mortar and pestle—but you may want to cover your mouth and nose. We sneezed for fifteen minutes after taking these photos!

Heartburn? Treat fire with fire!

Research shows that about 1 gram of cayenne powder in capsule form taken 3 times per day before meals is an effective treatment for heartburn. To make your own remedy, pour 1 cup of boiling water over ½ teaspoon of ground dried cayenne pepper and steep for 10 minutes. A teaspoon of this infusion can be mixed with water and taken 3 to 4 times daily. It's counterintuitive, but it works! Store the infusion in an airtight container in the refrigerator.

Excess weight? Melt the pounds away!

By consuming 10 grams of cayenne pepper with food daily, you're likely to eat less. And research shows that cayenne could also boost your metabolism to help you burn fat faster. However, 10 grams is equivalent to 2 teaspoons, and that's a lot of heat, especially if you're not into spices! Have no fear: you can make your own easy-to-swallow capsules. Start by purchasing a bag of 1000-milligram empty gelatin capsules from your local health food store.

Pick 30 fresh cayenne peppers and sun-dry them (see "Drying Herbs at Home" on page 365). Once dry, place the peppers in a blender, cover with the lid, and pulverize to a fine powder. Transfer the powder to a bowl and, using latex gloves, carefully (don't get the powder into your eyes or lungs!) fill the capsules. Take 5 capsules twice daily with food to enjoy a significantly reduced appetite and an increased metabolism.

» Fast Forward

Fast forward to the health food store to purchase Nature's Way cayenne pepper capsules or equivalent. Follow the instructions on the label.

! Cautions

Capsicum essential oil and cayenne pepper are both listed in the U.S. Food and Drug Administration (FDA) Generally Recognized as Safe (GRAS) list for use as spices in foods. But you can imagine that something this hot comes with a warning!

When taken orally, capsicum may irritate the gastrointestinal system, mouth, and throat. In some cases, heartburn, diarrhea, ulcer aggravation, and stomach pain can occur. Extremely hot varieties can also cause chemical damage to taste buds. Large amounts (over 20 grams a day) may cause kidney and liver damage. Inhaling it may cause shortness of breath and coughing.

When used topically as a cream, capsicum may cause burning, redness, and irritation, especially if it comes in contact with mucous membranes. Never use capsaicin cream on the same area more than 2 or 3 times a day. Even a weak cream will cause irritation if applied too often.

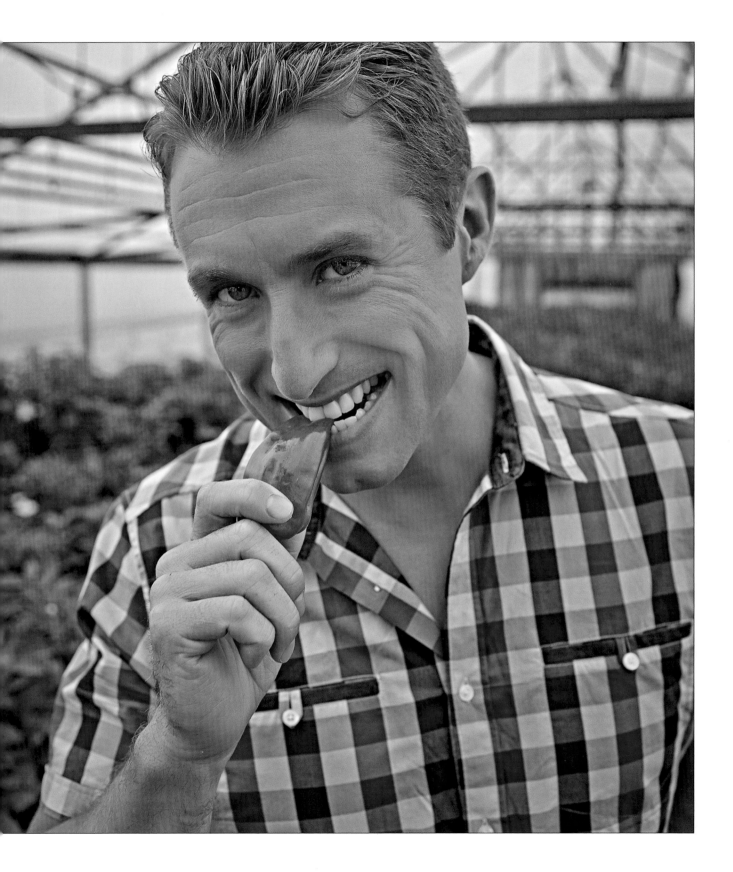

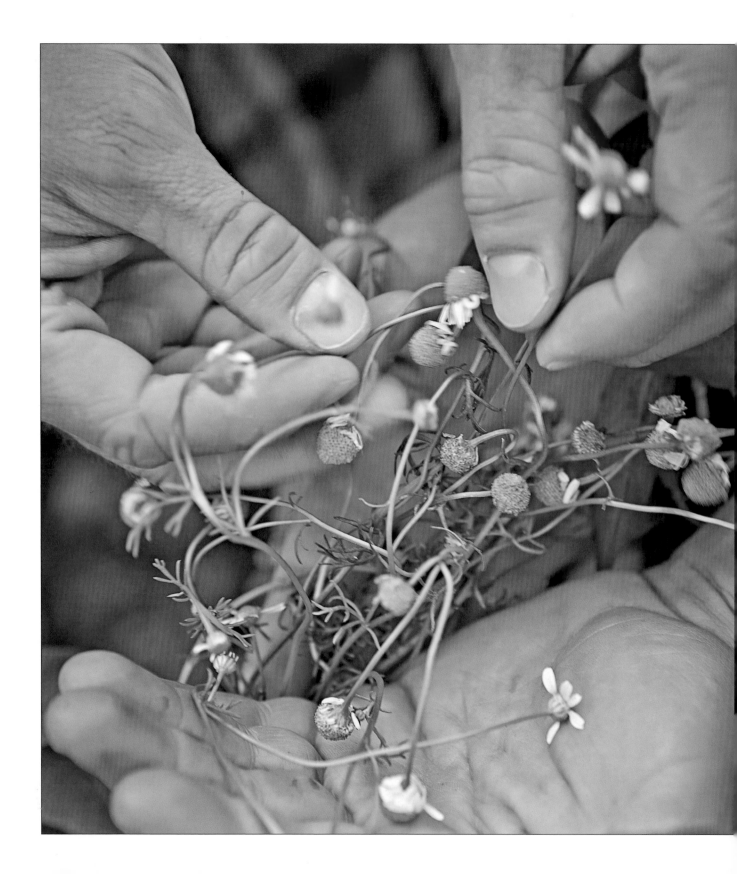

Chamomile

Chamomile is one of the most popular and widely used herbs in the world. Even if you're not into herbal medicine, you've probably had chamomile tea, and you must know about its calming properties. It has been used medicinally for thousands of years across many parts of Europe, where it enjoys a status similar to that of ginseng in Asia. As part of the *Asteraceae* family, the plant is related to daisies; its flower has a delicate, pretty white petal with a cone-shaped yellow centre. Chamomile gets its name from the Greek word for "earth apple" and, not surprisingly, features an aroma reminiscent of fresh apples. *Matricaria chamomilla* is sometimes called German chamomile. It should not be confused with Roman chamomile (*Chamaemelum nobile*), which is not typically used for medicinal purposes.

✚ Health Benefits

Chamomile is much more than just an herbal tea that helps put you to sleep: It's a popular treatment for numerous ailments, including anxiety, indigestion, skin infections, inflammation, eczema, infant colic, teething pain, and diaper rash.

Chamomile cream can be used for treating eczema. Chamomile's essential oil contains an ingredient called bisabolol, which has anti-inflammatory, antibacterial, antifungal, and ulcer-protective properties. The flavonoids in chamomile also act as a powerful anti-inflammatory.

Above all, chamomile has a reputation for being a mild relaxant. It's the go-to anxiety remedy, particularly when symptoms include sleeplessness and indigestion. Evidence indicates chamomile contains compounds that relax the nervous system.

One of chamomile's virtues is its ability to relax physical as well as psychological tension. Adding a chamomile infusion or essential oil to your bath after a stressful day—or to an anxious child's or teething infant's bath—will relax the nervous system and mind. Chamomile even eases muscle cramps: It goes to work on peripheral nerves and muscles and acts as an antispasmodic, relaxing the whole body. When the physical body is less stressed out, the brain takes that as a signal that it can relax—and vice versa.

🌱 Growing

Chamomile can be easily grown from seed or purchased as a transplant. It bears showy, daisy-like white flowers and is a great addition to herb, vegetable, and flower gardens, though it doesn't do well in containers. As an ornamental, chamomile attracts important pollinators like bees, birds, and butterflies. The plant

DIFFICULTY
Easy

HARDINESS
Annual (may self-sow)

TIME TO PLANT
Spring

TIME TO HARVEST
Early summer

LOCATION
Full to part sun

SOIL TYPE
Well-drained

thrives with minimal care—in fact, in some parts of the world it's considered a weed.

Common Varieties: Any cultivar of *Matricaria chamomilla*.

PLANT

Sow chamomile seeds directly in the garden after the risk of frost or purchase transplants from the garden centre. To get an early start, you can sow seeds indoors 4 to 6 weeks before last frost date and then plant in the garden mid-spring. Space the plants 7 to 15 cm (3 to 6 inches) apart in full sun. Chamomile will survive in most locations, but it will thrive in rich soils.

GROW

Chamomile thrives in cooler temperatures and will do well in spring, late summer, and fall, but may suffer in the peak heat of summer. Water deeply and infrequently. Chamomile is not only resistant to most insects and disease, it's also deer-resistant—a worry-free ground-cover herb!

HARVEST

Harvesting chamomile can be a painstaking task. Collect the blooms in early to midsummer by pinching them off the stems. Allow the dew to dry, and harvest during mid-morning on a sunny day. Use only blooms that are full and haven't discoloured; any discoloured flowers should be removed and discarded. Both the harvesting of full blooms and the deadheading will ensure good health and encourage additional flowers.

STORE

To dry chamomile, arrange the flowers in a single layer on drying screens. Spread them evenly to allow for increased airflow. Cover with cheesecloth and place out of direct light in a dry, well-ventilated area. If space allows, just leave them as is; otherwise, store in an airtight container.

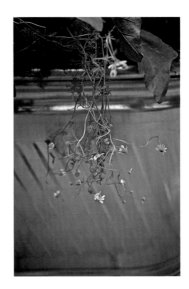

Many plants do better when they're grown along-side others. Chamomile is an ideal companion to basil, onions, cabbage, and cucumber, and some believe it increases the essential oil production of other herbs located nearby. That's how it was used here—to boost the plants around it, even if a container isn't its ideal spot.

⚙ Put It to Work

Upset stomach? Settle it with chamomile tea!
Place 3 grams of whole dried chamomile flowers into a mug. Fill the mug with boiling water, cover with a saucer, and steep for 10 minutes. Strain out the flowers or leave them in for a more robust flavour and stronger effect. Drink one cup 3 times daily between or after meals.

Hyper day? Chamomile nightcap and hit the hay!
If you need to "shut 'er down" early after a stressful day, you could just make a cup of hot chamomile tea using the simple recipe above. But why not get even more potency out of your "earth apples"? Letting the chamomile sit in vodka for a few days will get you zzz'ing much sooner!

What's more, one drink a day (but not more) is considered heart-healthy and may even slow down the aging process. Besides, we all know if you're not getting ample sleep you're contributing to heart disease and speeding up the aging process. Here's what you'll need for your chamomile nightcap:

1 cup dried chamomile flowers (about 20 flowers)
3 cups high-quality vodka (at least 80 proof)
1 cup liquid honey

Crush the chamomile flowers using a mortar and pestle or briefly pulse in a blender. Transfer the crushed flowers to a resealable glass jar (like a Mason jar) and add the vodka. Place wax paper over the jar and then screw the lid on tightly to seal it. Shake the jar well. Set aside in a cool, dark place for 4 days, shaking the jar vigorously every day.

After 4 days, cover the mouth of the jar with a coffee filter or cheesecloth and strain the liquid into a glass bottle with a lid (discard solids). Add the honey and shake well. Best served chilled, this liqueur keeps for months, though it will begin to lose its potency after 3 months. Sip 1 ounce about 30 minutes before your intended sleep time. Nighty night!

Irritating eczema? Use calming chamomile ointment!
This oil makes a soothing remedy for the symptoms of eczema.

½ cup freshly cut chamomile flowers
½ cup vodka (at least 80 proof)
3 cups vegetable oil

Using a sharp knife, roughly chop the chamomile. Combine it with the vodka in a resealable glass jar (like a Mason jar). Place wax paper over the jar and then screw the lid on tightly to seal it. Set the jar aside for 24 hours.

In a blender, combine the oil and the chamomile vodka infusion and blend at medium speed until smooth. Using muslin or fine

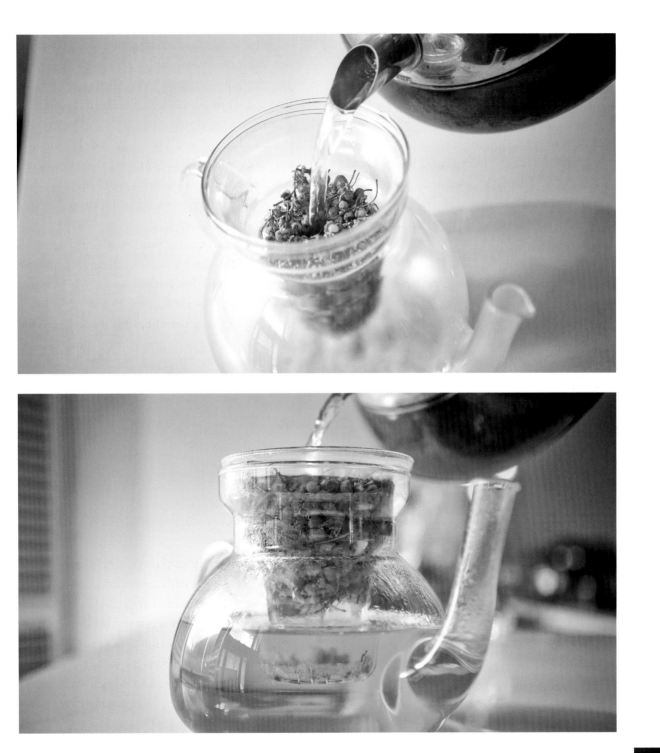

cheesecloth or a coffee filter, strain into a bowl (discard solids).

In a small heatproof bowl over a pot of boiling water (acting as a double boiler), heat the mixture over low heat for 2 hours or until all of the alcohol has evaporated (being careful not to burn the infused oil). Here's a tip: Test for any remaining alcohol by holding a flame next to the surface of the oil (a barbecue lighter will work). If it lights, there is still alcohol left that needs to be evaporated.

Transfer the oil to a sterile bottle with a tight-fitting lid. Apply to the affected area up to 3 times a day. The oil will keep in the refrigerator for up to 4 months.

» Fast Forward

Fast forward to the health food store to purchase Clef des Champs chamomile tincture or equivalent. Follow the instructions on the label.

! Cautions

Do not take chamomile orally when using blood-thinning medications (anticoagulants and antiplatelets), as it may increase the risk of bleeding.

Avoid chamomile if you're taking drugs that make you drowsy, as chamomile can strengthen their effects. These include anti-seizure medications such as phenytoin (Dilantin) and valproic acid; benzodiazepines; insomnia medications such as zolpidem (Ambien); tricyclic antidepressants such as amitriptyline (Elavil); or more than 1 ounce of alcohol.

Do not combine chamomile with sedative herbs such as valerian and kava.

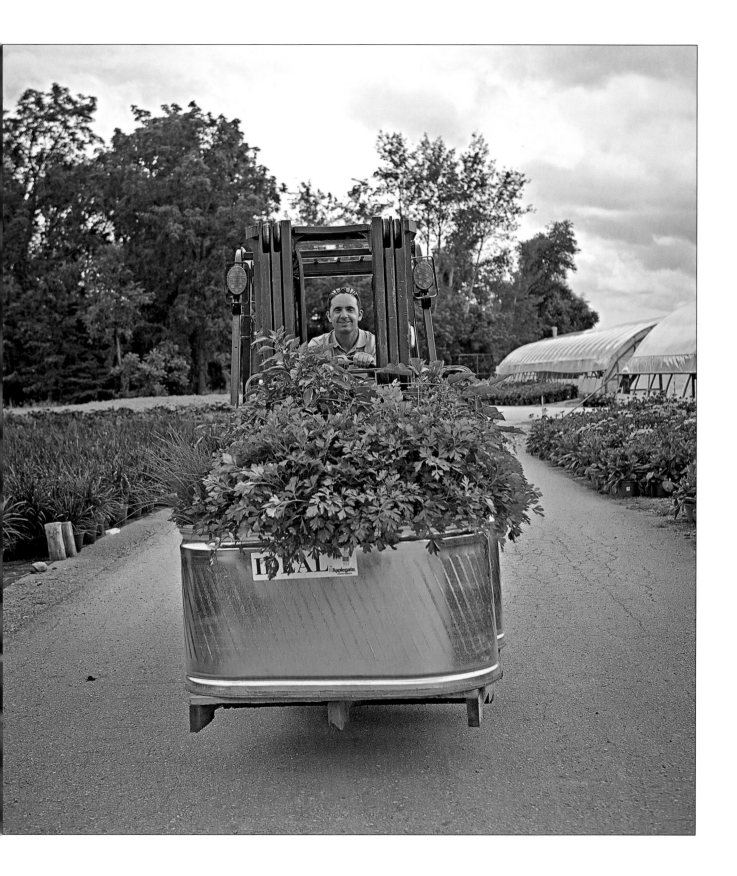

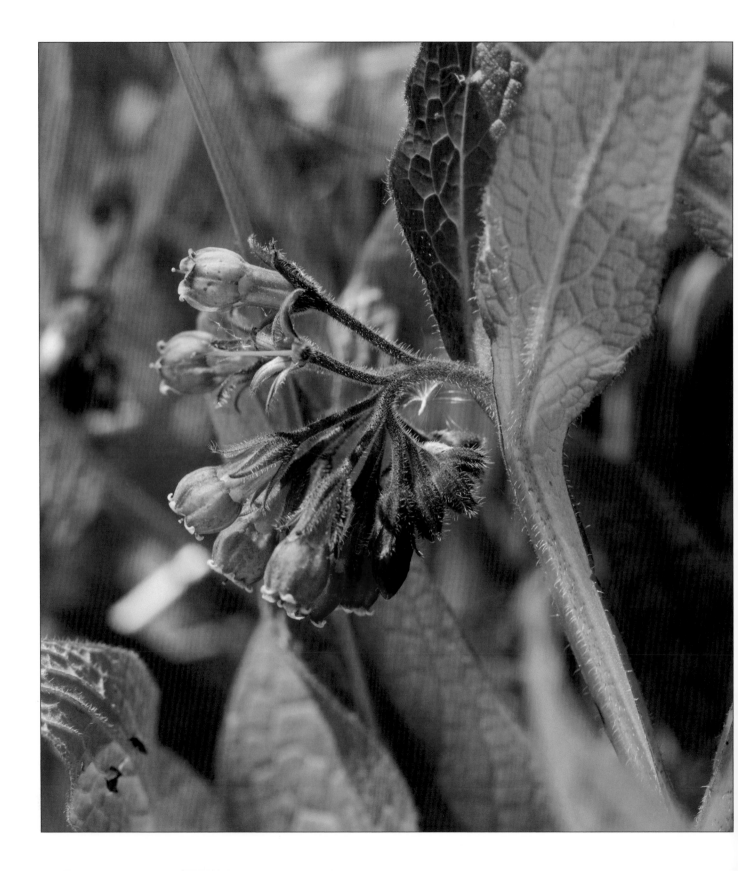

Comfrey

Comfrey is a member of the borage family (*Boraginaceae*), which also includes forget-me-nots. It is a large plant with broad, hairy leaves and purplish, blue, or white flowers. Native to Europe, it has long been cultivated for its remarkable healing properties and for use as an organic fertilizer. Its Latin name, *Symphytum*, is derived from the Greek *symphyo*, meaning to "grow together," and its folk names include bruisewort, boneset, and knitbone. Many herbal preparations now use a cultivar called Russian comfrey (*Symphytum × uplandicum*), which is a hybrid of common comfrey (*S. officinale*) and rough comfrey (*S. asperum*).

⊕ Health Benefits

Comfrey is nature's answer to the Band-Aid. In the past, its leaves were sterilized in boiling water and applied directly to wounds to reduce swelling and bruising, and even to promote rapid healing of broken bones. Comfrey's ability to help heal wounds comes from a compound called allantoin (present in both the leaves and roots), which is believed to reduce inflammation and promote new cell growth.

Modern science seems to back up traditional beliefs. In one study, for example, a 35% comfrey cream applied topically to ankle sprains was very effective at treating tenderness, swelling, and pain even when compared with anti-inflammatory pharmaceutical creams.

In the past, comfrey was taken orally for gastrointestinal, respiratory, and gynecological concerns; however, it is now known that the plant contains toxic compounds, and it is listed as "topical use only" in herbal and medical textbooks.

Growing

Comfrey is a hardy perennial that is extremely easy to grow: its vigorous roots will even break through clay. It blooms throughout the summer and spreads rapidly, so it will thrive in most gardens. But a word of warning: comfrey is a big plant that will easily grow ½ to 1 ½ metre (2 to 5 feet) tall and wide and can take over its location.

Common Varieties: Common comfrey (*Symphytum officinale*) and the hybrid Russian comfrey are the most common; Red Comfrey ('Rubrum') is a cultivar that tolerates shade.

DIFFICULTY
Easy

HARDINESS
Perennial in zones 4 to 9

TIME TO PLANT
Sow seeds directly into garden in early spring or purchase transplants in mid-spring

TIME TO HARVEST
Flowers in early to mid-summer, roots in fall

LOCATION
Full to part sun

SOIL TYPE
Most (will grow in clay)

PLANT

Comfrey should be located in the middle or at the rear of a garden, since this large plant has been known to shade out its neighbours. Comfrey is propagated from seed, root cuttings, crown divisions, and transplants. Plant it in mid-spring after the risk of hard frost, or directly sow seeds in the ground in early spring, as soon as soil is workable. Divide plants in early spring or early fall. For best results, locate common comfrey in full sun, in rich, well-drained soil, and space 30 to 60 cm (1 to 2 feet) apart.

GROW

The biggest challenge with growing comfrey is getting it established; after that it will take care of itself. Water deeply and infrequently, ensuring new transplants never dry out. Regular applications of general-purpose water-soluble fertilizer (20-20-20) or compost tea (page 175) will also help.

Once established (give it about a year), comfrey is extremely winter-hardy, drought-resistant, and unlikely to be bothered by diseases or insects, but inspect it occasionally and remove any brown side shoots as necessary. Ensure adequate airflow by not overplanting.

HARVEST

Harvest mature plants only: Wait for a plant height of at least 60 cm (2 feet) before cutting leaves. Harvest during mid-morning on a sunny day after the dew has dried. Wear gloves, as the plant's hairy leaves have been known to cause rashes.

Remove entire stalks by cutting to just above the base of the plant. You should not harvest more than a third of the plant at a time, but comfrey is an incredibly tough plant that will bounce back even after aggressive harvesting. In fact, it will produce additional growth and can be harvested up to 3 times per season.

STORE

Dry the stalks and leaves by hanging them upside down in a dry place out of direct light (see "Drying Herbs at Home" on page 365). Comfrey has dense foliage and will take longer to dry than other herbs. After drying, store the foliage in airtight containers out of direct light.

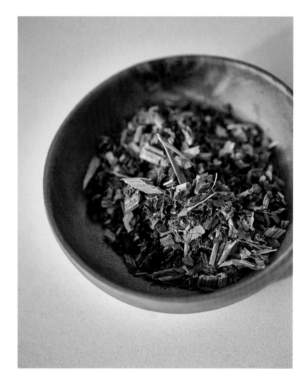

Put It to Work

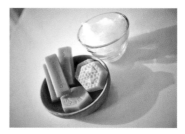

Breastfeeding blues? Comfrey brings re-leaf!

The soothing demulcent properties of comfrey leaves can help relieve sore nipples after breastfeeding. Demulcents are traditionally used to aid healing and soothe irritated tissue.

To prepare a poultice, dip 2 fresh comfrey leaves into a mug of boiling water. Lay them flat on a clean surface and allow to cool. While they are still wet, wrap each leaf in a layer of gauze. Apply to the nipples for instant comfort and relief. Holding a heating pad or hot water bottle over the application will keep the poultice warm and active longer. Leave on for up to 15 minutes.

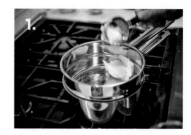

Before the baby breastfeeds again, the area should be rinsed thoroughly to remove any herbal residue.

IMPORTANT: Women planning to use herbs during pregnancy or breastfeeding should always seek the supervision of a qualified healthcare practitioner.

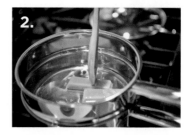

Joint or muscle trauma? Rub on some relief!

Comfrey cream should be in everyone's first-aid kit. It can bring comfort to aching arthritic joints and sore muscles without the strong smell of most topicals—and it's easy to make your own!

10 fresh comfrey leaves
¼ cup coconut oil
75 grams (5 tbsp) beeswax

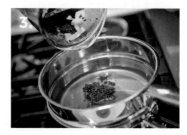

In a blender, purée the comfrey leaves with enough water to make a thick paste. In a small heatproof bowl over a pot of boiling water (acting as a double boiler), melt the coconut oil and beeswax, stirring occasionally (1, 2). Add the puréed comfrey and mix thoroughly (3). Transfer the mixture to a small glass jar with a

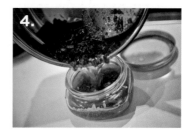

tight-fitting lid (4). Once the cream has cooled and solidified, apply it liberally to the affected area. The cream will keep in a cool, dry place for up to a year.

Roll an ankle? Sit down and get comfrey!

You don't have to be an athlete or weekend warrior to sprain an ankle—just walking over a curb or an uneven surface can end up in a painful ankle roll. It is always best to start treatment for this type of injury with ice, but after several minutes it's time to slip into something a bit more "comfrey." This poultice will work on more than just a sprained ankle: apply to any sprained, strained, bruised, or battered body part.

Collect about 20 fresh comfrey leaves. In a food processor, chop the leaves and add enough water to make a thick soup. Transfer the mixture to a bowl and add enough psyllium husk (unflavoured Metamucil) to make a thick and sticky "porridge."

Divide the mixture in half and spoon equal amounts into an old pair of socks. Flatten the poultice within the socks and seal the tops using elastic bands. Apply the socks to both sides of your hurt ankle and cover with plastic wrap to hold the socks in place and prevent leaking. Leave on for 15 minutes. Do not reapply more than hourly, and no more than 4 times in a day.

›› Fast Forward

Fast forward to the health food store to purchase Gaia Herbs Comfrey Compound or equivalent. Follow the instructions on the label.

! Cautions

Many countries, including Canada and the United States, have banned oral medicines containing comfrey. Comfrey (especially the roots) contains potentially dangerous pyrrolizidine alkaloids. Avoid ingesting comfrey, as these compounds are toxic to the liver.

Just as with calendula cream, do not use comfrey on deep, puncture-type wounds, as it can cause the skin to heal over and seal infection inside.

Comfrey should also be avoided if you are allergic or hypersensitive to any member of the borage family (*Boraginaceae*). If you have never used comfrey it may be prudent to first test your sensitivity by firmly rubbing a leaf on the skin of your inner wrist. If a rash or irritation appears immediately or within a few hours, discontinue.

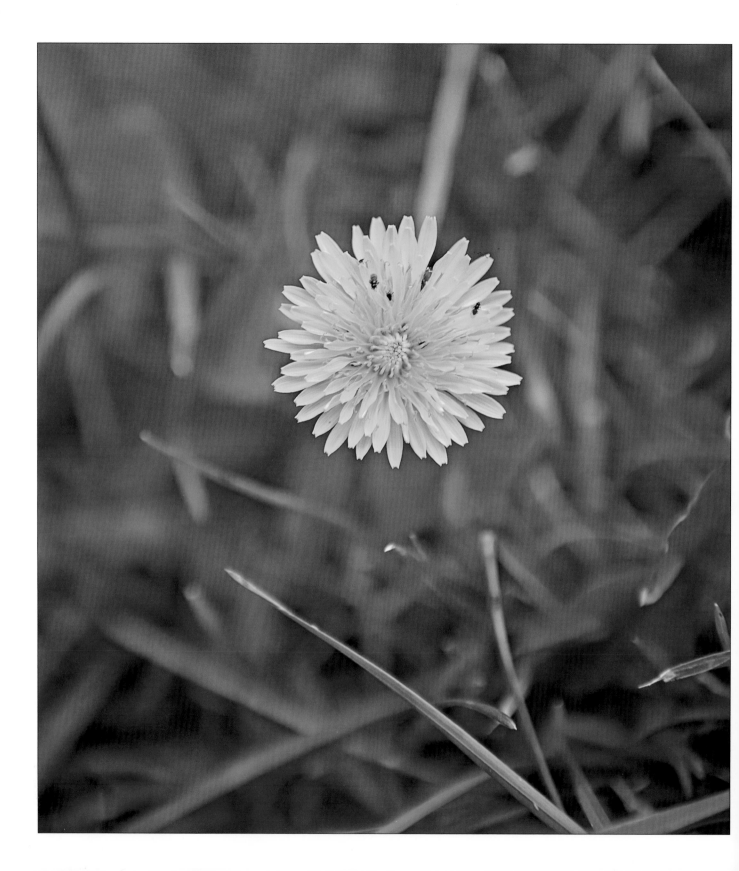

Dandelion

You either love dandelions or despise them. As a kid you probably enjoyed blowing the seeds from their globe-shaped heads—but your neighbours likely didn't share your enthusiasm when new dandelions popped up all over their lawns! Dandelions are now one of the most widespread weeds in the world. If you know about their medicinal virtues, however, you absolutely adore dandelions. They have long been used as an herbal remedy in Europe, North America, and Asia: Their Latin name, *Taraxacum*, means "disease remedy." The plant gets its common name from the French description of its sharply serrated leaves: *dent de lion* translates as "lion's tooth." The French have given this plant a funnier name that comes from its function as a diuretic: *pissenlit* or "pee in the bed."

Health Benefits

Dandelion leaves are eaten in salads, the flowers are made into dandelion wine, and the roots are roasted and ground to make a coffee substitute. The plant also has many traditional medicinal uses. The roots and leaves are used to treat gastrointestinal ailments. The European Scientific Cooperative on Phytotherapy (ESCOP) recommends dandelion root for improving liver and bile function and for treating indigestion and loss of appetite. In Canada, the Natural Health Products Directorate recognizes products containing dandelion for their role in treating appetite loss and indigestion, and as a diuretic.

In clinical practice dandelion is used to detoxify the liver and gallbladder, reduce side effects of medications metabolized by the liver, release stored water (edema), and relieve symptoms associated with liver disease.

Dandelion also contains inulin, a dietary fibre key to helping the good bacteria in your gut proliferate.

Growing

Dandelion is a weed loathed by people who want a lush green lawn, so it feels odd to talk about planting it. Just take a short walk and you will find dandelions growing in front yards, gardens, ditches, fields, forests—even the cracks in your driveway. Despite its lowly status, dandelion is an important plant for both culinary and medicinal use. Being Italian, my family made harvesting *ciccoria* an annual celebration: We would go in search of the perfect patch untouched by pesticide, dog urine, or human foot traffic!

Common Varieties: If you do decide to grow dandelion in the garden, there are several cultivars available in seed form

DIFFICULTY
Easy (it's a weed!)

HARDINESS
Perennial in zones 3 to 9

TIME TO PLANT
Early spring

TIME TO HARVEST
Early to mid-spring

LOCATION
Full sun

SOIL TYPE
Will grow anywhere

and, occasionally, even as transplants. In addition to the common dandelion (*Taraxacum officinale*), look for red-seeded dandelion (*T. erythrospermum*) and Japanese white dandelion (*T. albidum*).

PLANT

Dandelions will grow anywhere, and they will disperse their seeds far and wide. So "planting" them is really more about controlling where they end up. Prevent seeds from being distributed by removing the flower heads early on. Dandelions are known for their incredible tap roots—if even the slightest section of the root is left behind, another plant will grow.

GROW

Dandelion is disease- and insect-resistant, and it has a perennial taproot that makes the plant drought-tolerant, too. You will spend more time controlling it than encouraging it to grow!

HARVEST

Harvest dandelion leaves in early to mid-spring when foliage is young and before blooms appear—that's when they are tastiest. Harvest the flowers when they bloom in mid-spring (midday is best, after the morning dew has dried and the flowers are open).

The roots of mature plants can be pulled in late fall or early spring. Harvesting roots is best done after rain or when soil is moist, as tap roots will come up more easily. Use a dandelion puller—or in a pinch just grab a screwdriver, kitchen knife, or fork—to loosen the surrounding soil.

STORE

Wash dandelion leaves just before use. To store fresh leaves, wrap them in a paper towel and place in a resealable bag in the refrigerator for up to a week. Use freshly picked dandelion flowers in salads or make dandelion wine (pages 101–102).

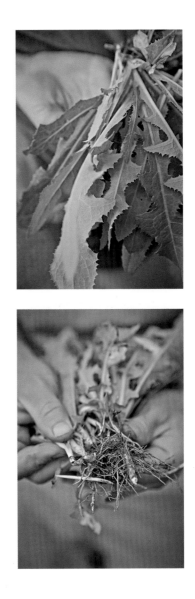

Dandelion roots can be dried or stored in the refrigerator or cold storage like any other root vegetable, such as carrots. To dry, scrub roots thoroughly. Using a sharp knife, cut lengthwise, ensuring uniform thickness (to speed drying). Spread in a single, even layer on a drying screen and set aside in a cool, dark place for up to 2 weeks or until brittle. Dried roots will keep in an airtight container for up to a year. Store fresh dandelion roots wrapped in paper towel in the refrigerator for up to 3 weeks.

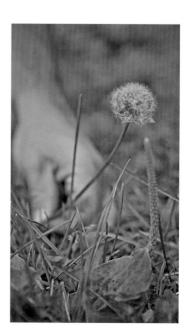

Put It to Work

Always bloated? Eat a prebiotic salad!
Dandelion is rich in inulin, a naturally occurring carbohydrate called an oligosaccharide (several simple sugars linked together). Inulin is a prebiotic—a nutrient that "feeds" the much-desired probiotic bacteria in your gut. If you're feeling bloated, try this prebiotic salad.

1 tsp mustard powder
3 tbsp extra virgin olive oil
Freshly squeezed juice of 1 lemon
½ red onion, chopped
Sea salt and freshly ground black pepper
1 bunch dandelion greens (about 10 oz)
2 medium tomatoes

In a salad bowl, whisk together the mustard powder, oil, and lemon juice. Add the onion and stir to combine. Season with salt and pepper to taste. Add the dandelion greens and tomatoes and toss to coat well. Serve immediately.

After you have eaten this salad at least 5 times in one week, try consuming an over-the-counter high-dose, broad-strain probiotic for a week. Don't stop eating the dandelion! With this regimen, regularity will return and your bloating is sure to disappear.

Feel the need to cleanse? Detox with *Tarax*!

Your liver may be overwhelmed: it's the organ that breaks down medications and removes metabolites from alcohol and fatty foods. Dandelion leaf and root are diuretics that can remove excess toxins and water from your body, helping purify your blood and leaving less work for your tired liver.

We're going to supercharge this detox with garlic and onion, boost it even more with lemon, and empower the immune system with shiitake and maitake mushrooms!

3 tbsp extra virgin olive oil
2 cloves garlic, very thinly sliced
2 cups chopped red onion
2 cups chopped shiitake mushrooms
2 cups chopped maitake mushrooms
10 cups dandelion greens
¼ tsp sea salt
Freshly ground black pepper
Freshly squeezed juice of 1 lemon

Heat the oil in a large wok or cast iron pan over medium heat and sauté the garlic and onion until translucent. Add the mushrooms and cook until slightly browned. Add the dandelion and salt, season with pepper to taste, and sauté for 1 minute, until the leaves are just wilted. Sprinkle with the lemon juice and serve.

Indigestion? Wine not try this!

Dandelion benefits not only the liver but also the gallbladder, its digestive associate responsible for bile production and breaking down dietary fats. If you want to help it do that important job, a glass of this aperitif is what you need!

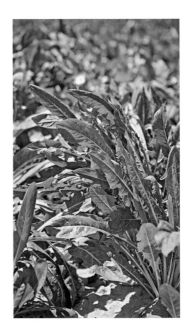

A field of commercially grown dandelion—or what your lawn might look like if you're not careful!

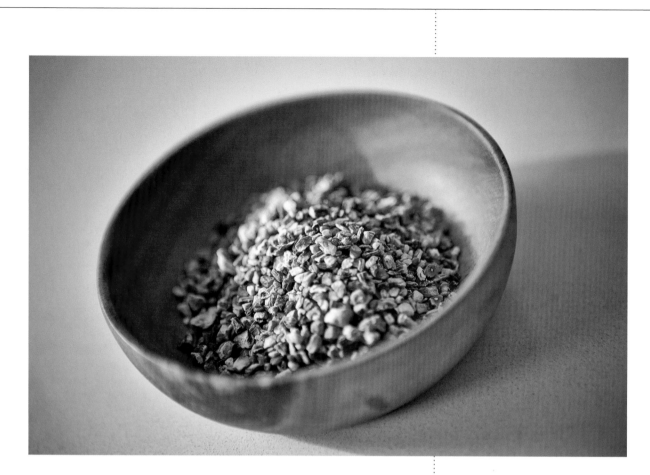

Dried dandelion root.

2 cups whole, young dandelion flowers
1 bottle your favourite red wine (preferably Cabernet)
½ tsp ground ginger
1 sprig fresh rosemary leaves

In a large bowl, cover the flowers in water and set aside to soak overnight. Remove the stems and leaves and any bugs and debris. Using a colander, drain then rinse the flowers under cold running water. Transfer the blossoms to a blender and add half the wine and the ginger and rosemary. Blend on high speed until puréed. Using a funnel lined with a coffee filter, strain the mixture back into the original half-filled wine bottle. Re-cork and refrigerate overnight before taking first dose.

Drink 3 to 4 ounces before dinner or heavy meals. One bottle will yield about 5 glasses, and the wine will keep in the refrigerator for up to a week.

Holding water? Drink diuretic tea

Dandelion helps to cleanse the entire urinary tract and naturally lowers blood pressure by stimulating you to urinate more. Use this tea only if you're not already taking diuretics or "water pills."

Pick and thoroughly wash 4 dandelions—flowers, leaves, roots, and all. Bring 2 cups of water to a boil in a saucepan. Add the dandelions and boil for 10 minutes. Turn off the heat and steep for 15 minutes. Using a fine-mesh sieve, strain the tea into a mug and sweeten with honey or stevia, if desired.

» Fast Forward

Fast forward to the health food store to purchase St. Francis dandelion tincture or equivalent. Follow the instructions on the label.

! Cautions

Herbicides are widely used against dandelions in urban areas. Never pick and use dandelions unless you can guarantee they have not been sprayed with poisons!

Dandelion is a strong detoxifier and may decrease the body's absorption of certain drugs, such as antibiotics. Because some medications are metabolized in the liver, dandelion might decrease how quickly the liver performs this task; it might also increase the effects and side effects of medications.

Don't use dandelion if you are already using another diuretic. Also, if you're taking lithium, dandelion might decrease how well the body gets rid of it.

Consult your pharmacist before combining dandelion with your prescription medications.

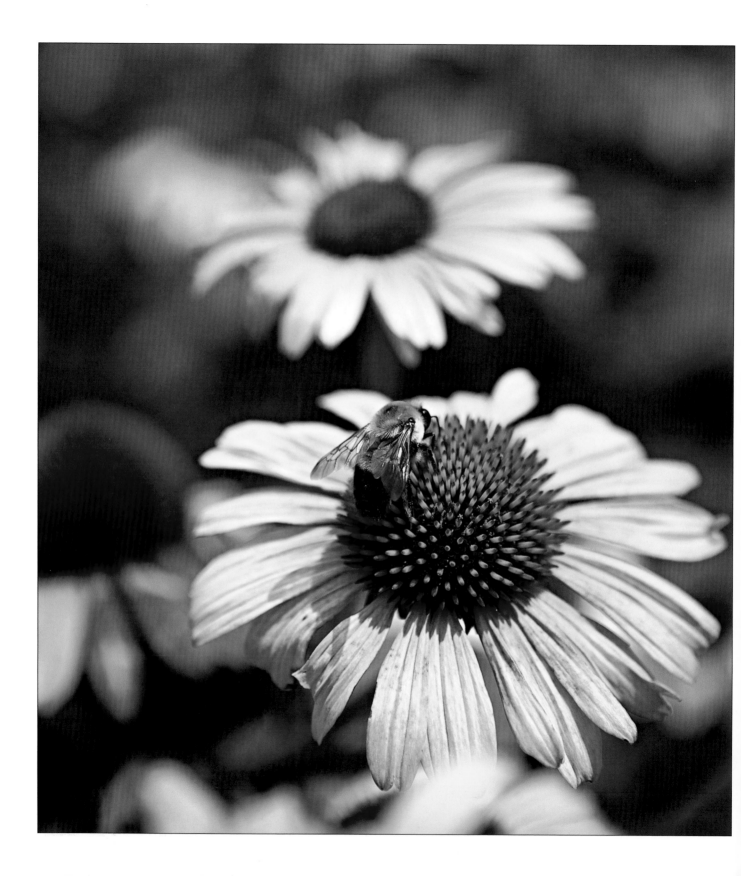

Echinacea

Echinacea—popularly known as coneflower—originated in eastern North America and is part of the daisy family (*Asteraceae*). If you look closely at the centre of each flower, you'll notice a spiny cone-shaped disc that resembles a sea urchin. That's where this plant gets its name: from the Greek *echino*, which means "sea urchin." Coneflower has long been popular in gardens, but it recently gained new popularity as an herbal remedy. An AC Nielsen MarketTrack report in 2010 showed Canadians spent more than $12 million on echinacea, with sales growing 7% each year. That makes it the fastest-growing remedy in the herbal category in Canada.

Health Benefits

In North America, Aboriginal peoples have used echinacea for hundreds of years, and it has enjoyed a dramatic resurgence in the 20th century. It is frequently taken at the onset of a cold or flu to reduce the duration of the illness and the severity of symptoms. It is also believed to boost the immune system by stimulating the body's white blood cells.

There is a growing body of research about its effectiveness. In one large study of 755 adults, researchers at Cardiff University found that both cold episodes and number of days with a cold were reduced by 25% in the group that took echinacea.

Research also suggests taking echinacea may increase red blood cell production and oxygen intake in healthy men, which may be linked to improved athletic performance. Combine this with the known immune-stimulating effects of echinacea, and it seems anyone who exercises at a gym, with its plethora of germs, should be taking this plant extract before and after workouts!

Growing

Coneflower is one of the most popular plants in the perennial garden—so popular that every year plant breeders introduce new colours, new sizes, and even new shapes. This showy low-maintenance flowering plant is extremely easy to grow and is a great choice if you're looking to decrease water use. Originally prairie plants, coneflowers are drought-tolerant and can be grown anywhere there is sun. They look great in borders, open meadows, and formal gardens and can be used indoors as a cut flower. As a bonus, they even attract bees and butterflies!

Common Varieties: *Echinacea purpurea*, or purple coneflower, is the most familiar species, but two others are also pop-

DIFFICULTY
Easy

HARDINESS
Perennial in zones 4 to 8 (some varieties hardy to zone 3)

TIME TO PLANT
Spring

TIME TO HARVEST
Flowers in summer, roots in fall

LOCATION
Full sun

SOIL TYPE
Well-drained

ular in herbal remedies: narrow-leaved purple coneflower (*E. angustifolia*) and pale purple coneflower (*E. pallida*).

PLANT

Mature transplants can be planted anytime during the growing season, but spring or early fall is ideal. Choose a location with lots of sun and well-drained soil. Remove the root ball from the pot and plant just deeply enough so the soil line remains unchanged. Water deeply and infrequently until established.

GROW

The term "low-maintenance gardening" was created for echinacea! Drought-tolerant and resistant to disease and insects, echinacea needs only an occasional watering, lots of sun, and regular removal of surrounding weeds.

For overall plant health, I recommend deadheading (removing spent flowers) often. However, you may want to let the flower heads go to seed if you want to plant more echinacea next spring. Harvest the seed heads in late summer after the flowers have dried. Store the seeds in envelopes in a dark, dry location indoors and sow them directly in the garden in early spring.

Echinacea plants can be divided in early spring or late fall.

HARVEST

Harvest echinacea flowers mid-morning after the dew has dried. Remove the entire stem back to the first leaves, then remove the flower tops from the stems.

Harvest the roots in fall. Lift the plants with a garden fork and cut away sections of the root with a sharp knife, leaving large sections behind so the plant will survive. Place the roots in the sun to dry them, then remove the soil with a brush. Cut root sections into 5 cm (2 inch) pieces for storage.

STORE

Dry both roots and flowers on drying trays or open screens in a dark, dry, well-ventilated place (see "Drying Herbs at Home" on page 365). Use separate trays for the roots and flowers and don't allow the pieces to touch one another. After drying, store the roots and flower petals separately in airtight containers in a cool, dark place.

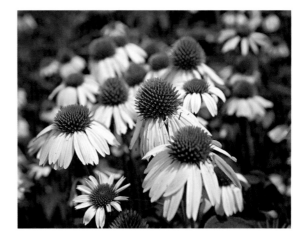

Some varieties of white echinacea, like 'White Swan' pictured here, pack the same medicinal punch as their purple cousins. But the purple varieties are far more common.

⚙ Put It to Work

Cold or flu? Echinacea is for you!

Rigorous trials have shown that echinacea extracts shorten the duration and lessen the symptoms of the common cold. Fresh-pressed juice and alcoholic tinctures of echinacea root are the forms most commonly studied and proven effective.

You can make your own tincture using the purple flower top and roots—that's where the powerful medicine is found. Dig up 4 mature echinacea plants, chop off the roots and flower tops, and discard the leaves and stems (all the green stuff). Wash the flowers and give the roots a good scrubbing.

Using a sharp knife, chop the flowers and roots into fine pieces. Loosely pack them into a resealable glass jar (like a Mason jar) until two-thirds full. Pour in enough vodka (at least 80 proof) to fill the jar. Place wax paper over the jar and then screw the lid on tightly to seal it. Label the jar, including the date prepared and the alcohol used. Set aside in a cool, dark place for at least 2 weeks, shaking the jar vigorously for 2 minutes every day.

After 2 weeks the tincture can be strained through a fine-mesh sieve (optional). Pour the tincture into a sterile dark-coloured glass container with a tight-fitting lid to protect it from light. The tincture will keep for at least a year stored in a cool, dark place.

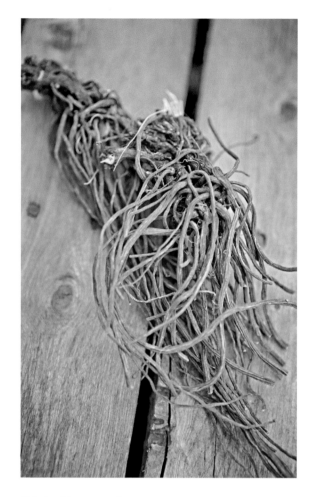

Dried echinacea root.

At the first sign of a cold or flu, dilute 1 teaspoon of the tincture in 1 ounce of water and gargle for 1 minute before swallowing. Repeat 3 times daily. You will feel your tongue get slightly numb or tingly—this is normal. It indicates the activity of some of the phytochemicals in the echinacea and will last only a few minutes.

Got gingivitis? Swish with this!

Gingivitis is chronic inflammation of the gums, causing them to bleed and swell. It is the most common type of gum disease and a common cause of tooth loss after age 35. Gingivitis is caused by plaque around the teeth. Flossing and brushing regularly can help treat and prevent it, but because recent research has linked gingivitis with heart disease, adding a third layer of protection is a good insurance plan. It turns out echinacea may help.

Open a new bottle of your favourite mouthwash and swish with the first dose (a capful, or about 1 ounce). Then pour 1 ounce of echinacea tincture (see opposite page) into the bottle. Continue to use the mouthwash as directed. Do not swallow.

Weekend warrior? Add echinacea to your water bottle!

Once you're into exercise, you typically can't stop. Some athletes and weekend warriors end up with a condition called overtraining syndrome, where performance begins to deteriorate and the immune system begins to malfunction. One sign is an increased incidence of upper respiratory tract infection after excessive exercise.

One way to help prevent the immune suppression caused by overtraining is adding echinacea to your water. Start by making echinacea tea. Boil 1 cup of water with ½ cup of freshly chopped echinacea flower and root for 10 minutes. Cool and strain through a fine-mesh sieve into 4 to 8 cups of water and consume as you normally would during exercise.

» Fast Forward

Fast forward to the health food store to purchase A. Vogel Echinaforce tincture or equivalent. Follow the instructions on the label.

! Cautions

Echinacea is a very safe herb that has very few side effects when taken orally. It was once believed long-term use was unsafe, but it has since been proven that it is safe for up to 4 months at a time at therapeutic ranges or year-round as a regular addition to your weekend water bottle.

You should avoid echinacea if you have an autoimmune illness, such as lupus, or other progressive diseases, such as tuberculosis or multiple sclerosis. Those who are allergic to flowers of the daisy family (*Asteraceae*) should not take echinacea.

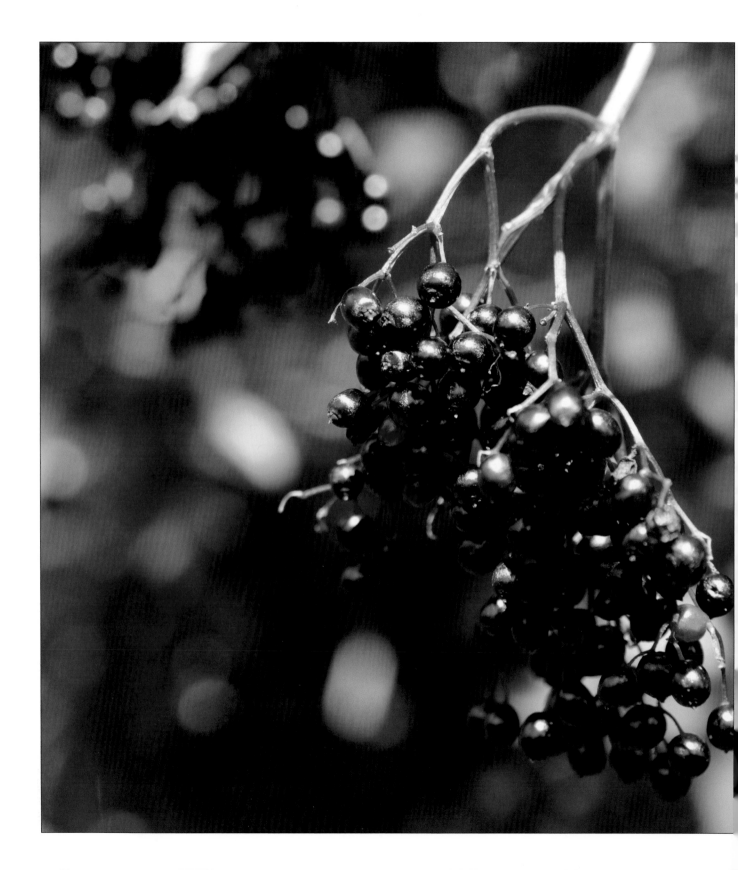

Elderberry

If you're a Harry Potter fan, you know one of the most powerful magical objects is the Elder Wand, which was fashioned from the wood of the *Sambucus nigra* shrub, native to the warmer regions of Europe and North America. Elderberries may not be magic, but they have long been applied to swelling and wounds, and have more recently been used as a treatment for cold and flu symptoms. The delicious purple-black berries are enjoyed in jams and jellies, and they make a popular type of wine.

⊕ Health Benefits

In the fall, elderberries turn a deep purple, showcasing their high concentrations of antioxidant flavonoids, anthocyanins, and quercetin, all believed to account for the medicinal actions of this plant's berries and flowers.

European herbalists traditionally used elderberry for pain relief and to promote the healing of injuries. They later learned from North American Aboriginal peoples that the plant was useful for infections, coughs, and other conditions, too.

Elderberry is one of your most powerful allies against influenza. According to Health Canada, the flu affects between 10% and 25% of Canadians every year (usually between November and April), and sends 20,000 people to the hospital, killing roughly 4,000. The good news is one study confirmed that people receiving a daily dose of elderberry syrup—packed with therapeutic phytonutrients—recovered faster than those receiving a placebo.

Additional uses include as a laxative for constipation, a stimulant for general immune function, and a treatment for chronic fatigue syndrome, allergic rhinitis, and sinusitis. Essentially, if anything from your nose to your throat to your lungs is infected or affected, turn to these berries.

🌱 Growing

Elderberry is an attractive landscape shrub and comes in a wide range of varieties. They are relatively easy to grow, but they are not suited to small spaces. Some varieties will grow well in pots, but these will not produce adequate fruit yields.

Common Varieties: Elder varieties are sometimes treated as distinct species, and other times as subspecies of *Sambucus nigra*. The Canada elder (*S. nigra canadensis*) is common in central and eastern North America. Popular cultivars include the

DIFFICULTY
Easy

HARDINESS
Perennial in zones 3 to 9

TIME TO PLANT
Spring or early fall

TIME TO HARVEST
Late summer

LOCATION
Full to part sun

SOIL TYPE
Moist, well-drained

cutleaf elderberry ('Lacinata') and Black Lace ('Eva'), which has purple-black foliage. Make sure that you don't plant dwarf elder (*Sambucus ebulus*) for medicinal purposes—it can be toxic.

PLANT

Plant elder in early spring. Although elderberries will thrive in almost any soil, they do best in loamy soil that is well-drained and rich in organic matter. Elders grow big: They average about 2 metres (6 feet) high and up to 3 metres (10 feet) wide, and some can get much larger. So leave plenty of space when planting—at least 1 to 2 metres (3 to 6 feet), or as indicated on the plant's tag.

Elders need to be cross-pollinated if they are to produce berries, so plant two or more cultivars close to one other.

GROW

Elderberry is not drought-tolerant. On average it requires between 10 and 20 mm of water per week. Water as needed, and use mulch to maintain moisture and reduce the risk of plant loss.

In late winter or early spring, prune away any dead, broken, or weak stems. During the growing season remove weeds surrounding the plants. Avoid heavy pruning for the first couple of seasons; wait until they are established.

Elderberries are loved by many creatures, especially birds. Apply garden netting in midsummer, before berries ripen, to save some fruit for you!

Inspect plants often and be on the lookout for white powdery mildew on the leaves; if you spot mildew, remove and discard the infected branches.

HARVEST

The shrub will produce some berries during its first season, but yields will increase during the second and third years. Berries will ripen sporadically over a 2-week period in late summer to early fall. To harvest them, use a fork to tease the ripe berries off their

When designing gardens or containers that are functional and attractive, look for plants with more than one season of interest. Plants like elderberry offer multiple periods of display, from flowers to foliage to fruit! White blooms appear in spring, giving way to purplish berries in the fall. Varieties such as Black Lace 'Eva' (below) also feature show-stopping dark foliage throughout the growing season.

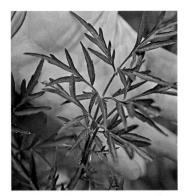

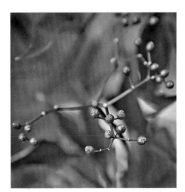

stems. Only harvest fully ripe berries, which will be plump and almost black in colour.

STORE

Wash elderberries just before use. Store fresh berries loosely in a container, cover with plastic wrap, and refrigerate for up to a week. To freeze, wash berries in cold water and pat dry. Arrange in a single layer on a baking sheet and freeze. Once frozen, transfer to resealable bags. You can preserve berries in jams and jellies. Elderberries can also be placed in a dehydrator and dried.

Put It to Work

No flu for you? Take this triple tincture!

North Americans spend about $2.9 billion on over-the-counter cold and flu remedies every year, but some may be unsafe, especially for children. Many include the cough suppressant dextromethorphan (DXM) and an expectorant called guaifenesin, two chemicals worth avoiding. Elderberry extract can address both of these treatments naturally!

To make this remedy you'll need to keep an eye on your elderberry plants throughout the growing season. In spring, when the shrub is blooming, collect 2 cups of the flowers and wash them thoroughly. Bring ½ cup of water to a boil in a large saucepan and add the flowers. Boil for 10 minutes, turn off the heat, and let cool. Drain.

Purée the boiled flowers in a blender. Pour into a small resealable glass jar (like a Mason jar; it should be filled about halfway). Fill the jar with vodka (at least 80 proof) to make a tincture. (To make a children's formula, substitute vinegar for the alcohol.) Place wax paper over the jar and then screw the lid on tightly to seal it. Set aside in a cool, dark place. Vigorously shake the jar daily until it is time to harvest the berries.

In the fall, collect 3 cups of fully ripe berries. Wash the berries. Place 2 cups of the berries in an airtight container and place in the freezer. Place the remaining 1 cup of berries in a blender and add the prepared flower tincture. Blend on medium speed until smooth. Pour into a clean jar large enough to hold the entire contents. Seal and set aside in a cool, dark place for 2 weeks.

After 2 weeks, cover the mouth of the jar with a coffee filter or cheesecloth and strain the beautiful dark purple liquid into a glass bowl. Carefully squeeze out all the liquid from the coffee filter (discard solids).

In a blender, blend the infusion with 1 cup of the frozen berries until smooth. Return the mixture to the jar. To sweeten, add 5 tablespoons of manuka honey.

For a super-concentrated, flu-busting elderberry elixir, repeat the process with the remaining cup of frozen elderberries 2 weeks later.

Take 1 teaspoon 3 times daily through cold and flu season. Store the tincture in a cool, dark place.

Always getting sick? Stick to this syrup!

Some people seem to succumb to every virus that goes around. Elderberry is suspected to boost the immune system as well as coat viral particles so they can't infect cells as readily. If you're always coming down with something, consider taking this immune-boosting syrup right through the winter.

4 cups water
Freshly squeezed juice of ½ lemon
1 cup elderberries (fresh or frozen)
1 tsp ground cinnamon
3 tsp ground ginger
½ cup liquid honey

In a saucepan over medium heat, combine the water and lemon juice. Add the berries, cinnamon, and ginger and bring to a boil. Reduce the heat, cover, and simmer for 1 hour, being careful not to overboil. Remove from heat and set aside to cool. Strain through a fine-mesh sieve into a resealable glass jar (like a Mason jar). Add the honey and mix thoroughly. If desired, add ½ cup of echinacea tincture (see opposite page). Take 1 tablespoon daily to support and strengthen your immune system. The syrup will keep in the refrigerator for up to 3 months.

≫ Fast Forward

Fast forward to the health food store to purchase Clef des Champs elder tincture or equivalent. Follow the instructions on the label.

! Cautions

Make sure elderberries are fully ripe and fully cooked before you use them: Unripe raw berries are poisonous. Other plant parts (including the leaves, stems, and root) may also contain toxic constituents related to cyanide and may cause nausea, vomiting, and diarrhea.

Avoid elderberry if you have any allergy to plants in the *Adoxaceae* family, which also includes viburnum. There are some reports of allergies in children playing with toys made from fresh elder stems.

Because elderberry helps to heighten immune response, people with autoimmunity disorders and those taking immunosuppressant drugs should avoid it. High doses of elderberry may have diuretic (urine-producing) effects, so those already taking diuretics or "water pills" should avoid it. Elderberry may also lower blood sugar, so additional blood tests may be necessary in those with diabetes or hypoglycemia.

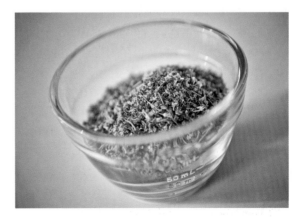

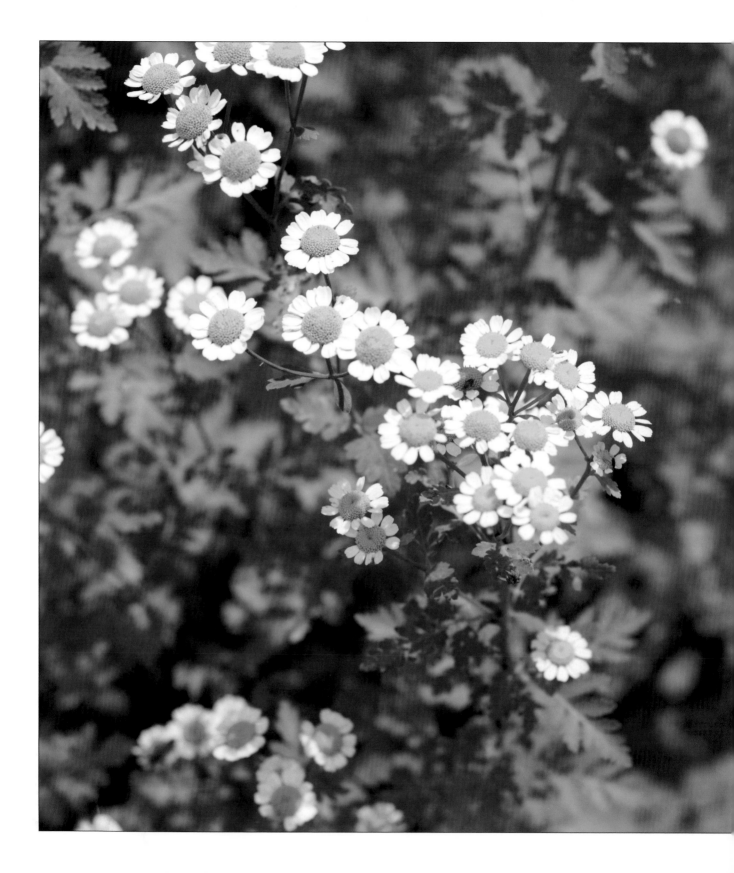

Feverfew

Feverfew is a member of the daisy family (*Asteraceae*) and features clusters of small white-petalled flowers with yellow centres. The plant gives off a strong, bug-deterring odour reminiscent of camphor. Feverfew is native to Europe but is also widespread throughout North America and Australia. The plant's common name comes from the Latin for "fever reducer," as that was one of its traditional uses. It's also known as featherfew or bachelor's buttons.

⊕ Health Benefits

Feverfew was used in ancient Greek medical practice as a remedy for inflammation and menstrual discomforts. Over the years, traditional herbalists have also used it to treat arthritis and aches and pains. As its name suggests, the herb was traditionally used to treat fevers, but this is no longer the case.

Today feverfew is commonly taken orally for the prevention of migraines. It is believed to reduce inflammation and prevent blood vessel constriction in the head and neck, and research suggests feverfew may reduce the incidence of headache attacks in patients who experience chronic migraines.

The plant's most active ingredient is believed to be parthenolide, a compound that has anti-inflammatory properties.

🌱 Growing

A close relative of chrysanthemums, feverfew has been grown in gardens for centuries. While it's mainly grown for medicinal purposes, this tender perennial is cherished for its foliage and its mounds of showy daisy-like flowers, which typically bloom from July to early fall.

Common Varieties: *Tanacetum parthenium* has many cultivars, including 'Aureum', 'Flore Pleno', 'Golden Ball', 'Plenum', 'Snowball', and 'Wild'.

PLANT

Sow seeds indoors 8 to 10 weeks before last frost date. Plant the seedlings (or transplants from the garden centre) outdoors after the risk of frost. Choose a location with full sun and well-drained soil, or grow them in containers. Space plants 30 cm (12 inches) apart. Water deeply and infrequently until established.

DIFFICULTY
Easy

HARDINESS
Perennial in zones 5 to 9

TIME TO PLANT
Spring (or start seeds indoors 8 to 10 weeks before last frost date)

TIME TO HARVEST
Early summer (foliage)

LOCATION
Full sun

SOIL TYPE
Moist, well-drained

What's in a plant's name? It can be confusing to identify plants if they have several common names, nicknames, marketing names, or regional names. The only reliable way to ensure you get the plant you're looking for is to pay attention to the Latin name. Whether it's called feverfew, featherfew, or bachelor's button, the scientific name is *Tanacetum parthenium*. Look for it on the tag.

GROW

You can successfully grow feverfew with very little effort: it's an insect- and disease-resistant plant. Deep infrequent watering, regular weeding, the occasional application of fertilizer, and frequent deadheading are the keys to success. When deadheading, consider removing some buds to promote leaf growth—but don't strip all of the flowers! Feverfew will easily self-sow if you leave some flowers to dry on the plants.

In late fall or early spring, cut the plant back to the ground while it is dormant.

HARVEST

Harvest when in bloom or when foliage has matured. Wash the plants the day before harvesting by watering their foliage in the morning. The next morning after the dew has dried, cut the foliage, stems and all, removing no more than half the plant at a time. Use a sharp, clean knife and do not tear the stems.

STORE

Dry feverfew by hanging stems in a dark, dry place for up to 2 weeks (see "Drying Herbs at Home" on page 365). Space them out to increase airflow and minimize rot. After drying, store feverfew in an airtight container out of direct light.

Put It to Work

Prone to migraines? Say hello to feverfew Jell-O!

Feverfew may be nature's answer to unbearable migraine pain, but the research seems to suggest you'll need to take it every day for it to be most effective. You also require about 100 milligrams per day for 4 to 6 weeks before it starts to really work. I admit this can be something of an ordeal. What's more, it tastes horrible. And you need to take it in the whole-leaf form, which is particularly foul-tasting. You've been warned.

Fortunately, there is a solution that makes this remedy more palatable. This recipe is adapted from herbalist James Green.

You'll need two BPA-free ice-cube trays. For each cube in your trays harvest 2 large feverfew leaves. Wash and place them in a blender. Boil enough water to fill one-and-a-half trays and add the boiling water to the blender. Pulse until well combined, with the leaves evenly dispersed in the boiling water.

In a bowl, add a box of Jell-O powder (I recommend a citrus flavour to mask the taste of the feverfew) (1). Pour the feverfew mixture into the bowl and stir for 2 to 3 minutes (2), making sure that the gelatin is fully dissolved. Add an additional ⅛ cup of very cold water and stir well.

Fill each compartment in both ice-cube trays with the Jell-O mixture (3). Refrigerate for about 2 hours to set. The texture will be squishy (4).

Consume one Jell-O cube every day. You won't love them, but you will love not having headaches!

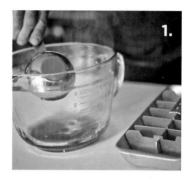

» Fast Forward

Fast forward to the health food store to purchase Genestra feverfew capsules or equivalent. Follow the instructions on the label.

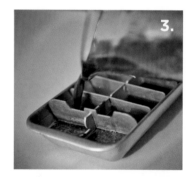

! Cautions

Known side effects of feverfew are usually mild. Ulcers in the mouth, swelling of the lips, tongue irritation, and bleeding of the gums (primarily from chewing the leaves) as well as loss of taste have been reported, but all are reversible. In rare instances, sensitivity to light, nausea, abdominal bloating, and heartburn have also been recorded.

If you have been taking feverfew regularly for more than a week, do not stop abruptly or you may experience headache, fatigue, anxiety, and sleeplessness, or stiffness of the muscles or joints.

Pregnant women should not take feverfew.

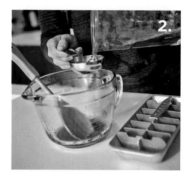

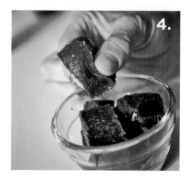

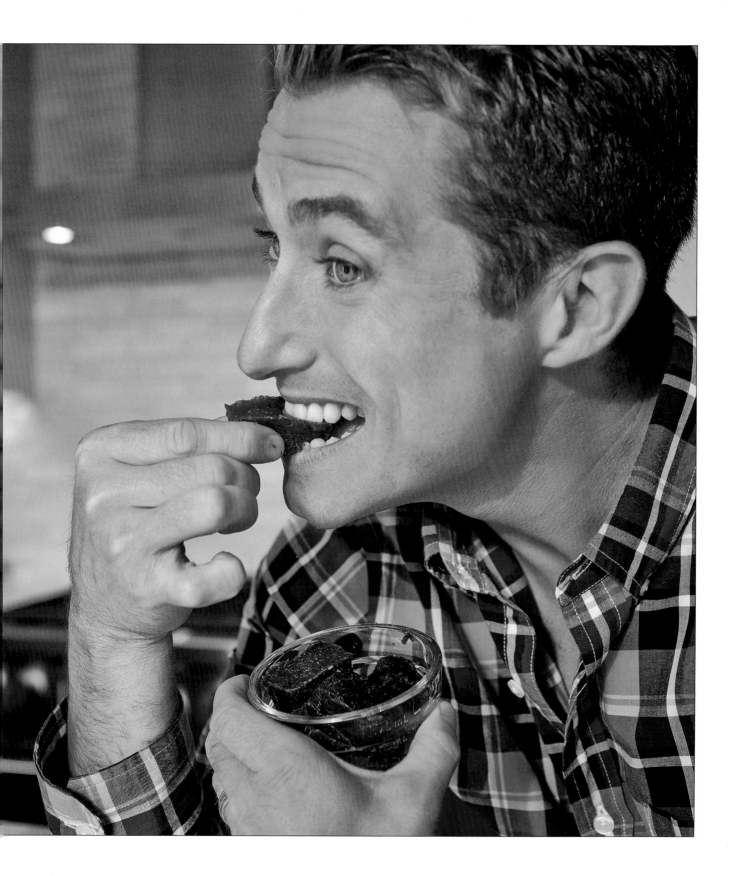

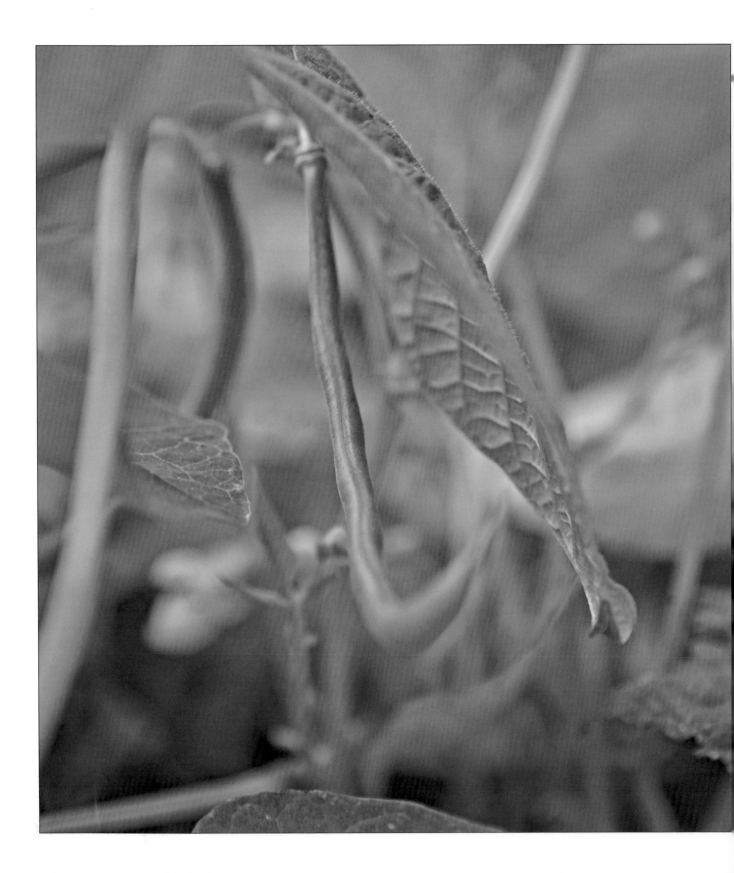

French Bean

If you feel like being chi-chi, you could call this humble member of the *Fabaceae* family a "French bean." But chances are you know it as the humble string bean, field bean, garden bean, haricot bean, or snap bean. It turns out, however, this common bean has some amazing and uncommon health benefits. The common bean is widely cultivated around the world. Different cultivars vary in shape and come in many colours: Navy beans, pinto beans, kidney beans, and wax beans are all varieties of this species.

Health Benefits

Beans are an economical source of protein and starch, and they're high in fibre and low in fat. The common bean is loaded with micronutrients, including iron, potassium, beta carotene, thiamine, riboflavin, and other B-complex vitamins.

Beans have garnered attention recently as a potential weight-loss aid. White kidney beans, in particular, have been promoted as "starch blockers" that can slow the absorption of carbohydrates, resulting in fewer calories entering the system. Starch blockers have also been suggested as an aid to managing blood sugar in people with type 2 diabetes.

You know the saying, "Beans, beans, they're good for your heart…"? It turns out research suggests beans really can reduce the risk of heart disease. As a source of dietary fibre, they reduce lipids. The French bean might also bind cholic acids and fat, which reduces fat absorption. The pods also contain compounds that can help manage cholesterol and improve immune balance.

Growing

French beans are quick to germinate, fun to harvest, and in the right conditions very easy to grow. I often recommend beans as a starter plant for children who want to experience the growth of new seedlings, because they provide instant gratification! Space will determine the type of bean you grow; some need lots of space, and others need staking. If you have minimal space, some can even be grown in a pot.

Common Varieties: *Phaseolus vulgaris* is available in countless varieties, but the main categories are pole beans (climbing) and bush beans (mounding). Pole beans don't have a large footprint, but they require a trellis or some other support, as they will

DIFFICULTY
Easy

HARDINESS
Annual

TIME TO PLANT
Late spring, after risk of frost

TIME TO HARVEST
Early summer

LOCATION
Full sun

SOIL TYPE
Well-drained, rich in organic compost

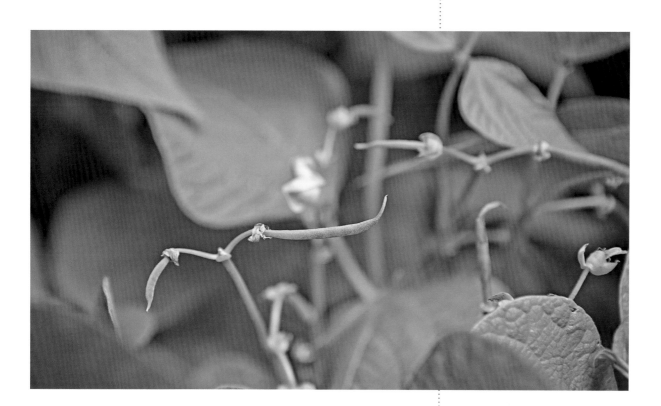

grow 2 to 3 metres (6 to 10 feet) tall. For small-space gardens, I recommend bush beans; they need at least 1 metre (3 feet) per plant but require no staking.

PLANT

Sow seeds directly in the garden after all risk of frost. Prior to sowing, soak the seeds in warm water for 12 to 24 hours to help them germinate. Plant the seeds in well-drained, rich soil where they will get lots of sun. Sow seeds 5 cm (2 inches) deep, 10 cm (4 inches) apart, in rows separated by 30 to 45 cm (12 to 18 inches). If you're planting pole beans, you'll need to make sure you have enough room to support them.

You can occasionally purchase transplants, but remember beans are frost-sensitive plants and cannot be placed in the garden until that risk has passed.

GROW

You will face a few challenges when growing beans. First, they hate low temperatures, so if you get a cold snap in late spring you must cover them at night to protect them from frost.

Pole beans must also be secured to stakes, obelisks, wigwams, or trellises. As they grow, you will need to train them around these supports.

Both bush and pole beans will be threatened early on by everything from slugs and snails to cutworms, squirrels, deer, and rabbits. Consider placing a collar around the base of the young plants (this can be something as simple as a Styrofoam cup with the bottom removed). You may have to do some additional plantings if you lose some seedlings, so save some extra seed.

Monitor during the growing season for aphids, and apply insecticidal soap as a preventive measure. Water deeply and infrequently, never allowing plants to completely dry out, and keep the area weed-free. Mulch well and fertilize twice a month using an organic compost tea (page 175) or water-soluble general-purpose fertilizer (20-20-20).

HARVEST

Beans typically mature in about 60 days. Harvest them in early to midsummer when pods reach a length of 10 cm (4 inches). They should be plump in appearance and should easily snap. Harvest mid-morning while plants are cool. After harvest continue to water and fertilize; you may be rewarded with an additional harvest, though the yield will be reduced.

STORE

Wash beans just before use. They will keep in resealable bags in the refrigerator for up to a week. Freeze young pods only. Wash them in cold water, pat dry, and place in resealable bags in the freezer.

Experienced gardeners know the three S's of germinating seeds: soaking, scarification, and stratification. For seeds with hard shells like beans, a simple overnight soak will help speed the process of germination. Sometimes seeds also need to be "scarified," which involves taking a file or some sandpaper and rubbing the outer coating until you can see the inner part of the seed. Seeds that need "stratification" should be placed in a cold space (such as the refrigerator) for up to 3 months to mimic an outdoor dormancy period.

Put It to Work

Need to clear the air? Try this bean soup!

If you want to drop some weight or lower your cholesterol, try eating soup at least 3 times per week. Soup is one of the best ways to get the necessary servings of vegetables you need to stay healthy. If you eat this homemade bean soup every day for lunch for 3 months and otherwise maintain a healthy diet and exercise routine, we promise you will see the results! (Feel free to switch up this recipe, so long as the major ingredient is French beans.)

4 cups water
1 cube chicken bouillon
1 tbsp extra virgin olive oil
10 cloves garlic, minced
1 sweet onion, chopped
4 cups chopped French beans
4 egg whites
1 tsp sea salt
¼ tsp freshly ground black pepper
½ tsp Italian seasoning

In a large saucepan, bring the water to a boil. Add the bouillon, reduce the heat to a simmer, and stir until dissolved completely.

Meanwhile, in a skillet over medium heat, heat the oil. Add the garlic and onion and sauté for about 5 minutes, until the onions are translucent. Add the beans and sauté for 15 minutes or until the beans are soft. Transfer the bean and onion mixture to the broth, bring to a boil, and boil for 10 minutes. Reduce the heat to a simmer and stir in the egg whites. Add the salt, pepper, and Italian seasoning. Using a regular or immersion blender, purée until smooth.

On a diet? Here's a snack!

If you're trying to shed some pounds but getting cravings between meals, the solution is a snack that will provide energy and also aid in your weight-loss goal: French bean spread. The hot pepper will give you an additional metabolic boost. You can enjoy this high-protein, low-carbohydrate, spicy, metabolism-boosting snack 3 to 4 crackers at a serving.

1 cup chopped French beans
½ Spanish onion
1 clove garlic
10 black olives, pitted
1 hot red pepper, seeded
6 sprigs fresh tarragon leaves
3 tbsp extra virgin olive oil
Sea salt and freshly ground black pepper
12 brown rice crackers
1 tbsp finely diced red bell pepper
2 tbsp crushed walnuts

In a saucepan, cook the beans in boiling water for 2 minutes. Drain and rinse under cold running water.

In a food processor, purée the cooked beans, onion, garlic, olives, hot pepper, tarragon, and oil. Season with salt and pepper to taste.

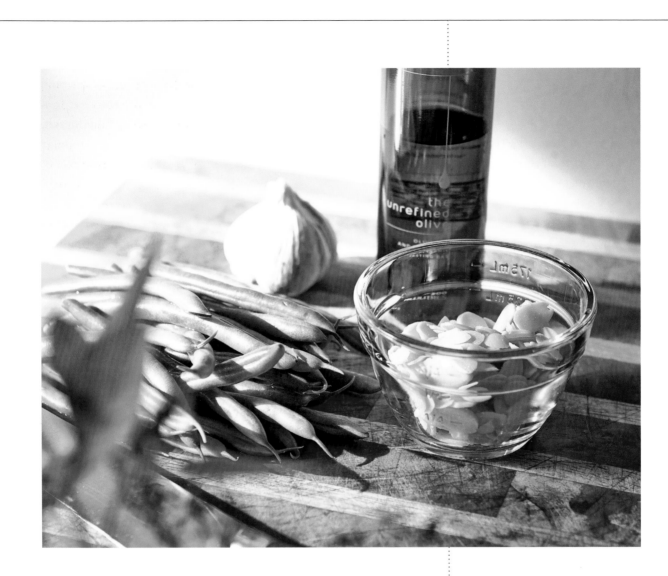

Spread the bean paste onto the rice crackers. Garnish with the red pepper, the crushed walnuts, and a sprinkling of black pepper.

Bean meaning to lose weight? Eat these on the side!
If you're on a high-protein diet, it's always a challenge to come up with a side dish that is low-carb, high-fibre, and still tasty. This is it! Plus it contains additional protein, not to mention carb-blocking potential.

2 lb French beans
1 tbsp extra virgin olive oil
½ tsp garlic powder
1 tsp crushed dried chilies (or to taste)
Sea salt and freshly ground black pepper
1 tbsp apple cider vinegar
½ cup pine nuts

In a large saucepan, bring 1 cm (1/2 inch) water to a boil. Add French beans, cover, and steam for 5 to 10 minutes or until bright green but still crunchy. Drain and rinse with cold water.

In a skillet, heat the oil over medium heat. Add the cooked beans and sauté for 5 minutes. Add the garlic powder and chilies, and salt and pepper to taste.

Transfer to a serving bowl, add the vinegar and pine nuts, and toss to coat well.

» Fast Forward

Fast forward to the grocery store to purchase fresh, canned, or frozen French beans.

! Cautions

Beans are safe when consumed frequently for 2 or 3 months. Large amounts of fresh bean husks or their extract may not be safe, since the raw husks contain chemicals that can cause stomach upset, vomiting, and diarrhea. Cooking, however, destroys these chemicals.

Many people who have trouble digesting beans simply eat too many at one time. This is usually not an intolerance: It just means enzymes need time to ramp up in your digestive system. If you haven't been eating beans, you'll want to begin by eating no more than ¼ cup per day for the first week to minimize gas, bloating, and digestive upset. Here's a tip: Always rinse beans really well. This may help to cut down on gas for many people.

If you have irritable bowel syndrome or inflammatory bowel disease, ask your healthcare provider if significantly increasing beans in your diet is reasonable.

If you have diabetes and intend to incorporate large amounts of French beans into your diet, you need to monitor your blood sugar even more closely. The dose of your diabetes medications may also need to be adjusted by your healthcare provider.

There is some concern that beans may interfere with blood sugar control during and after surgery. If you are having major surgery, avoid beans for at least 1 week prior.

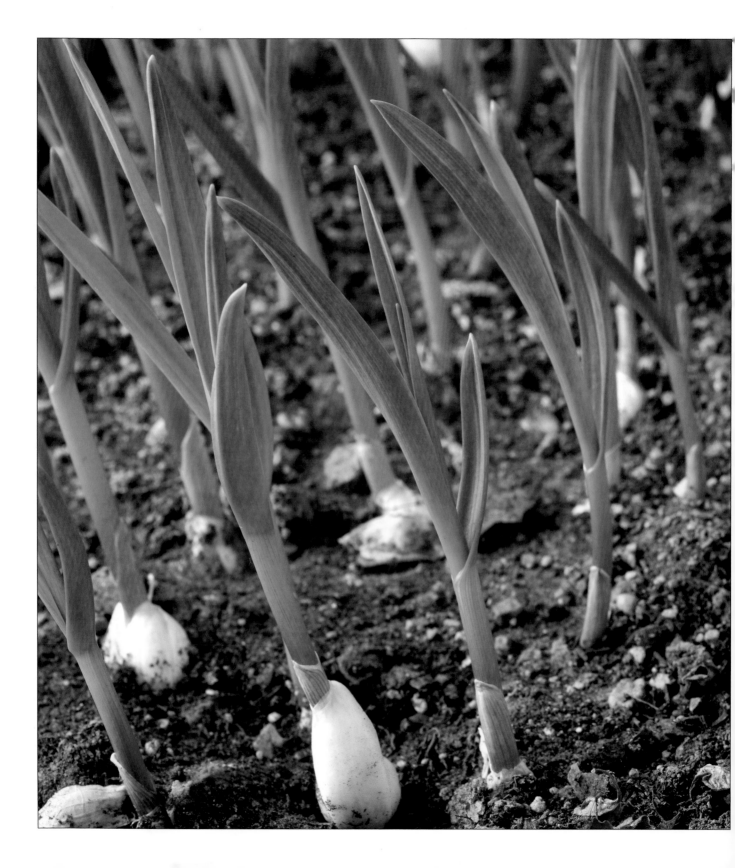

Garlic

Garlic is one of the world's most common culinary herbs. It's an essential part of cuisine throughout Asia, the Middle East, northern Africa, Europe, and parts of South and Central America. China produces more than 13.5 million tons of garlic a year—that's enough to fill 5,500 Olympic-sized swimming pools! Garlic is a species from the genus *Allium*, which also includes onions, shallots, leeks, and chives. The bulb—made up of multiple cloves—is the most prized feature, but other parts of the garlic plant are also edible.

Health Benefits

Everyone should eat a fresh clove of garlic every day. That way we'd all be used to the smell and we'd all be healthier! Garlic may reduce the risk of developing heart disease, high blood pressure, and elevated cholesterol, as well as diseases with an underlying inflammation (that's most diseases).

What makes garlic so special is a sulphur compound called alliin, which interacts with an enzyme called allinase to produce another compound called allicin. If that's too many *a*'s, *l*'s, and *i*'s to even think about, not to worry! The important thing is that when the garlic bulb is crushed or ground, it releases a high concentration of the stuff that can keep your ticker healthy. Allicin also has antibacterial and antiviral properties.

Garlic is loaded with compounds that can boost the immune system, plus a host of antioxidants. It's definitely worth enduring a bit of bad breath to put all that in your body!

Growing

Garlic is a must-grow plant and has been for millennia. There are two main types: hardneck and softneck. Hardneck varieties are hardier, so they're the best choice for colder climates, which means most locations in Canada and the northern United States. Softneck garlic is best grown in warmer climates and is the choice of commercial producers in California—that's what you'll see most often in grocery stores.

Hardneck garlic varieties produce 4 to 12 cloves in the traditional shape, while softneck varieties produce 10 to 40 cloves layered on top of each other like the petals of an artichoke. If you've already got garlic planted, how do you tell the difference? Simple: Hardneck garlic produces a flower stock, while softneck doesn't. As a bonus, softneck garlic is easier to braid.

DIFFICULTY
Easy

HARDINESS
Varies; check the label

TIME TO PLANT
Late summer to early fall

TIME TO HARVEST
Late summer to early fall the following year

LOCATION
Full sun

SOIL TYPE
Well-drained loam—clay or sandy soil won't work at all

Garlic is helpful to other plants in the garden: The same compounds that make your breath stink also repel aphids if you plant it close to your beautiful roses.

Common Varieties: Hardneck varieties include 'Asiatic', 'Creole', 'Porcelain', 'Purple Stripe', 'Glazed Purple Stripe', 'Marbled Purple Stripe', 'Rocambole', and 'Turban'. Popular softneck varieties include 'Artichoke' and 'Silver Skin'.

PLANT

Garlic is easy to plant, but it takes a little planning. For optimum results plant it in the fall so it has time to set roots before freeze-up. After the first frost, separate the cloves from the bulb and plant them pointy side up. (The most common garlic goof is planting the entire bulb instead of individual cloves!) The cloves will rest during the winter, grow again through spring and summer, and be ready to harvest in late summer as mature bulbs.

Garlic can be planted on its own in rows or in your garden between flowering plants. If you're planting in rows, space cloves 15 cm (6 inches) apart and leave 20 cm (8 inches) between rows. It's important to loosen the soil where you'll be planting, so dig down about 20 cm (8 inches) and then level the soil out again. Use your fingers to push each clove down to a depth of 5 cm (2 inches), making sure the pointy side faces up (basal side down).

When you separate the individual cloves before planting, keep the protective papery husk around them. Each clove will yield a whole bulb of garlic. The larger the clove, the larger the eventual bud will be.

GROW

Just after the first hard frost, mulch your garlic with 10 to 15 cm (4 to 6 inches) of clean straw to insulate against the winter frost–thaw cycle. Then put your feet up for the winter while your garlic rests!

In early spring, your garlic will start to grow immediately: Watch for the green spikes. When all risk of killing frost has passed, carefully remove the straw mulch.

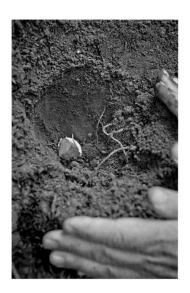

Make sure to plant individual cloves pointy side up.

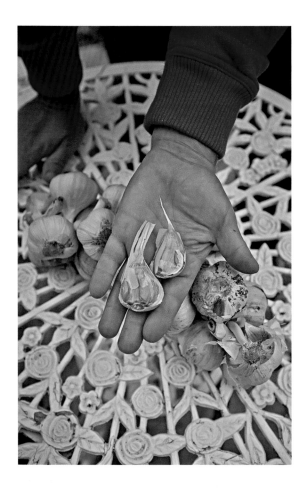

Garlic doesn't normally need fertilizer, but if your soil lacks nutrients, early spring is the time to apply it. Garlic enjoys nitrogen-rich soils, so an organic manure tea or granular fertilizer with a high first number would be ideal. Blood-meal (12-0-0) is one of my favourites. During the growing season, water deeply and infrequently.

Always remove any yellowing or sickly-looking garlic. Garlic is disease- and insect-resistant for the most part and will not require the use of insecticides or fungicides.

Hardneck garlic produces "scapes" midway through the growing season. These are curled flower heads that should be removed early on to encourage bulb growth and help increase bulb size. Simply snap them off—but don't throw them away. Scapes are a culinary delight! Many feel they provide the same health benefits as the bulbs.

HARVEST

When it comes to harvesting garlic, timing is crucial. In late summer, you'll notice the green leaves start to turn yellow and brown from the bottom up. When the bottom 3 or 4 leaves have yellowed and the top 5 or 6 leaves are still green, it's time to harvest.

Gently lift one bulb out to ensure it has swelled to mature size (check the package). If so, lift out the remaining bulbs with a garden fork. Trim the dangling bottom roots to 1 cm (½ inch) and brush off any soil, then braid the leaves in groups of 3 to 6 bulbs and hang them in a shaded location with good air circulation and no danger of frost. The bulbs need to dry for at least 2 weeks before eating or storage.

STORE

Depending on which variety you grow, garlic can be stored for 6 months to a year from the date of harvest. Store it in a cool, dry, dark location with a temperature between 0°C (32°F) and 20°C (68°F). Never store garlic in a refrigerator.

Put It to Work

Heart help? Juice this!

Most people cook with their garlic. But if you want the most powerful effects, you gotta juice it! To make your own heart-healthy, cholesterol-lowering, immune-boosting, blood-pressure-controlling, detoxifying juice, process the following in a vegetable juicer:

> *4 large carrots*
> *1 small beet*
> *½ Granny Smith apple*
> *2 large kale leaves*
> *1 handful fresh parsley*
> *1 to 2 cloves garlic*
> *1 ½-inch piece gingerroot*

You can adjust the amount of ginger and garlic to taste. It's best to start with small amounts and then increase them if you can handle it, but use no more than 4 cloves of garlic or it will be far too strong to drink and may cause stomach irritation and nausea.

Got an earache? Oil it!

Few things are more unpleasant than a painful ear infection. There are two main types: otitis externa (in the external ear canal) and otitis media (in the inner ear, beyond the eardrum). Garlic oil is a highly effective remedy for relieving the inflammation, pain, discomfort, and itching associated with both types.

Garlic has proven very useful for swimmer's ear (external ear), mild otitis media (the antimicrobial oils from the garlic can bypass the tympanic membrane into the inner ear), and non-specific dermatitis of the external ear canal. It is also excellent for removing excess earwax. (Normal amounts of earwax are actually protective, so speak to your doctor before removing it.)

In a double boiler (or a heatproof bowl placed over a saucepan of boiling water), gently warm 4 tablespoons of olive oil and 2 cloves of minced garlic over low heat for 1 hour. Strain the oil through cheesecloth and store it in a resealable glass jar (like a Mason jar) in the refrigerator.

Any remedy placed inside the ear should be warmed to a comfortable temperature first, so place the jar in your pocket or against your belly 10 minutes before applying. Then, using a dropper, place 4 drops into the affected ear. Cover your ear with a very warm, wet cloth and lie on your opposite side for 10 minutes. After 10 minutes, gently pat your ear dry with a cloth.

Yeast infection? Try this!

Bakers don't add garlic to bread while the dough is still rising because it would kill the yeast and flatten the bread. This antifungal property can also be used to treat a vaginal yeast infection.

Women who experience frequent yeast infections are familiar with the slight itchiness that comes and goes at the onset. That is when you want to start treatment.

Strip a clove of garlic by peeling off the cover. Cut it lengthwise into 4 pieces. Line up the 4 pieces end-to-end at one of the long edges of a sterile 5 x 10 cm (2 x 4 inch) piece of gauze and roll it up. Sew each end shut and tie a string around one end for easy retrieval.

Place the gauze into the vagina (like a tampon) before bed. Don't be surprised if you taste garlic in your mouth—that's quite normal. (Don't worry, this cannot enter the uterus through the cervix, nor can it get lost, especially if the string remains intact.)

Repeat this for 2 to 3 nights or until itchiness is gone (no more than 5 nights consecutively). If the infection persists or complicates, see your physician or gynecologist for conventional treatment.

» Fast Forward

Fast forward to the health food store to purchase CLM's Allimax capsules or equivalent. Follow the instructions on the label.

! Cautions

Because garlic can thin the blood, it might enhance or even contradict the effects of certain prescription medications, including anticoagulant and antiplatelet drugs such as warfarin, aspirin, clopidogrel, and enoxaparin. Discontinue your daily regimen of garlic at least 1 week prior to having surgery, including dental surgery.

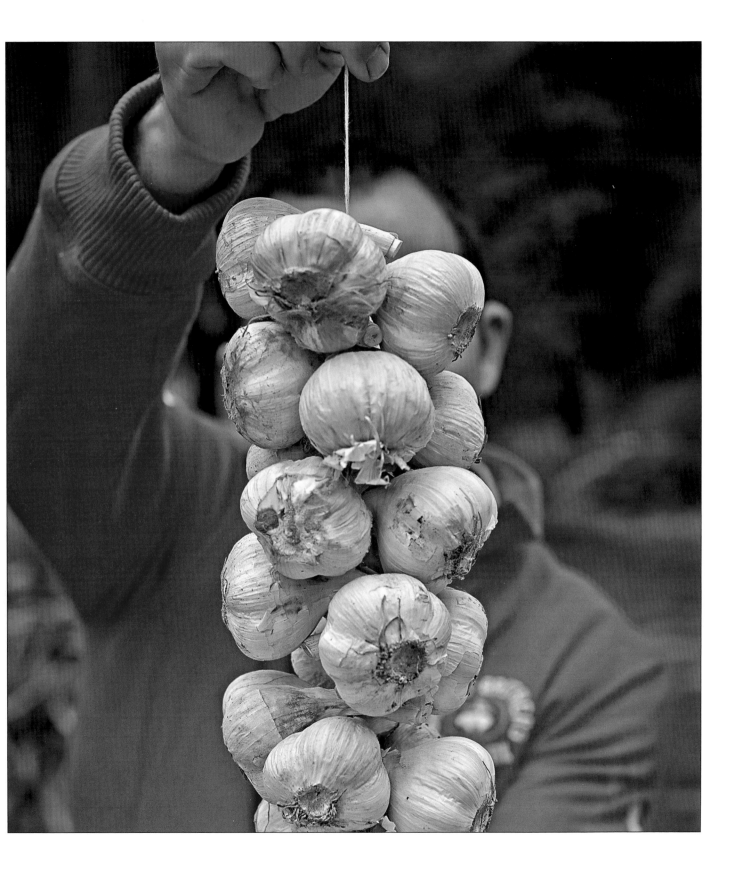

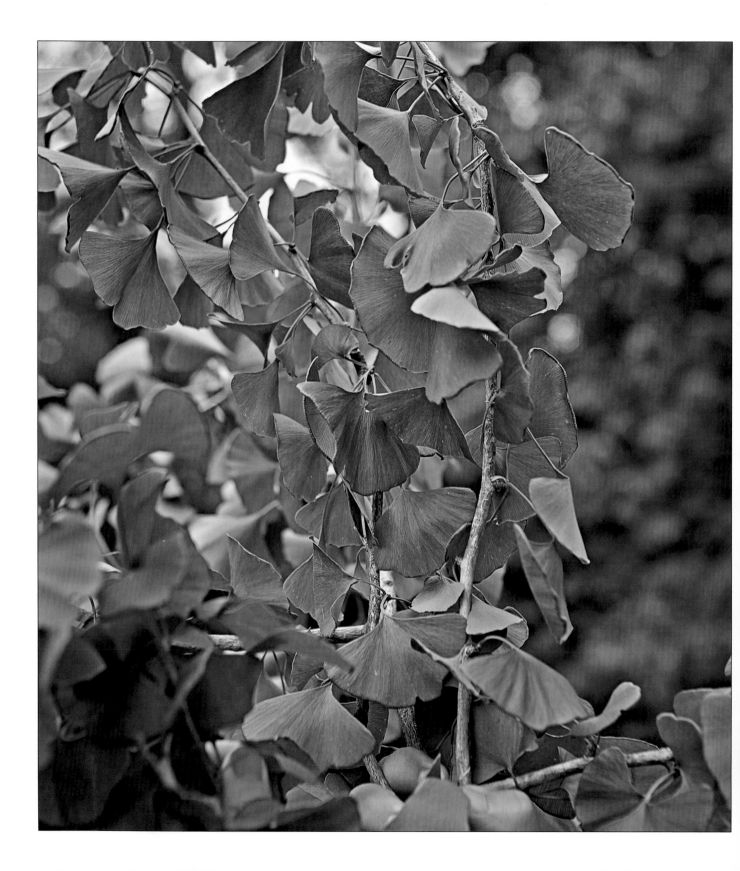

Ginkgo

The ginkgo is one of the planet's oldest and longest-lived trees. The species is a living fossil, largely unchanged for some 300 million years. A highly unusual tree with unique, fan-shaped leaves, it can get very tall (up to 35 metres/115 feet or more), but it grows extremely slowly. Some trees are believed to be more than 1,000 years old. *Ginkgo biloba* originated in China, where it has been used in traditional medicine for thousands of years, but is now grown in many places around the world.

Health Benefits

Ginkgo is a "brain herb" that improves memory and age-related mental decline. It improves blood flow to the far corners of the brain, mainly due to its anticoagulant effects. It also encourages release of a powerful natural chemical called nitric oxide that helps to open up the blood vessels of the brain for better circulation and better cognitive function.

Some of the nutrients in ginkgo leaves are powerful antioxidants, including the terpenes and proanthocyanidins. These compounds protect brain nerve cells, allowing them to communicate better and improving cognition and alertness. They may also increase synthesis of an important memory chemical called acetylcholine.

Ginkgo also helps with problems related to the eye. Macular degeneration and diabetic retinopathy—diseases that severely impede sight—are related to decreased circulation to the optic nerve, as well as inflammation and blockage of the tiny blood vessels in the eye. By opening up these blood vessels and decreasing the stickiness of blood platelets, ginkgo helps feed the optic nerve with blood nutrients and oxygen.

The circulatory benefits are not limited to the eyes. Ginkgo also helps improve blood flow to the extremities and improves peripheral vascular disease, which afflicts those with diabetes, Raynaud's, and Buerger's disease. And if that wasn't enough, it may also help circulation to the genital region to aid in erectile dysfunction.

Growing

The ginkgo—or maidenhair tree—is a slow-growing shade tree that has survived ice ages, wars, and even the pollution of cities. Some are hundreds of years old, and the oldest ginkgo fos-

DIFFICULTY
Easy

HARDINESS
Perennial in zones 3 to 9

TIME TO PLANT
Early spring or early fall

TIME TO HARVEST
Late spring to early summer

LOCATION
Full sun

SOIL TYPE
Well-drained; will not tolerate wet soils

sils date from a period before flowering plants even existed! If you are looking for instant gratification, ginkgo won't give it to you, but if you desire an attractive specimen offering vibrant yellow fall colour and edible foliage, then this is your tree. On the downside, ginkgo is a messy tree that often drops its leaves, so don't place it close to your deck or pool unless you like to clean.

Gingko trees are either male or female. Female trees produce a fruit that smells awful when crushed, so choose male plants for your garden (this should be clearly labelled on the plant tag).

Common Varieties: There are many cultivars of *Ginkgo biloba* offering different mature heights and foliage colour. Varieties include 'Autumn Gold', 'Jade Butterflies', 'Fairmount', and 'Pendula'. Smaller varieties such as 'Chi-Chi', 'Troll', and 'Horizontalis' are suitable for containers.

PLANT

Plant ginkgo in early spring or early fall when frequency of rain is greater, and days are warm but nights are cool. That combination is ideal for root establishment of any shade tree or container-grown shrub. Locate in full sun.

Dig a hole twice the depth of the root ball and two-and-a-half times the width. Improve the soil by removing any clay or sand and add loam and manure. Backfill the hole while ensuring the root ball is just above ground level. If your gingko came from the nursery in a container, remove it and score the roots before placing it in the planting hole; with field-dug gingko, just place it into the hole and remove the burlap. Firmly tamp down the amended soil around the root ball.

Stake your new tree and water it deeply. Then get comfortable and wait!

GROW

Gingko is a slow grower—sometimes painfully slow. New plants will take several months to root, and you will not notice growth until the second or third season. But slow and steady wins the race! Gingko is a salt-tolerant, pollution-tolerant tree that will endure pretty much everything you throw at it once it's established, including periods of drought.

Most garden varieties of gingko won't grow more than 5 to 8 metres (16 to 26 feet), but I have seen some very mature specimens reach 12 to 20 metres (40 to 65 feet) high by 6 to 12 metres (20 to 40 feet) wide.

Remember, soil settles! One of the biggest failures with new trees and shrubs is planting too deep. This increases the chances your plants will drown during the growing season, especially in clay soils. You should plant trees and shrubs above ground level in clay soils. Even in well-drained soils, large plantings like shade trees should be slightly above ground level; root balls will settle in and drop slightly after watering because the soil will compact.

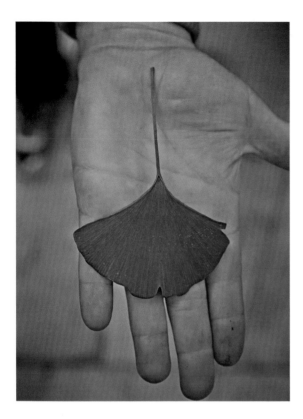

HARVEST

Harvest the foliage when the tree has fully "leafed out" in late spring or early summer. The goal is to get tender leaves before they mature; old leaves are tough and may lack potency. Be selective: Prune inward-facing or arching branches first, as this will increase airflow and benefit overall tree health. Strip all of the leaves from the branches you just pruned. If you need more leaves, be sure to remove random leaves, never stripping entire branches at one time. Do this midday when it's cool and dry.

You may be able to enjoy a harvest even if you don't have a gingko on your property.

Gingko often can be found in native forests and are a popular roadside planting—there may even be one on your street.

STORE

Gingko leaves can be eaten in salads, brewed in teas, or made into extracts. The leaves can be used fresh or dried. Wash fresh leaves just before use. Store fresh leaves in resealable bags in the refrigerator for up to a week. To dry gingko, place the leaves on a drying tray or baking sheet in a well-ventilated area out of direct light for up to 2 weeks, until brittle (see "Drying Herbs at Home" on page 365). After drying, store the leaves in an airtight container and use for teas.

Put It to Work

Drawing blanks? Try this tincture!
The best way to put ginkgo to work is to make an alcohol tincture. It's super-easy! Just pick 2 cups of ginkgo leaves, wash them, and place in a resealable glass jar (like a Mason jar). Cover with about 2.5 cm (1 inch) of vodka (at least 80 proof). Place wax paper over the jar and then screw the lid on tightly to seal it. Set aside in a cool, dark place for 4 weeks, shaking the jar daily.

After 4 weeks, strain the mixture through a fine-mesh sieve, ensuring you press out all the liquid from the ginkgo. Take 1 teaspoon daily for improved cognitive function and memory.

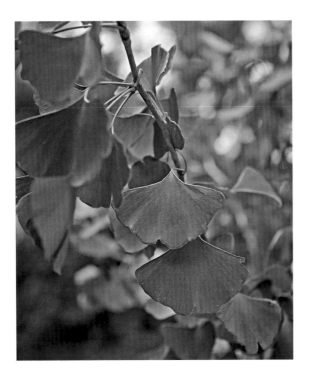

This formula will keep in a cool, dark place for up to a year.

Bad memory? Don't forget about this tea!

Place 5 coarsely chopped fresh ginkgo leaves or 1 heaping tablespoon of dried ginkgo in a mug with 1 cup of boiling water. Cover with a saucer and steep for 15 minutes. Sweeten with manuka honey to taste. To achieve the same effects of 1 teaspoon of tincture, you'll need to drink at least 3 to 4 cups of this tea per day.

Mental fatigue? Toss back some brain-boosting gel shots!

If your issue is forgetfulness or lack of mental energy, what are the chances you'll remem-ber to take the tincture or tea? We've got the solution: ginkgo gel shots. You'll need 7 shot glasses. We recommend one shot a day, and you can make a week's worth in advance so they'll be in plain sight in the refrigerator and you won't forget!

Place 7 tablespoons of ginkgo tincture (see opposite page) into a small mixing bowl. Add 1 ounce (a shot glass full) of Jell-O powder (your choice of flavour) and ½ cup of boiling water. Mix well. Pour evenly into each of the 7 shot glasses and refrigerate. "Shoot" one per day for optimal memory.

» Fast Forward

Fast forward to the health food store to purchase PhytoPharmica's Ginkgo Phytosome capsules or equivalent. Follow the instructions on the label.

! Cautions

This plant has a powerful anticoagulant effect, and there have been reports of internal bleeding in those who took ginkgo. Do not combine gingko with anticoagulant drugs such as warfarin or aspirin, ibuprofen, or any other type of non-steroidal anti-inflammatory drug (NSAID) that has blood-thinning effects.

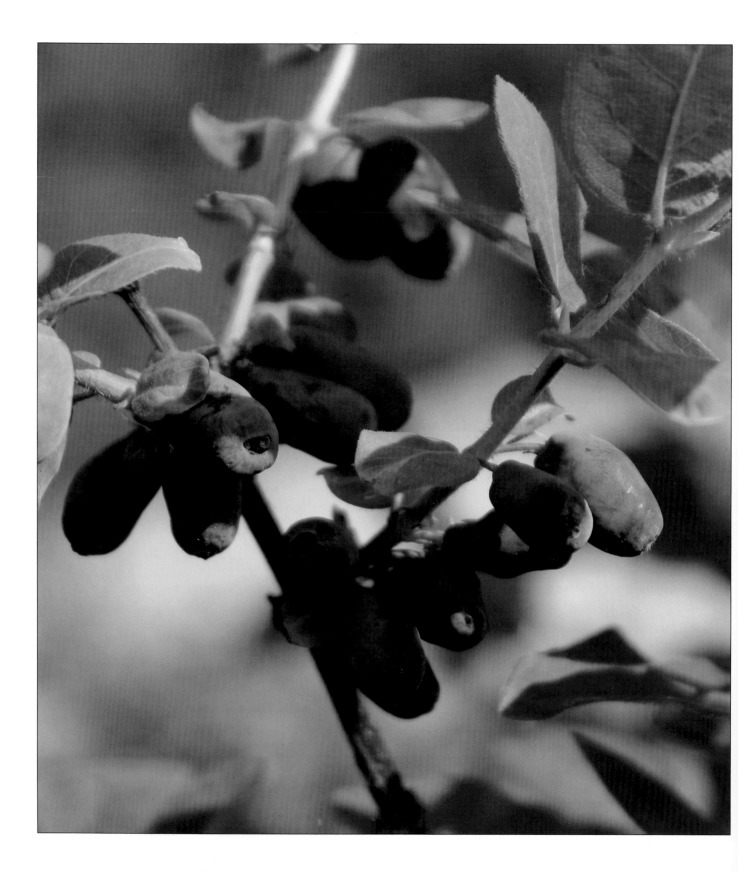

Haskap

Haskap—also known as blue honeysuckle or honeyberry—was known to the ancient Japanese as "the fruit of longevity." It originates from the island of Hokkaido— Japan's northernmost island territory—and was introduced to Canada in the 1950s as an ornamental. By the late 1990s, scientists had developed hardy varieties with tasty fruits that are now prized for their health benefits. Haskap fruit is similar to blueberries in colour, but it is elongated and slightly cylindrical—more like a mini plum. The plant is not a close cousin of blueberries or cranberries; it is more closely related to the tomato.

⊕ Health Benefits

Blueberries are well known for containing polyphenol antioxidants, but Haskap berries have five times the amount, making them an antioxidant superfood.

Polyphenols provide the fruit with natural protection against ultraviolet radiation, fungal attack, and other pathogens. In humans, these antioxidants help prevent heart disease, cancers, cardiovascular diseases, diabetes, osteoporosis, and neurodegenerative diseases.

The phenolic content in this berry is directly associated with its colour and flavour. The skin of red grapes also contains high concentrations, which helps explain red wine's colour and its antioxidant properties. But the flesh of most red grapes is actually white. Haskap berries, on the other hand, have flesh that is reddish-purple. That means the berries have high phenol content throughout, and not just in the skin, giving Haskap a higher antioxidant score and superior health benefits.

🌱 Growing

Haskap is the rising star of the berry industry in North America. The fruits are packed with antioxidants, and the plant is extremely well suited to northern climates. It was cultivated in Siberia in the 1950s, and more hardy varieties were developed by the University of Saskatchewan. Not only does it survive Canadian winters, but it is the first berry to flower and the first to bear fruit. Haskap is also fast-growing and high-yielding.

Common Varieties: The most popular Haskap varieties are 'Indigo Gem', 'Indigo Treat', 'Tundra', 'Borealis', and 'Honey Bee'. Most varieties are not self-pollinating, so they need to be planted alongside a complementary variety. For example, 'Honey Bee' can pollinate the other types.

DIFFICULTY
Easy

HARDINESS
Perennial in zones 2 and above

TIME TO PLANT
Early spring

TIME TO HARVEST
Spring to early summer

LOCATION
Full to part sun

SOIL TYPE
Well-drained

PLANT

Haskap can be planted anytime during the growing season, but early spring is ideal (as soon as the soil is workable). Locate the plants in full sun out of direct wind, and ensure the soil is well-drained. While Haskap will grow in average soils and can tolerate slight acidity, it will thrive in soils rich in organic matter or amended with composted manure. Plant 1 metre (3 feet) apart and water deeply and infrequently. Mulch to minimize weed growth and keep the roots cool.

GROW

Haskap will thrive with occasional watering, some weeding, and infrequent fertilizing with compost tea (page 175) or general garden fertilizer (10-10-10). Haskap are resistant to disease, insects, and deer, but your biggest challenge is birds, especially cedar waxwings. Apply netting, install noisemakers, and even put up a plastic owl to discourage birds from eating your prized crop.

After harvest, continue watering and weeding, and watch out for powdery mildew. Treat as necessary with a fungicide and ensure good airflow around plants.

Haskap can get quite large: The mature shrub is about 1 metre (3 feet) wide and 1 to 2 metres (3 to 6 feet) tall. While the plant is dormant in late winter or early spring, prune out older and/or dead branches. When the shrub becomes very dense, central branches should be removed. Be careful never to prune more than 25% of the entire bush in a season.

HARVEST

Haskap is the first berry you can harvest in spring, but don't be fooled: The berries will appear deep in colour and plump, but they still may not be ready for harvest for up to 10 days. If there is any green still inside the berry, it's not fully ripe. Ripe berries will naturally fall when you shake the bush.

The birds and the bees play a big role in the garden. Many plants that produce fruits, berries, and nuts require pollinators. In some cases (such as hollies) the plants are actually male and female. But with Haskap you need more than one cultivar in order to produce fruit. You don't need to plant them in even numbers; one pollinator can be effective for up to eight producing plants.

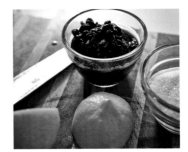

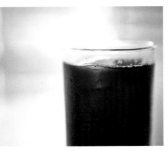

Frozen Haskap berries; Haskap juice.

STORE

Wash Haskap berries just before use. They can be stored in an airtight container in the refrigerator for up to 10 days, or frozen. Haskap can also be preserved in jams, jellies, and wines.

Put It to Work

Not getting your antioxidants? Get syrupy about Haskap!

The trend today is all about eating healthier without abandoning taste. Haskap syrup is not only an antioxidant powerhouse, but it can single-handedly make pancakes healthier and tastier, sweeten a shake, and even give you partial justification for eating vanilla ice cream!

> *6 cups Haskap berries (fresh or frozen)*
> *3 tsp freshly squeezed lemon juice*
> *2 cups water*
> *6 cups granulated sugar*

In a blender, combine the berries and lemon juice and blend on high speed until smooth. Pour into a large pot. Bring to a boil and, one cup at a time, stir in the sugar until completely dissolved. Reduce the heat and simmer for 15 minutes, stirring often. Remove from the heat and let cool. Strain through a cheesecloth into a bowl (discard solids). Using a funnel, pour the syrup into a sterilized narrow-neck pouring jar (like an old syrup jar) with a tight-fitting lid. The syrup will keep in the refrigerator for up to 2 weeks.

Got gout? Haskap smoothies daily!

Gout is a form of inflammation that occurs when crystals of uric acid accumulate in a joint (most commonly the big toe) and cause sudden pain. People with gout either overproduce uric acid or are less efficient at eliminating it.

If you suffer from gout you should closely watch your purine intake. Purines are compounds found in high-protein foods such as poultry and meat (especially organ meats), beer (and alcohol in general), and seafood. Gout can also be triggered by too much sugar, so limit soft drinks sweetened with high-fructose corn syrup or sugar and sugary drinks—stick to water!

Antioxidants and vitamin C will help a gout flare-up tremendously. Thankfully, Haskap is full of both. Drink this smoothie daily to reduce uric acid.

> *1 cup Haskap berries (fresh or frozen)*
> *½ cup strawberries (fresh or frozen)*
> *½ cup raspberries (fresh or frozen)*
> *2 cups coconut milk*
> *½ cup plain Greek yogurt*
> *1 tsp chia seeds*
> *8 ice cubes*
> *Liquid honey*

In a blender, combine all of the ingredients (sweeten with honey to taste) and blend on high speed until smooth.

Can spinach salad get any healthier? Yes!

Spinach is chock full of micronutrients, includ-

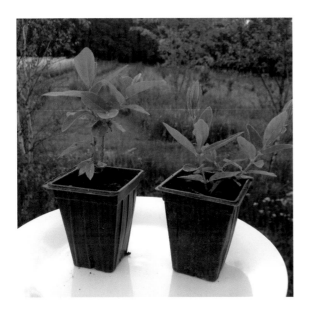

ing powerful antioxidants and phytonutrients hard to find in other foods. Dress it up with Haskap and you have the dream team of disease prevention!

> ½ cup puréed Haskap berries (fresh or frozen)
> Freshly squeezed juice of 2 lemons
> ½ cup extra virgin olive oil
> 1 tbsp liquid honey
> Sea salt and freshly ground black pepper
> ¼ tsp turmeric powder
> 6 cups baby spinach
> ½ Spanish onion, chopped
> 1 cup chopped pecans
> ¼ cup fresh coriander leaves

In a blender, combine the Haskap berries, lemon juice, oil, honey, salt and pepper to taste, and turmeric and blend on high speed until smooth.

In a salad bowl, toss the baby spinach with the dressing. Sprinkle with the onion and pecans and garnish with coriander.

» Fast Forward

Fast forward to Haskapa.com to purchase Haskap products.

! Cautions

Haskap is a new crop, so very little research has been done to assess risks or possible drug interactions.

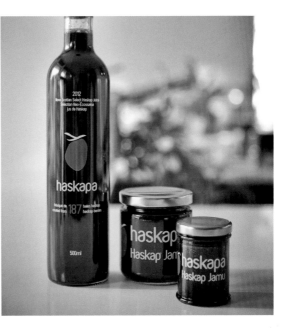

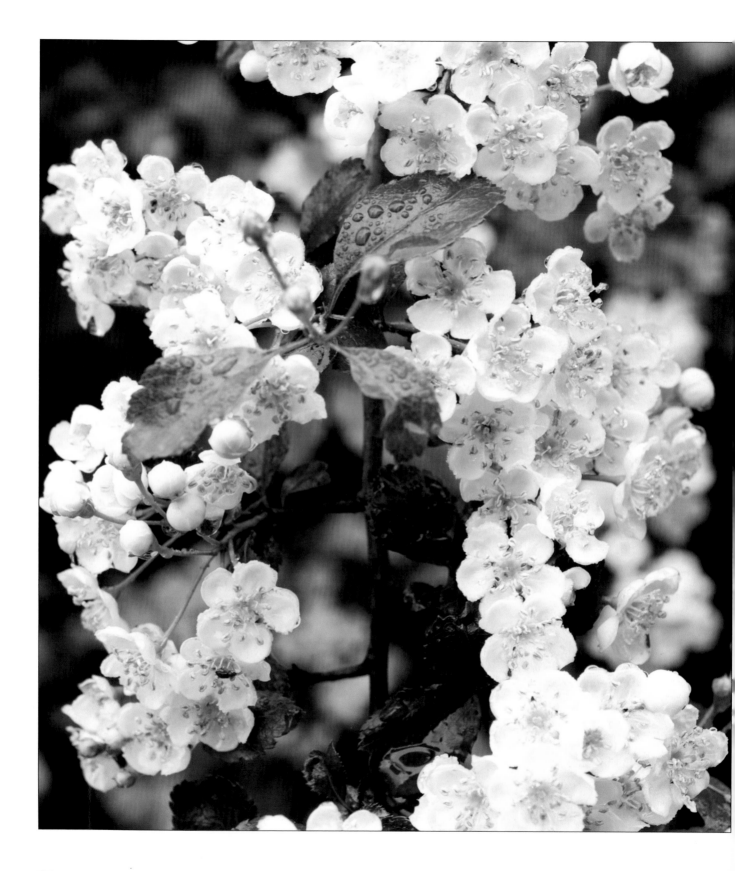

Hawthorn

Hawthorn, sometimes called hawberry, is part of the rose family (*Rosaceae*). The plant has thorny branches and produces white flowers followed by small berries called "haws." They are usually red when ripe, but may also be black. Hawthorn leaves are shiny and grow in a variety of shapes and sizes. There are many species, though the common hawthorn (*Crataegus monogyna*) is the one most likely to be used for medicinal purposes.

Health Benefits

Hawthorn has been used since the first century as a treatment for heart disease. This superberry is best known for its ability to bolster the connective tissues of the cardiovascular system and as a remedy for congestive heart failure. When the heart is unable to provide sufficient pump action to maintain blood flow, hawthorn may be able to improve the cellular integrity of the heart muscle and help with any inflammation in the blood vessels.

Research and trials show symptoms such as shortness of breath and fatigue improve significantly with hawthorn treatment, and there is a substantial benefit from using hawthorn extract as an adjunctive treatment for chronic heart failure.

Flavonoid compounds called procyanidins help normalize blood pressure and enhance circulation during exercise. Taken daily, hawthorn may improve athletic performance.

Until recently the berries were more commonly transformed into heart tonics. Today, herbal preparations are more likely to use the leaves and flowers, which contain more of the active flavonoid properties than the berries.

Growing

Hawthorn comes in many shapes and sizes, from small shrubs to massive trees. It's a versatile landscape plant, but it isn't easy to grow. Hawthorn doesn't transplant well; because it's a member of the rose family it has the same insect and disease challenges. In the wild, hawthorn bushes are easy to find: Their bark is scaly and greyish brown, and their leaves start out bright green and darken with age. Their white flowers appear in mid-spring, followed in the fall by bright red berries and spectacular fall foliage.

Common Varieties: There are many species of hawthorn, including the common hawthorn (*Crataegus monogyna*), English

DIFFICULTY
Medium

HARDINESS
Perennial in zones 4a to 7b

TIME TO PLANT
Early spring or early fall

TIME TO HARVEST
Fall

LOCATION
Full sun

SOIL TYPE
Well-drained

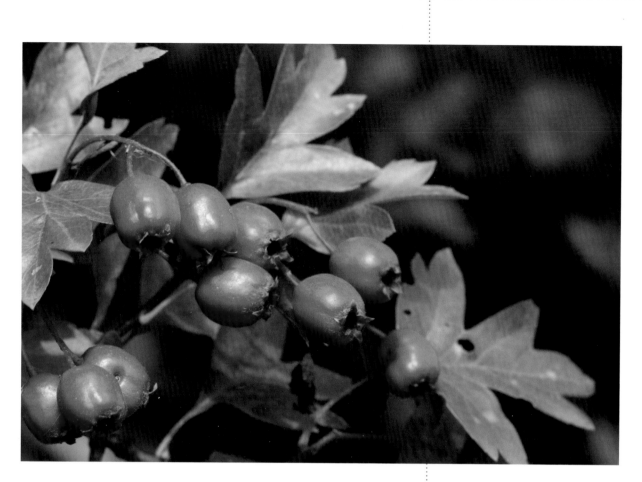

hawthorn (*C. laevigata*), Chinese hawthorn (*C. pinnatifida*), and downy hawthorn (*C. mollis*). Cockspur hawthorn (*C. crus-galli*) has particularly showy foliage in fall.

PLANT

Look for container-grown hawthorn at your local nursery, but it may be a special request, as it's generally not readily available. Hawthorn is best transplanted when young; once established it doesn't like to be moved.

Plant hawthorn in a sunny location with rich, well-drained soil in early spring or early fall. Don't plant it too deeply: Ensure the top of the root ball is just above the soil level of your planting hole. Transplant fertilizer is recommended at the time of planting to reduce shock. Water deeply and keep moist until established.

GROW

Hawthorn is hardy and can grow in a wide range of environments, but it always seems to struggle with insects and diseases. Be on the lookout for leaf spot (purple spots dot the leaves), stem rust (orange spots form on the stems and the leaves fall off), and fire blight (the leaves shrivel and appear to be scorched). Common insects include aphids, cankerworms, and gypsy moths. Each can be controlled through applications of insecticidal soaps, horticultural oils, and sulphur. Do your best to catch them early.

Prune hawthorn in late winter or early spring while the plant is dormant and buds have not yet cracked. Remove dead and/or diseased wood, including stems that appear weak. After removing diseased stems, wipe your pruners with bleach to minimize spread of diseases. In fall, rake and discard any diseased leaves to reduce the risk for next season.

Fertilize in spring for increased health; use a root feeder or water-soluble fertilizer (25-10-10).

HARVEST

While the berries are most cherished, hawthorn blossoms can be used in salads, and the leaves can be chewed or used as a garnish (note that the berries' seeds are toxic: see page 157). Hawthorn is even a desired carving wood for sculptors.

Collect the red (some appear black) berries in fall, starting around early October. Berries should appear plump and brightly coloured at their peak. Harvest by plucking berries or pulling on the ripened bunch.

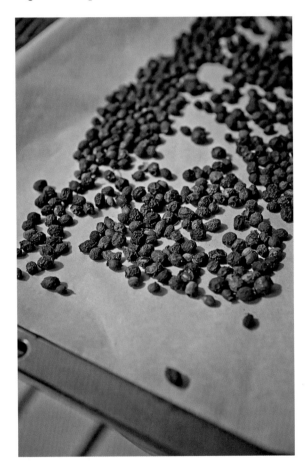

Dry your own hawthorn berries on a baking sheet in a very low oven for several hours.

STORE

Wash hawthorn berries just before use. Store in an airtight container in the refrigerator for up to a week. To freeze, wash berries and pat dry. Arrange in a single layer on a baking sheet and freeze. Once frozen, transfer to resealable bags. You can also preserve hawthorn berries in jellies or jams. Dry berries on a drying tray or baking sheet or using a dehydrator.

Put It to Work

Intense workouts leave you tired? Enjoy a recovery fruit leather!

Enjoy a hawthorn berry snack after an intense cardiovascular workout. The flavonoids will help your heart recover, while the antioxidant power of this rolled-up snack will sweep up the mess left behind from the physical stress.

Pick 2 cups of hawthorn berries. In a saucepan over medium heat, combine berries with 1 cup of water and simmer for 15 minutes. Let cool. Using the back of a spoon, press the berries through a fine-mesh sieve into a bowl (discard solids). Pour the strained pulp evenly onto 2 baking sheets lined with wax paper. Spread it about 3 mm (⅛ inch) thick. Bake at 38°C (100°F) or lowest temperature setting for 20 to 25 minutes. Cool for 10 to 15 minutes to set. The fruit leather is ready when it can be easily peeled off the trays.

Using a sharp knife, cut the fruit leather into roughly 7.5 x 15 cm (3 x 6 inch) pieces. Peel and place the pieces onto a fresh piece of wax paper of equal size and tightly roll it up. Store in an airtight container for up to 1 month.

History of heart disease? Take this cardio tonic!

An ounce of prevention is worth a pound of cure—especially when we're talking about heart disease. Hawthorn flowers and berries each have powerful cardio-protective compounds. For your heart to get the best of both, make this two-part tincture.

The beautiful white flowers blossom in the spring, so that's when you'll gather enough blooms to fill a large resealable glass jar (like a Mason jar) half full (press them down firmly to pack tightly). Cover the flowers with at least 2.5 cm (1 inch) of vodka (at least 80 proof). Place wax paper over the jar and then screw the lid on tightly to seal it. Shake the jar well. Set aside in a cool, dark place for 4 weeks, shaking the jar vigorously for 2 minutes every week. After 4 weeks, using a fine-mesh sieve or cheesecloth, strain the liquid into a sterile glass bottle (discard the flowers) and set aside until ready to use.

When it's time to harvest berries in the fall, collect 3 cups. In a saucepan over medium heat, combine the berries with 1 cup of water and simmer for 15 minutes. Let cool. Using the back of a spoon, press the berries through a fine-mesh sieve into a bowl (discard solids).

In a blender, combine the berry pulp with the prepared flower tincture and purée. Pour the mixture into a wide-mouthed glass jar (a

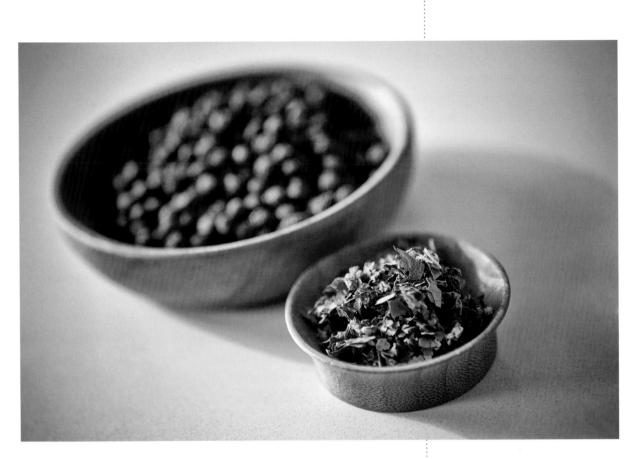

large Mason jar is best). The high concentration of pectin in the mixture may cause it to nearly solidify over time, so a jar with a wide opening is key to being able to fit a spoon inside. Cover the mouth of the jar with cheesecloth or a coffee filter and set it aside in a cool, dark place for 4 weeks.

After 4 weeks, you should be left with a jar full of deep red jelly. Spoon the jelly into a bowl lined with cheesecloth, gather up the cloth, and squeeze out the liquid (this may be difficult). Alternatively, run the jelly through a juicer or juice press (discard solids). Transfer the liquid to a sterile glass jar with a tight-fitting lid.

Take 1 tablespoon daily to support heart tone and prevent cardiovascular disease. The tincture will keep indefinitely stored in a cool, dark place.

Need a heart-healthy breakfast? Top it with oatmeal hawthorn compote!

In a saucepan over medium heat, combine 1 cup of hawthorn berries with ½ cup of water and bring to a boil. Let it reduce to about half its volume. Using the back of a spoon, press the berries through a fine-mesh sieve into a bowl (discard solids). Stir in ¾ cup of sugar until completely dissolved. The compote will keep in an airtight container in the refrigerator for up to 2 weeks.

Enjoy a bowl of steel-cut oatmeal with ¼ cup of plain low-fat yogurt and 2 tablespoons of this compote.

» Fast Forward

Fast forward to the health food store to purchase Wise Woman Herbals Crataegus Hawthorn extract or equivalent. Follow the instructions on the label.

! Cautions

Avoid eating the white seeds of hawthorn berries, as they contain amygdalin, a compound that changes to hydrogen cyanide in the stomach.

Avoid if you have a known allergy or sensitivity to hawthorn or any of its components.

The elderly or individuals at risk for low blood pressure should be cautious when using hawthorn, as should those with cardiovascular disorders or those taking heart drugs (such as digoxin), blood pressure drugs, cholesterol-lowering drugs, or herbs or supplements with similar effects.

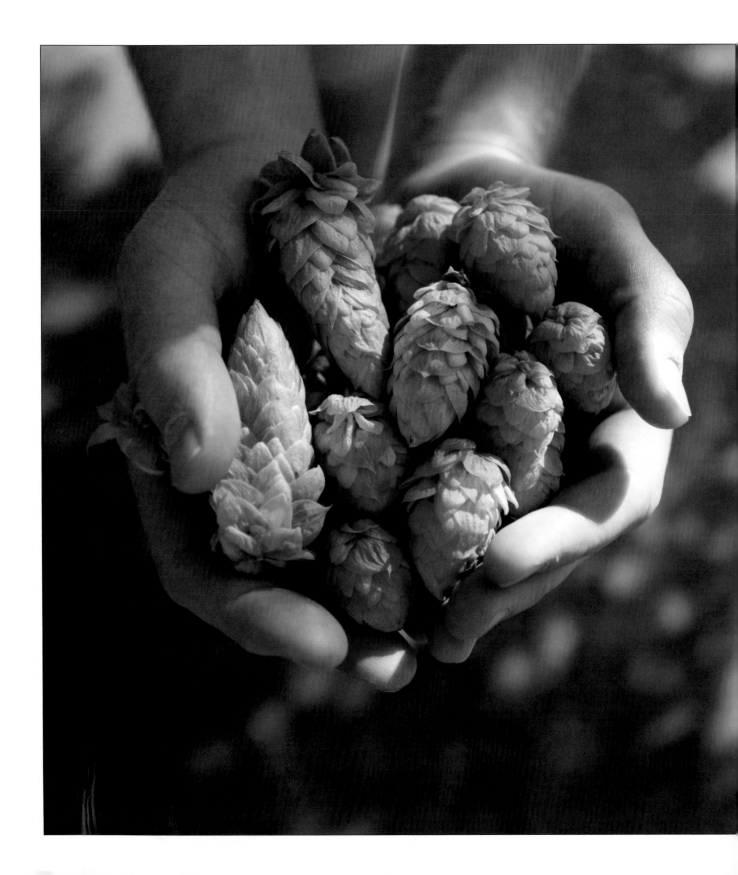

Hops

Hops are seed cones from the *Humulus lupulus* plant, which is part of the hemp family (*Cannabaceae*). Hops are native to Europe, Asia, and North America, and today are cultivated primarily in the United States, Germany, and England. Most people know that hops are widely used to make beer, giving it a characteristic aroma and bitter flavour, but not many know hops are also used to preserve beer. Hops flower essential oil is used in perfumes, cereals, beverages, and tobacco.

⊕ Health Benefits

The Cherokee have long known that hops cause drowsiness. Historically, they used hops as a sedative and an analgesic. Traditional Chinese medicine also uses hops to treat insomnia, restlessness, indigestion, intestinal cramps, and lack of appetite.

Hops can regulate and balance hormonal activity so may have effects on hormone-sensitive conditions such as breast cancer, uterine cancer, cervical cancer, prostate cancer, or endometriosis. Their bitter properties have appetite-stimulating effects shown to be helpful in treating anorexia.

Because hops sedate gently without narcotic side effects, they are a safer and milder alternative to addictive sedatives. By soothing the smooth muscle of the gastrointestinal tract, hops relax the "second brain" or the enteric nervous system. That, in turn, relaxes the central nervous system.

Hops are known to cause "man boobs" because of their estrogen-like compounds. Female hop pickers can even experience interruptions in menstruation due to the constant contact with the plant.

🌱 Growing

Hops have been gaining popularity with home gardeners and beer lovers. If you lack time and space, however, hops aren't for you! The hops plant is an aggressive vine that can easily reach over 5 metres (16 feet) and requires time-consuming pruning and staking. The vine will die in winter, but the rhizomes (roots) survive, so hops grow on new wood every year.

Common Varieties: Beer lovers may recommend some of these popular varieties: 'Cascade', 'Centennial', 'Willmette', 'Chinook', 'Amarillo', 'Golding', or 'Saaz'.

DIFFICULTY
Medium

HARDINESS
Perennial in zones 3 and above

TIME TO PLANT
Spring or late summer

TIME TO HARVEST
Late summer to fall

LOCATION
Full sun

SOIL TYPE
Well-drained, slightly acidic

PLANT

Hops are grown from rhizomes, which are a type of root (technically an underground stem) that will be familiar to anyone who has seen a piece of gingerroot. Hop rhizomes are available online or at select garden centres and some craft brewers. Purchase them in early spring and plant them when the soil is workable and after the risk of hard frost.

For great results, plant rhizomes in rich, well-drained, and slightly acidic soil (pH 6.5 to 7.5). Remember, hops grow quickly and will require heavy staking. You need a lot of space, and you don't want to shade out surrounding plants.

Hops generally do best when planted in direct sun with the soil mounded in rows. The rhizomes don't require much depth; they should be planted approximately 5 cm (2 inches) deep with the eyes facing up, spaced 0.5 to 1 metre (1 ½ to 3 feet) apart. Water deeply immediately after planting. If you're planting more than one variety, leave some distance between them—they will mix with each other! Build and install stakes shortly after planting or while the plant is dormant to minimize root disturbance.

I can't stress this enough: You need to build proper stakes for hops. Build them big and build them strong! I recommend even using steel rebar. Just one vine can yield up to 1 kg (2.2 lb) of hops: That adds up to a lot of weight over the entire plant, and when they're wet they weigh even more.

GROW

Hops require patience: You won't see good yields in the first few seasons. Once the plants mature, prune half the new vines that first appear in early spring (always prune the weakest vines and leave the thick ones). This will put more energy into the rhizome, and the more energy, the more hops! Prune again when vines measure 30 cm (12 inches) during the growing season. To minimize disease and insect infestation, remove the lower sections of growth and foliage. Tie vines during the growing season.

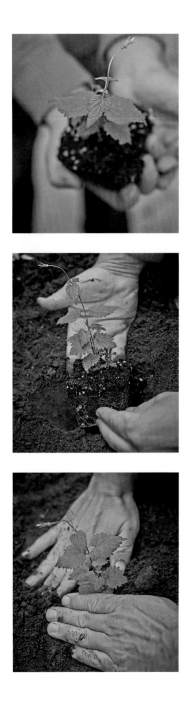

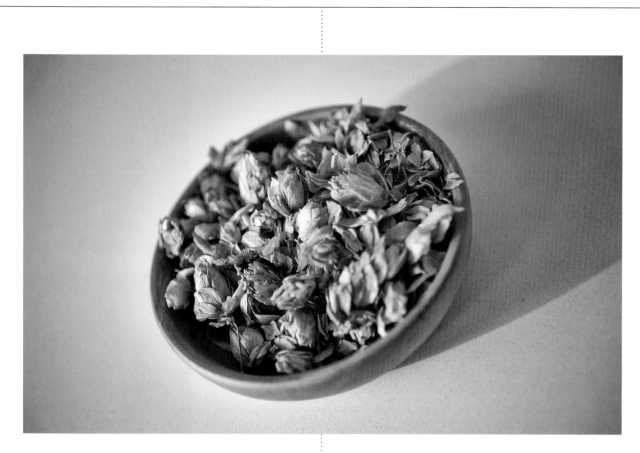

Dried hops.

Hops benefit from mulch, which reduces competition from weeds and maintains moisture. Hops should be watered often; never allow them to experience periods of drought.

When planted in soils rich in organic matter (compost or manure), hops will not require fertilizer. In poor soils use compost teas (page 175), organic fish emulsion, or a general-purpose water-soluble fertilizer (20-20-20).

To minimize mould, avoid overhead watering, increase airflow around plants (do not overplant), and water in the morning so foliage dries quickly. Tilling the soil surrounding hops in early spring can kill overwintering spores.

Monitor the plants often for aphids and spider mites and treat by applying insecticidal soaps, or attract or purchase ladybugs to eat the aphids!

HARVEST

Hops are ready to harvest when their aroma is strongest: Crush a cone and take a sniff. Late in summer, the cone will develop a dry, almost papery feel. Some browning of the lower sections is a good sign of ripeness. As they ripen you will also notice the cones become softer to squeeze, compared with the green, hard appearance and feel they have when young.

Be careful: Your greatest hop yields will be on vines closest to the sun. You could use an extension ladder to get to them, but that's an accident waiting to happen. Untie the vines and bring them to you instead of you going to them!

STORE

Hops can be used fresh, but it's best to dry them in a dehydrator or oven, or on drying trays in the direct sun. Sun-drying takes a few days, so make sure rain isn't in the forecast. How do you know when they're dry? The stems will break instead of bending. Once they're dry, store hops in airtight containers out of direct light.

Put It to Work

Counting sheep? Do it over a hop pillow!
When "Mad" King George III suffered from insomnia, his prime minister, Henry Addington, recommended he sleep on a pillow filled with hops. It worked! And it has worked for countless other kings and paupers since. If you have a problem falling asleep at night, this remedy may work for you, too!

Harvest the hops in the fall when they begin to feel slightly papery and are turning amber. At this point they are producing a bitter resin called lupulin, which imparts most of the medicinal virtues of the plant. Pick enough to fill a plastic shopping bag and dry them in the sun. Fill a pillowcase with the dried hops and sew the end closed. Place this inside the case of your regular pillow so you actively breathe in the magical sleep charm overnight. (If sleeping right on top of the crunchy hops isn't to your liking, flip the pillow over so that they are on the bottom. You'll still get a good dose of the active sedative.)

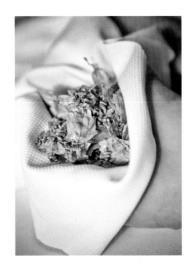

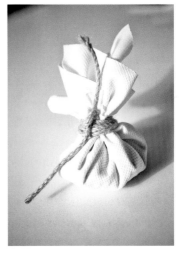

If you don't have enough hops to fill a pillowcase, you can make a small sachet to slip inside your normal pillowcase. Here we've added lavender for an extra-soothing scent.

Hops tend to lose their potency in 45 to 90 days, so for maximum effectiveness you'll want to refill the pillowcase before the end of 3 months. For most people the pillow will be enough, but if not, try a teaspoon of hops tincture (see below) just before you lie down.

Difficulty falling asleep?
Try this hops primer!
If you have ever felt relaxed after having a beer, it wasn't just the alcohol. It's all in the hops! This tincture can deliver a far more potent effect, but without the calories and with a fraction of the alcohol.

Tightly pack about 15 to 20 hops into a resealable glass jar (like a Mason jar) and fill to the top with vodka (at least 80 proof). Place wax paper over the jar and then screw the lid on tightly to seal it. Shake the jar well. Set aside in a cool, dark place for 2 weeks, shaking the jar vigorously every day or two.

After 2 weeks, using a fine-mesh sieve or cheesecloth, strain the liquid into a sterile, preferably dark-coloured, glass jar with a tight-fitting lid (discard solids).

Take 1 tablespoon with an ounce of lukewarm water 20 minutes before bed. The tincture will keep indefinitely stored in a cool, dark place.

⏩ Fast Forward

Fast forward to the health food store to purchase Metagenics Kaprex tablets or equivalent. Follow the instructions on the label.

❗ Cautions

Hops are a very safe remedy. Just use caution and don't consume before driving or operating heavy machinery, as drowsiness is likely. Some people report an allergic skin rash after handling the dried flowers; this is most likely due to a pollen sensitivity.

Don't take hops or use the hops pillow if you suffer from depression.

Hops have a mild influence on estrogen and can cause menstrual irregularities.

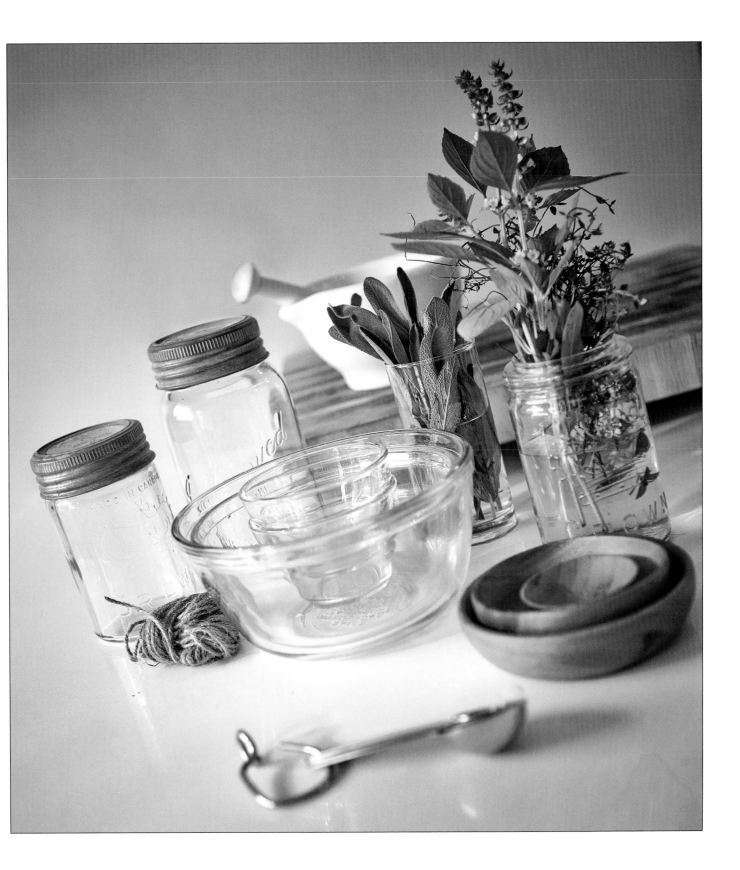

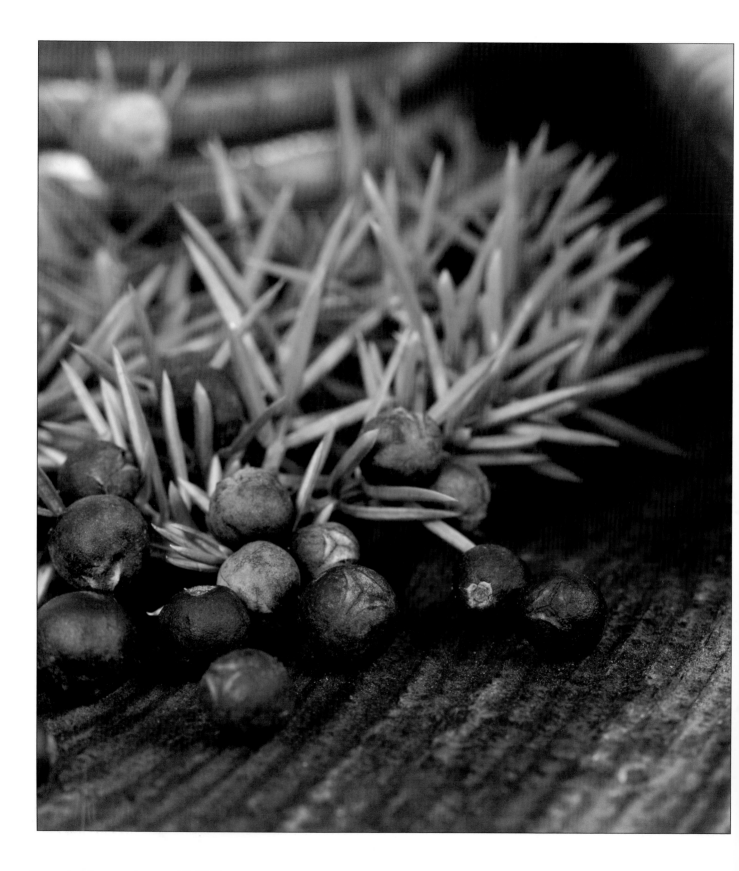

Juniper

If you like gin, you're already familiar with the essence of juniper. The berries, which are found amongst the prickly leaves of the bush, give off the strong and distinctive aroma that defines gin. These "berries" are actually fleshy cones that ripen to blue-black and show up only on the female plant. Junipers are in the cypress family (*Cupressaceae*), and they're widely distributed around the world. There are dozens of species, but the berries used in gin and in herbal remedies are usually taken from the common juniper, *Juniperus communis*.

✚ Health Benefits

In ancient Rome, coating the body with a juniper berry extract was protection against being bitten by snakes, being poisoned, and contracting the plague. It was even considered a remedy for feeble-mindedness.

Beginning in the 20th century, juniper was often prescribed as a diuretic for treating water retention, to relieve kidney and bladder problems, and externally for muscle aches and pains, arthritis, and even eczema.

Juniper berries contain flavonoids, tannins, and many volatile oils that laboratory research has shown to be effective as diuretics in animals. These compounds work by irritating the kidney lining, thereby increasing fluid loss by increasing urine flow.

🌱 Growing

This popular landscape shrub comes in many different shapes, sizes, and colours—spreaders or upright pyramidal forms, blue needles or gold needles—and some even provide fall colour. Junipers can really enhance a landscape by offering winter interest and colour all year long, but not all of them are suitable for medicinal purposes. Some produce berries that are bitter, and a few are even poisonous. Know what you are eating!

Common Varieties: The best berries come from *Juniperus communis*, which is common in the wild. Other edible species include *J. drupacea*, *J. phoenicea*, *J. deppeana*, and *J. californica*. Avoid *J. sabina* and *J. virginiana*, which are toxic.

PLANT

Junipers can be planted throughout the growing season, but for best results plant them in early spring as soon as the ground is

DIFFICULTY
Easy

HARDINESS
Perennial in zones 3 to 8

TIME TO PLANT
Early spring or early fall

TIME TO HARVEST
Fall

LOCATION
Full sun

SOIL TYPE
Well-drained; will survive rocky soils

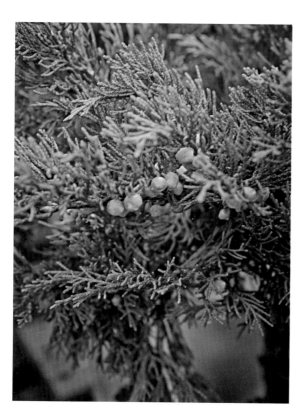

There are over 50 known varieties of juniper worldwide. From short to long needle, upright to spreading, most junipers will produce berries, whose colour can range from red to orange to blue.

Every landscape needs some evergreens, and junipers fit the bill. Not only do they provide four seasons of colour and interest, but the taller varieties also help block winds and will provide cover for birds during harsh weather.

GROW

Junipers are easy: Once they're established they take care of themselves. But I do recommend a few things that can help.

First, prune them annually in early spring before buds appear: Remove any dead or broken branches and selectively remove others to improve airflow. Never remove more than a third of the plant at one time. Junipers can be lightly pruned again in early summer, but avoid pruning in late summer or fall.

Ensure junipers are well watered in fall; this will minimize winter burn. In areas of high winds, cover junipers with a burlap screen in late fall or early winter. You may also want to tie upright varieties with twine to protect them from damage caused by heavy snow loads.

Junipers rarely have a problem with insects or disease. In residential settings, the browning of lower needles is often the result of dog urine. You don't want to eat the berries if that's the case!

HARVEST

In late summer or early fall, look for plump, bluish to black berries. Lay a bed sheet under your juniper, wear gloves, and give the bush a shake. The ripest berries will quickly fall onto

workable, or in early fall. Both seasons are ideal for establishing roots before harsh weather like dry summers or extremely cold winters.

Select healthy plants! Look for needles with no signs of browning. Junipers have both male and female plants, and berries only appear on the females. The sex is never marked on the plant tag, so if you're plant shopping in the fall, look for plants with berries already on them.

Locate in full sun and soil that is well drained—junipers hate being too wet!

the sheet. Hand-pick the remaining ripe berries, but don't harvest the green ones. You may want to come back and repeat this process later on if green berries remain.

Junipers can be easily found in the wild, so if you don't have the space to grow your own, just forage! Always make sure you can identify the species of juniper to make sure the berries are safe.

STORE

Wash the berries by soaking them in cold water to remove bugs and debris. Drain and spread them on drying trays or baking sheets, leaving space between the berries. Place them in a dry location out of direct light for up to 3 weeks. Monitor and remove any rotten berries (they'll turn brown or have holes in them). After drying, store in airtight containers in a cool, dry place.

Put It to Work

Retaining water? Expel it with juniper berry!
Edema is swelling caused by fluid retention—often in the feet, ankles, and legs, but it can involve your entire body. Because it can represent a more serious underlying condition, it requires attention from your physician. When it isn't too serious, a natural remedy like juniper berry may help.

Gather about 2 cups of ripe juniper berries and wash them gently with cold water. Place them in a large resealable jar (like a Mason jar). Cover the berries with at least 2.5 cm (1 inch) of brandy (at least 80 proof), seal tightly, and shake the jar well. Set aside in a cool, dark place for 1 week, shaking the jar daily.

After a week, transfer the contents to a blender and blend on low until smooth. Return the mixture to the glass jar and replace the lid. Set aside in a cool, dark place for 4 more weeks, shaking vigorously once a week.

When the 4 weeks are up, place a fine-mesh sieve over a bowl lined with cheesecloth. Pour in the berry pulp and allow the tincture to drain into the bowl. Gather up the edges of the cheesecloth and squeeze to extract as much liquid as you can (discard solids). Pour the tincture into a sterile jar and seal.

Take 1 teaspoon with water twice daily between meals. The tincture will keep indefinitely in a cool, dark place.

Joint or muscle pain? Juniper packs can help!
If your joints ache from an arthritis flare-up, if your muscles are sore from intense activity, or if you're just feeling like a rusted Tin Man, then these juniper oil packs may help.

In a small heatproof bowl over a pot of boiling water (acting as a double boiler), heat 2 cups of castor oil. When the oil is hot, add 1 cup of juniper berries and stir. Cover, reduce the heat to low, and simmer very gently for 3 hours. Check occasionally to make sure there is enough water in the pot and that the formula isn't burning. After 3 hours, the castor oil will

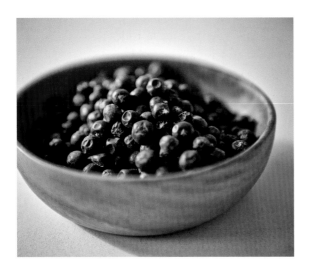

Dried juniper berries.

be infused with the juniper berries and your home will smell like a fresh forest!

Strain the berry mixture through a fine-mesh sieve into a glass bowl (discard solids). Add 1 cup of Epsom salts and stir well. While the mixture is still hot (but not hot enough to burn skin), dip a piece of flannel cloth into it. Let excess oil drip away. (Take care not to spill this oil on clothing—it will stain!) Carefully apply the soaked flannel directly to the area where there is pain, cover with a towel, and wrap with plastic wrap. (You can also apply a hot water bottle or heating pad.) Leave on for 10 minutes.

Remove the dressing and clean the area with baking soda and water. If desired, apply an ice pack for 7 minutes.

To store, place the flannel cloth into the bowl with the oil and cover with plastic wrap or a tight-fitting lid. The oil will keep in the refrigerator for up to 30 days.

» Fast Forward

Fast forward to the health food store to purchase Herb Pharm's juniper tincture or equivalent. Follow the instructions on the label.

! Cautions

Taking juniper for longer than 6 weeks could result in kidney damage. Strictly avoid in pregnancy and do not use if you experience any inflammation of the kidneys.

Don't exceed the recommended doses—doing so may lead to kidney and skin damage. Overdose symptoms include blood in the urine, increased heart rate, high blood pressure, convulsions, and non-menstrual uterine bleeding.

Juniper may also lower blood sugar levels, so those with diabetes or low blood sugar, and those taking drugs, herbs, or supplements that affect blood sugar should avoid it.

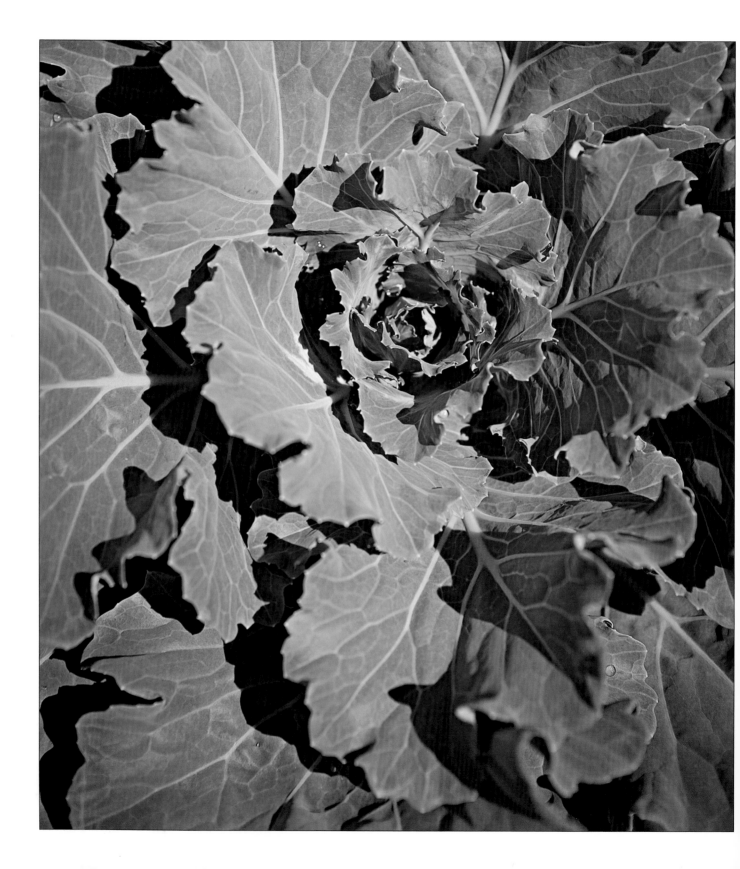

Kale

Kale is closely related to cabbage, broccoli, cauliflower, and Brussels sprouts—in fact, these foods are all cultivars of the same species. Kale comes in various shapes and forms—some edible and others ornamental—all flaunting green or purple leaves. Unlike its cabbage cousins, the central leaves of kale do not form a tightly packed head. Kale and its *Brassica* brothers have been grown for more than 2,500 years and are now a staple in many regions of the world.

Health Benefits

Kale may as well wear a cape. It isn't the new greens superhero for nothing! It's got more calcium by weight than milk, more vitamin C than an orange, more than 100% of your daily requirements of vitamin A per cup, up to 1,000% of your daily requirements for vitamin K per cup, and is a great source of alpha-linoleic acid (an omega-3 fatty acid that is healthy for your brain and heart). If those aren't superpowers, then what are?

You need vitamin K so that in case of an injury your liver can make the necessary platelets your body needs for blood to clot and heal the injury. A vitamin K deficiency is rare, but people are vulnerable if they have chronic malnutrition, celiac disease, or ulcerative colitis. Also, some drugs (including antibiotics, salicylates, or anti-seizure medications) may kill the friendly gut bacteria necessary for helping you get sufficient vitamin K. But have no fear: A cup of kale and you're getting your vitamin K hit as well as providing fibre to enhance the growth of good bacteria which in turn make more vitamin K.

Vitamin A is imperative for many biological processes, including vision and cellular growth. Research suggests vitamin A may prevent certain forms of cancer, aid in growth and development, and improve immune function. The recommended dietary allowance (RDA) is 900 micrograms (3,000 IU) for men and 700 micrograms (2,300 IU) for women. Less than a cup of kale has you covered.

Finally, kale is a source of Diindolylmethane (DIM), a compound believed to have anti-cancer properties, particularly against breast cancer and other cancers affected by estrogen.

Growing

Kale is an easy-to-grow member of the cabbage family (*Brassicaceae*). It's extremely tolerant of cold weather, which makes it a

DIFFICULTY
Easy

HARDINESS
Annual

TIME TO PLANT
Early spring or late summer

TIME TO HARVEST
Summer or fall

LOCATION
Full to part sun

SOIL TYPE
Well-drained, rich

popular fall ornamental, but isn't a fan of hot temperatures. Kale is known as a "cool crop" that enjoys cool nights with average daytime highs well below 25°C (80°F). In fact, the texture of kale will become almost woody in warm weather. Kale can be grown in the garden or in a pot, and with the wide range of leaf colours and textures, it's become popular to plant it for its looks and not its taste!

Common Varieties: Tuscan kale is my favourite. Other varieties include Scotch kale, Siberian kale, Japanese kale, and rape kale.

PLANT

You have many options when growing kale: You can purchase transplants in both spring and fall, sow indoors in late winter (start 8 to 10 weeks before last frost date), or direct-sow in the garden in spring. Purchasing transplants is easiest, and it gives you a jump-start on the season, though purchasing seeds will give you the greatest selection of varieties and will ensure your plants are organically grown from the start.

Plant kale in a location with lots of sun and soil that is well drained and rich in organic matter. Kale can be planted directly in flower gardens, placed in rows in vegetable gardens, or used as a foliage plant in containers. (When planting in containers use potting soil.) Ideal spacing for most kale varieties is about 30 cm (12 inches).

GROW

Kale is a cool-loving crop that thrives in spring, late summer, and fall. Kale will survive the heat of deep summer, but you may find the flavour lacking.

Water deeply and infrequently, keep weed-free (I recommend mulching), and only fertilize when planted in containers or poor soils. Fertilize with compost tea, fish emulsion, or general-purpose garden fertilizer (20-20-20). Kale will do exceptionally well without fertilizer if your soil is rich in compost or amended with manure.

Compost tea is a natural organic fertilizer. While there are many recipes, one of the easiest is to simply take a handful of your homemade organic compost, place it into cheesecloth, tie the ends, and then sink the "tea bag" into a pail of water. Allow it to steep for 24 to 48 hours before using.

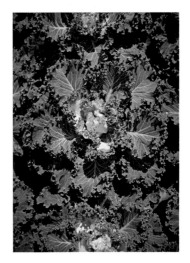

Many people assume that good-looking ornamentals aren't edible—but they're wrong! Dig into that container on your front step.

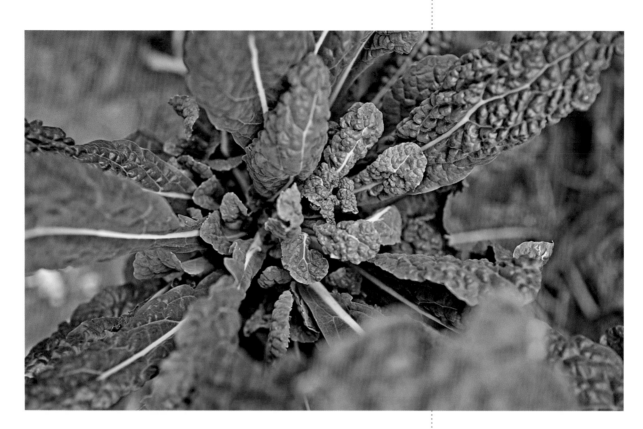

Dinosaur kale—one of many available varieties.

Increase watering during dry periods and monitor for insects and disease: Kale are victims of moths, cabbage worms, cabbage loopers, and cutworms. Cut off infected leaves and spray occasionally with insecticidal soaps. I've never had a kale demolished by cabbage worms; however, I have accidentally eaten a few of them! To prevent cutworm, make collars from paper cups and place them around the base of the plant.

HARVEST

Once mature, kale can be continually harvested. Harvest kale mid-morning or late afternoon, never during the heat of the day. Collect the outer leaves when the plant measures approximately 20 to 25 cm (8 to 10 inches) high, or approximately 30 to 40 days from planting transplants.

When harvesting the entire plant, cut the stem 5 cm (2 inches) from the ground. Shoots will re-sprout from the stem, offering an additional harvest later in the season. The youngest leaves are the most tender. You will find kale's flavour sweetens after frost arrives.

STORE

Harvest as needed; store only when required. To store, place kale loosely in a breathable bag and refrigerate for up to a week.

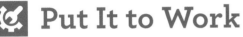

Put It to Work

Dull day? Brighten it up with a rainbow salad!

If you're going to pick up just one healthy habit, it should be eating a rainbow of antioxidant-rich vegetables every day. Green "leafies" are one of the most important groups, and that makes kale key!

Make a "rainbow salad" with thinly sliced kale; red, orange, and yellow bell peppers; and red onion. Top with blueberries, sprinkle with slivered almonds and mini bocconcini, and add your favourite salad dressing—I think poppy seed goes best!

Craving carbs? Try sautéed kale with pasta!

In a skillet, sauté some chopped kale with some extra virgin olive oil. Add onion, garlic, black olives, sun-dried tomatoes, shiitake mushrooms, and pine nuts. Cover and set aside. Cook gluten-free penne pasta until al dente, according to package instructions. Strain the cooked pasta and add to prepared kale mixture. Sprinkle with feta cheese and enjoy.

Looking for a side? How about naked kale?

Overcooking kale can destroy its health-protective powers, but sautéing it gently can release some of its nutrients. The best way to take advantage of kale is to "shock heat" it. Quick cooking preserves the nutrients, texture, colour, and flavour.

8 cups chopped kale, ribs removed
2 to 3 cloves garlic, minced
2 tbsp extra virgin olive oil
Sea salt and freshly ground black pepper
1 tbsp red wine vinegar

In a skillet over medium heat, heat the oil. Add the garlic and sauté for 1 minute, until soft. Add the kale and cook for 5 minutes, until tender-crisp. Season with salt and pepper to taste, and sprinkle with vinegar.

Want a healthy crunch? Try kale chips!

Slice kale into small chip-size pieces. Toss on a baking sheet with a drizzle of extra virgin olive oil and a pinch of sea salt. Bake in a preheated 175°C (350°F) oven for 15 minutes for a crispy treat.

Huge health craving? Jurassic kale salad!

Dinosaur kale, also called *lacinato* or *cavolo nero*, is a very dark green variety with huge leaves. It's ideal for this Jurassic salad!

6 cups chopped dinosaur kale (midribs removed)
Freshly squeezed juice of 1 lemon and 1 lime
4 tbsp extra virgin olive oil
1 tsp vegetable bouillon
2 cloves garlic, crushed
Pinch hot red pepper flakes
Sea salt and freshly ground black pepper
⅔ cup grated Pecorino, Asiago, or Parmesan cheese
¼ cup pitted and chopped kalamata olives
2 tbsp minced red onion
½ cup slivered almonds or pine nuts

In a large saucepan, bring 4 cups of water to a boil. Add the kale and boil for 20 to 30 seconds. Strain in a colander and immediately rinse under cold running water. Drain well and transfer to a salad bowl.

In a small bowl, whisk together the lemon and lime juices, oil, bouillon, garlic, salt, and a generous pinch of hot red pepper flakes (or to taste). Season with salt and pepper to taste. Pour the dressing over the cooked kale and toss well. Add two-thirds of the cheese and the olives and red onions. Toss to combine.

Let the salad sit at room temperature for at least 5 minutes to absorb the flavours. Add the almonds, toss again, and top with the remaining cheese. Refrigerate and serve cold.

» Fast Forward

Fast forward to the health food store to purchase organic raw kale chips.

! Cautions

One cup of kale can contain up to 10 times the Recommended Daily Allowance (RDA) of vitamin K. If you are taking anticoagulants such as warfarin, consult your doctor before adding it to your diet—too much vitamin K may pose problems.

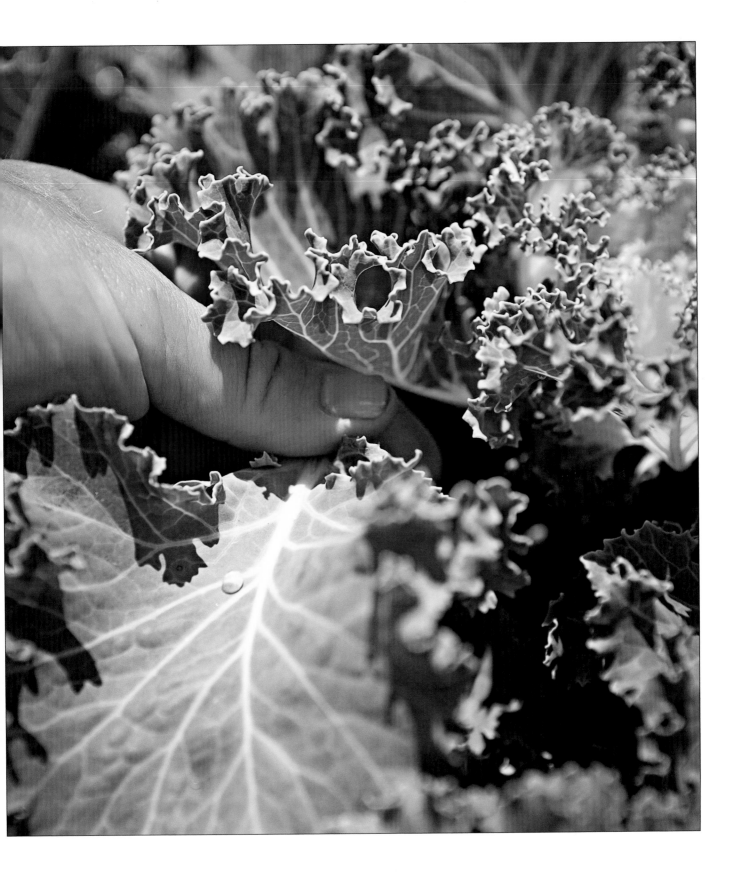

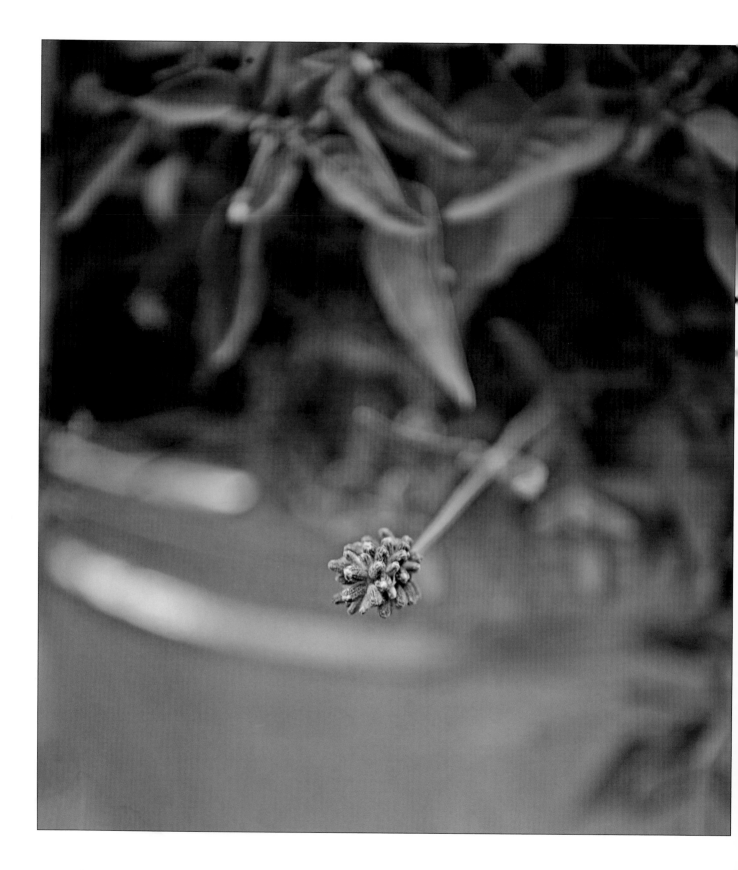

Lavender

Native to the Mediterranean, lavender is well known for its sweet, penetrating aroma. Many soaps, perfumes, detergents, and cleaning agents contain lavender, and the association of lavender with cleanliness goes back some time. The Romans used lavender oils for bathing and scenting the air. Indeed, the Latin root *lavare* means "to wash." Today lavender is probably best known for its use in aromatherapy. Its essential oil is extracted from the plant's tiny purple flowers.

Health Benefits

Lavender has been used therapeutically for pain, infection, relaxation, and sedation for many centuries. It is believed to have strong anti-anxiety effects, and there is some promising research to back this up. The active constituents of lavender are its volatile oils and hundreds of other compounds, including perillyl alcohol, camphor, limonene, tannins, and flavonoids.

Besides its relaxing effects, lavender also possesses antibacterial properties. Studies have shown that it acts against certain strains of strong bacteria, including methicillin-resistant *Staphylococcus aureus* (MRSA) and vancomycin-resistant *enterococci*, both of which can be spread in hospitals.

Growing

My mother loves lavender! Perhaps it's the fragrance, or her love of French provincial decor, of which lavender is a big part. I think anyone can love lavender for both its functional and aesthetic appeal. It's a beloved perennial used in formal borders, planted in groupings, or arranged in rows in herb and vegetable gardens, and adored for its showy bluish-purple flowers and fragrant foliage.

The biggest challenge with lavender is finding the perfect spot; where winters are harsh and summers are humid, lavender will struggle. But in the right location it will survive and thrive for many seasons.

Common Varieties: *Lavandula angustifolia* (sometimes called English lavender) is the most popular perennial variety. Hybrid varieties (*L. × intermedia*) are also called lavadins. Not all lavender cultivars are the traditional purplish blue; others are white, pink, or purple.

DIFFICULTY
Medium

HARDINESS
Perennial in zones 5 to 9 (some varieties are annual)

TIME TO PLANT
Spring

TIME TO HARVEST
Summer (in flower)

LOCATION
Full sun

SOIL TYPE
Well-drained, slightly alkaline (will not survive in acidic soils or clay)

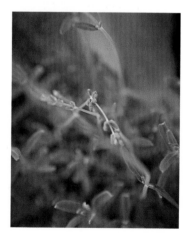

PLANT

Select varieties hardy for your region, or look for annual varieties (which may be other *Lavandula* species) for containers. Look for healthy plants free of browning leaves, with deep silvery-green foliage and no flowers. Transplants in bloom have been forced and will not provide the best results in the first season.

Plant in spring after the risk of frost. Select a site with well-drained soil, lots of sun, and shelter from harsh winds, especially in winter. Airflow during the growing season is vital to minimize disease, so ensure adequate spacing between plants.

Lavender hates having "wet feet." That's a gardening term for roots that stay wet for lengthy periods. In clay soils, where drainage is poor, lavender is almost impossible to grow. Plant it instead in raised beds or containers.

GROW

Lightly prune lavender in early spring, removing any dead or sickly looking stems. Water deeply and infrequently, ensuring the plant dries between waterings. Keep free of weeds. Lavender is an arid plant that hates humidity, so it may struggle in hot, sticky summers.

Lavender will thrive in poor soils (rocky or sandy) and rarely requires fertilizer. When amending soil to increase drainage, do not add too much peat moss, as this will increase acidity.

In colder areas, cover in late fall or early winter with clean straw or leaves free of any disease. Remove this covering in early spring after snow has melted.

HARVEST

Timing is key when harvesting lavender. Both the blooms and the buds contain essential oil, but if you harvest while the plant is in full bloom, most of the flowers and buds will drop from the stems after drying. It's best to harvest when only about a quarter to half of the flowers on a stem are in bloom.

STORE

Tie lavender into bundles and hang in a dry place, out of direct light (see "Drying Herbs at Home" on page 365). After drying, discard the stems and leaves and store the flower heads in airtight containers.

Put It to Work

Ready to use lavender? Stock up on the essential oil!

This essential oil forms the basis for all the lavender treatments that follow. Make a large jar so you'll always have some on hand.

Place 2 cups of fresh lavender buds in a big bowl. Use the back of a large serving spoon to crush them and begin releasing the oils. Do not overcrush the buds (they do not need to become mushy).

Dump the buds into a resealable glass jar (like a Mason jar). Pour in enough vodka (at least 80 proof) to cover the lavender completely. Place wax paper over the jar and then screw the lid on tightly to seal it. Set aside in a cool, dark place for at least 2 weeks, shaking the jar vigorously once daily to release the oil. The longer you let the lavender flowers steep, the more oil you will extract.

After 2 weeks, using a fine-mesh sieve lined in cheesecloth or a coffee filter, strain the mixture into a clean jar (discard solids). Place a clean cloth or coffee filter over the jar and let it sit for about 10 days to allow all the alcohol to evaporate. You'll be left with pure essential lavender oil.

Agitated? This smells like relief!

Add a few drops of lavender oil to a piece of cotton cloth and pin it inside your jacket or pants. You'll smell it throughout the day! Studies of those who suffer severe dementia in nursing homes found that lavender aromatherapy may help decrease agitated behaviour. The theory is that this will not only calm you down, but also calm those around you!

Burnt? Lavender is soothing and antibacterial!

Early research suggests lavender oils may have antibiotic activity, and that pain intensity and unpleasantness may be reduced after treatment with topical lavender therapy. If you've suffered a minor burn from cooking or by open flame, add 5 drops of lavender essential oil to ½ teaspoon of olive oil or vegetable oil (as a carrier) and apply to the wound up to 3 times daily.

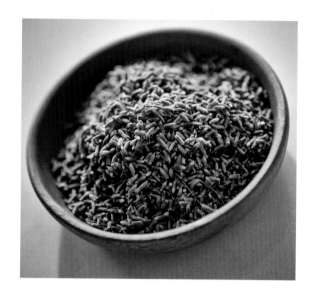

Suffer anxiety? Try lavender aromatherapy!

The traditional use for lavender oil is as aromatherapy for relaxation. Several small studies report that it helps to relieve anxiety. Add a few drops to your pillow before bed or simply rub a drop behind each ear like a perfume: The scent will make its way to your olfactory bulb, where it will have a positive and relaxing effect on your nervous system.

Decreased mental alertness? A few drops are all you need!

Research demonstrates that lavender oil helps maintain mental alertness and thus prevents deterioration of performance. Try adding a drop on the back of each hand when you're at your computer. Waving your hands around on your keyboard is enough to deliver the medicinal effects of the scent.

Poor sleep due to back pain? Get dual action relief!

Using lavender oil along with acupressure for short-term relief of lower back pain has been proven effective. Apply 2 drops of lavender on the back of each hand at the web between the thumb and index finger (this is known as the LI4 acupressure point). Find the highest point of the muscle when the thumb and index fingers are held together. Next, squeeze the point using the thumb and index finger of your opposite hand. While you press and massage deeply on the point, try to relax and breathe deeply for counts of five, hold for counts of seven, and breathe out through pursed lips for counts of eight.

» Fast Forward

Fast forward to the health food store to purchase NOW's lavender oil or equivalent. Follow the instructions on the label.

! Cautions

Avoid lavender if you have an allergy or are hypersensitive to any part of the plant.

Don't use lavender if you have a history of seizures, bleeding disorders, eating disorders (anorexia, bulimia), or anemia (low levels of iron).

You should not use lavender if you are using sedatives, blood thinners, cholesterol-lowering drugs, seizure drugs, antidepressants, or herbs or supplements with similar effects (like valerian, ginkgo, or garlic).

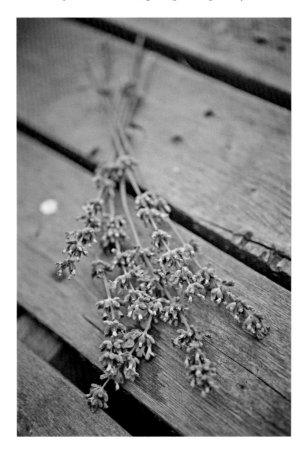

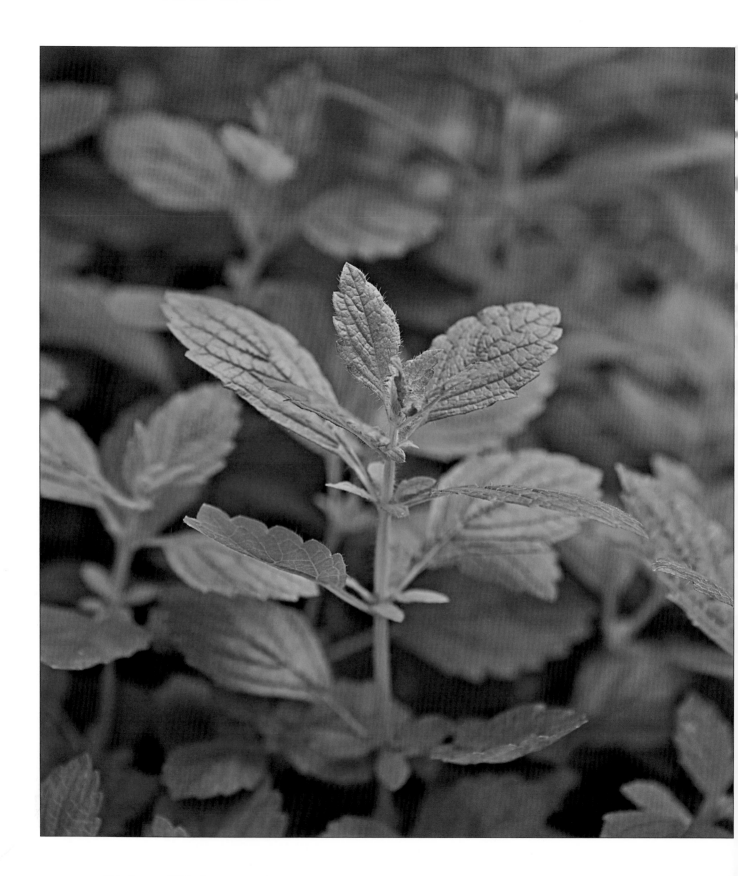

Lemon Balm

Lemon balm is a perennial herb and a garden staple. Native to southern Europe, it is now grown all over the world for brewing teas and garnishing salads—it even makes a beautifully scented addition to flower arrangements. The leaves of lemon balm have a gentle lemon scent with a hint of mint, and the flavour hits the palate like citronella hits the nose. Its genus name, *Melissa*, is from the Greek for "honey bee"; when in bloom, its small white flowers are full of nectar that entices bees. But this plant should not be confused with *Monarda didyma*, or bee balm (see page 35).

✚ Health Benefits

Lemon balm supplements are made from the leaves. The essential oils contain terpenes and tannins, both of which may play a role in the herb's relaxing and antiviral effects. Lemon balm also contains eugenol, which calms muscle spasms, numbs tissues, and kills bacteria.

Several clinical studies have looked at lemon balm for its calming, sleep-enhancing, and relaxing properties. It has been shown to help restlessness and improve sleep quality. Double-blind, placebo-controlled research shows that lemon balm significantly improved mood while increasing calmness and alertness.

Lemon balm can improve your digestive system, balance immunity, help you sleep more soundly, manage stress and anxiety, and even increase concentration. In fact, it's currently being researched in botanical medicine for its range of effects on improving cognition, and even shows promise in the role of Alzheimer's disease management.

Some research shows lemon balm may even help manage Graves' disease, where the immune system affects the thyroid gland. It can also be useful for the symptoms associated with cold sores (herpes simplex virus), anxiety, depression, cognitive performance, and even digestive complaints (colic, dyspepsia, colitis, and irritable bowel syndrome).

🌱 Growing

Lemon balm is one of the simplest herbs to grow. It's closely related to mint, and it's a similarly vigorous grower that can take over your garden if left unchecked. You can start it from seed if you want, or simply pick up a few transplants from your garden

DIFFICULTY
Easy

HARDINESS
Perennial in zones 4 and above

TIME TO PLANT
Early spring, or start from seed 6 to 8 weeks before last frost date

TIME TO HARVEST
Summer, before flowers appear

LOCATION
Full to part sun

SOIL TYPE
Well-drained

centre. If you spot it in a friend's garden, ask for a division; your friend will probably be glad to remove some!

Common Varieties: Available in several varieties, including those with golden and variegated foliage.

PLANT

To grow from seed, sow indoors 6 to 8 weeks before last frost date in a pot filled with seed-starting soil and placed in a brightly lit window. Scatter the tiny seeds directly onto the surface of the soil and do not cover them—that's the trick to starting lemon balm from seed! Keep the soil evenly moist until the seeds germinate in about 10 to 14 days. When your seedlings have 3 to 5 leaves, thin them out and transplant the stronger ones into individual pots. Bring them outside after all risk of frost has passed.

When planting your own seedlings or transplants from your garden centre, just look for a sunny spot. Consider planting lemon balm in a sunken container with drainage holes in your garden to keep it from taking over. Remember to give each plant some room: Within a short time transplants will take up 45 to 60 cm (1½ to 2 feet) of space in the garden. Water immediately after planting.

If you're dividing an existing lemon balm to move to your own garden, choose an overcast day in early spring and remove clumps of the plant with a garden fork. Don't be scared of hurting it—this hardy perennial can take abuse. Separate the roots into smaller sections and place into pots or directly into the garden.

GROW

Lemon balm doesn't require frequent fertilizing, and once it's established it just needs occasional watering—but don't overwater!

The biggest challenge with lemon balm is keeping it from spreading into other areas in your garden. Remember, 2 plants can quickly become 20 if not maintained, so make sure to weed out extra plants.

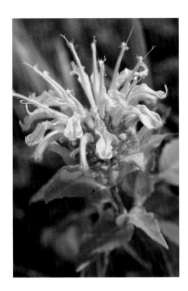

Don't make the common mistake of confusing bee balm (above) with lemon balm.

After a period of hot, humid days with cool nights, you may see hints of white powder on the foliage. This is a sign of powdery mildew, which is easily controlled by removing infected leaves and improving airflow around plants by thinning. Divide large clumps when necessary.

HARVEST

Like most herbs, lemon balm should be harvested before the plants start flowering in summer. If you miss that window, just pinch off any flowers that form to promote additional growth.

Harvest in the morning after the dew has dried, but before the heat of the day kicks in; late-day harvesting may reduce lemon balm's storage life. The most flavourful, oil-rich stems are the youngest, or the top third, of the plant.

When your plants appear weak and tired, give them a good kick in the butt by cutting them back to about 10 to 15 cm (4 to 6 inches). Then watch them grow again!

STORE

Lemon balm is always best used fresh, so harvest frequently during the growing season. If you harvest too much, cut the stems and place them in a glass of water on your countertop. Keep them out of the refrigerator or the leaves will blacken.

To dry, tie lemon balm into bundles and hang in a dry place, out of direct light (see "Drying Herbs at Home" on page 365). Dried lemon balm will last for up to a year stored in airtight containers.

To freeze, purée leaves and stems in a food processor and freeze in mini BPA-free ice-cube trays. Once frozen, transfer the cubes to a resealable plastic bag.

Put It to Work

Got digestive issues? Cook with lemon balm!
Lemon balm is a versatile culinary herb. The fresh leaves can be picked right off the plant and used as a garnish, chopped and tossed into a salad, or added to virtually any dish to give it a lemony zest. It's the perfect addition to a sweet, spicy, or tangy dish such as a curry or chutney. Consider pairing it with bay leaves, mint, rosemary, and thyme.

When adding lemon balm to a soup or roast, do so at the end of cooking. Otherwise, the important ingredients can evaporate. (This is true of any fresh herb that contains essential oils.)

Sleep issues? Make a tea!
If you want to keep things really simple, make a lemon balm tea. Add about 1 rounded tablespoon of dried lemon balm leaves to a mug of boiling water. Cover with a saucer, steep for 15 minutes, and then strain. Add honey and a slice of lemon, if desired.

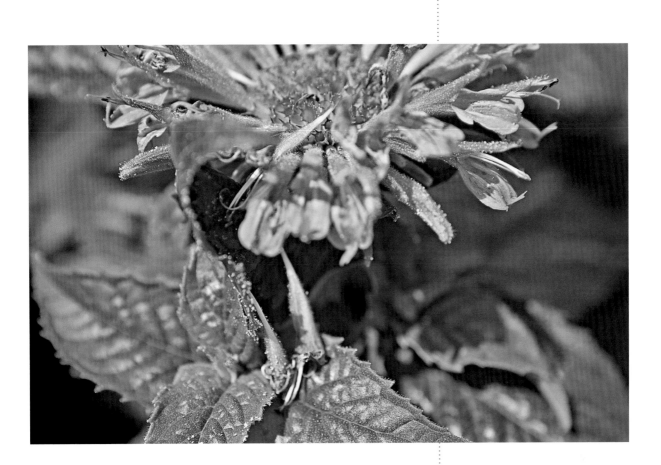

Have a cold sore? Make an infusion!

Cream containing lemon balm essential oil is becoming a popular treatment of cold sores (herpes simplex virus). In one study, those who applied lemon balm cream to their lip sores experienced significant improvement after only 2 days.

To make an at-home remedy with a similar effect, add 4 teaspoons of crushed fresh lemon balm leaf (use a mortar and pestle) to 1 cup of boiling water. Cover with a tight-fitting lid and steep for 15 minutes. Let cool, then use cotton balls to apply the tea concentrate to the affected area 3 to 4 times per day.

Anxious? Have a balm bath!

Add lemon balm to your next bath for an uplifting and relaxing aromatherapy experience. Simply add 4 teaspoons of crushed fresh lemon balm leaf (use a mortar and pestle) to 1 cup of boiling water, cover with a tight-fitting lid, and steep for 15 minutes. Strain. Pour the tea concentrate directly into the bath.

Memory deficient? Take this tincture!

If you're looking to use lemon balm to improve cognition, help balance immunity (in the case of Graves' disease), or as a more powerful sleep aid, you'll need a stronger concentration than tea can provide. Here's how to make a tincture.

Gather enough lemon balm leaves to tightly pack a large resealable glass jar (like a Mason jar). Using a mortar and pestle, crush the leaves to release the essential oils. Return the leaves to the jar and top with vodka (at least 80 proof; it should completely cover the leaves). Place wax paper over the jar and then screw the lid on tightly to seal it. Shake the jar well. Set aside in a cool, dark place for 3 to 4 weeks, shaking the jar vigorously every day. (You many need to add more vodka after a few days to keep the leaves completely submerged; the leaves will absorb some of the alcohol.)

After the 3 to 4 weeks are up, add more fresh, macerated lemon balm leaves and set aside for another 3 to 4 weeks, shaking the jar vigorously every day. Repeat a total of three times. Strain through a fine-mesh sieve into a sterile glass jar with a tight-fitting lid.

To help with cognition or Graves' disease, take 30 drops in water twice daily between meals. As a sleep aid, take 1 tablespoon before bed on an empty stomach. The tincture will keep for up to three years stored in a cool, dark place.

» Fast Forward

Fast forward to the health food store to purchase Clef des Champs lemon balm tincture or equivalent. Follow the instructions on the label.

! Cautions

Lemon balm is thought to be safe when applied to the skin, taken orally as a supplement, or when consumed in amounts normally found in foods.

Use cautiously if you have diabetes or low blood sugar, or if you're taking agents that affect blood sugar. Also be cautious if you have low blood pressure or you're taking agents that lower blood pressure, or if you're using central nervous system depressants, sedatives, or selective serotonin reuptake inhibitors (SSRIs).

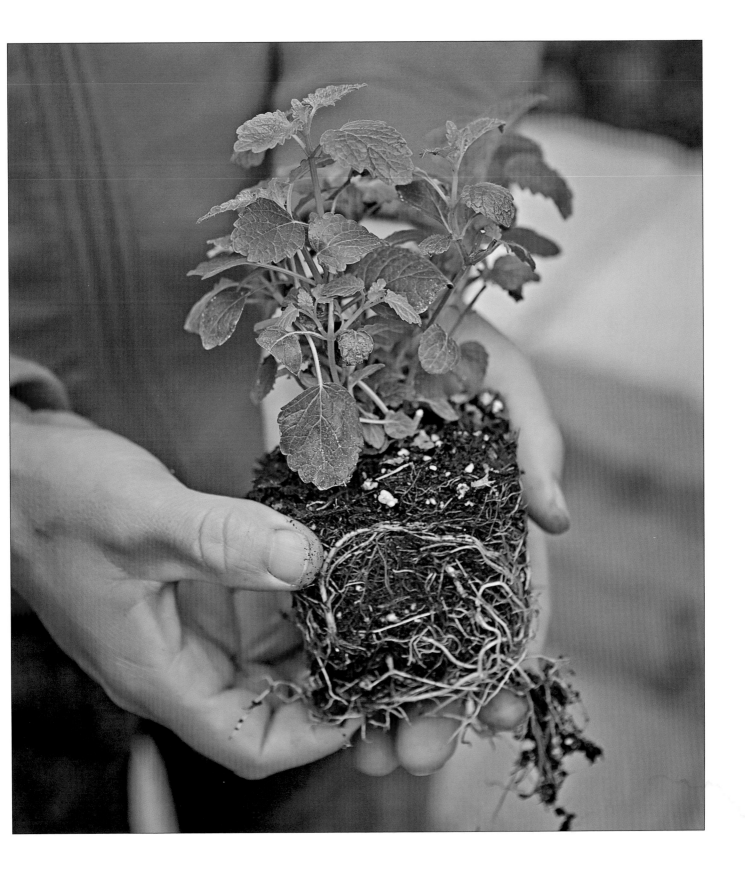

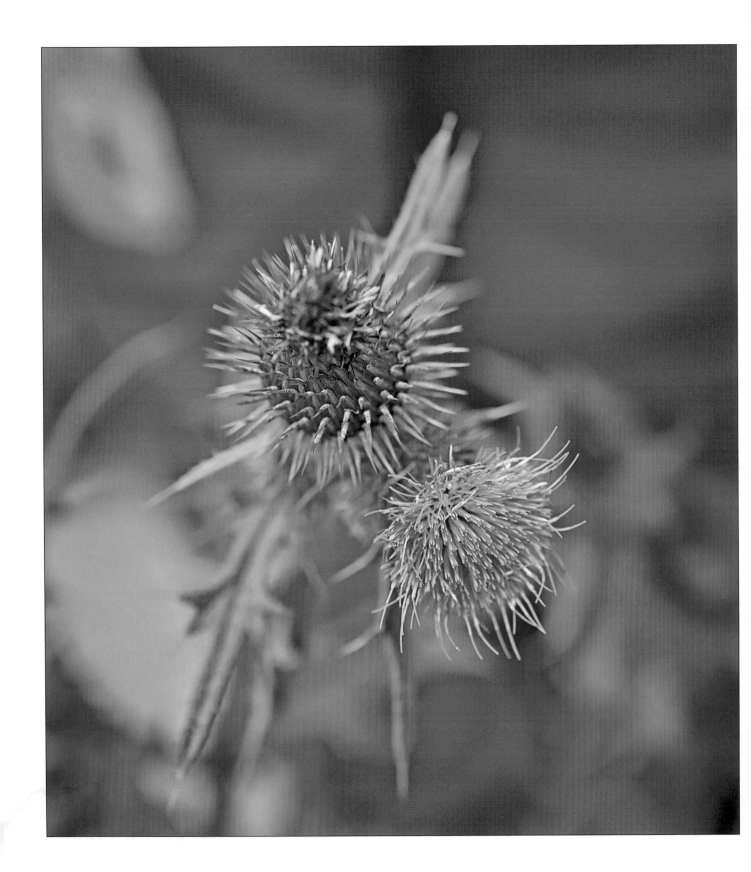

Milk Thistle

Milk thistle is part of the daisy family (*Asteraceae*). It originated in Europe, but is now grown widely in Asia and the Americas. Although it is considered a common weed in many areas, it is also cultivated for its seeds, which are perhaps the most common botanical extract found in health food stores today. This prickly plant features wide leaves with prominent blotchy white veins that emit milky white sap when crushed. Folklore has it that the Latin name *Silybum marianum* is derived from the belief that the Virgin Mary's milk once fell upon the herb, bestowing on it the ability to improve lactation in nursing mothers.

Health Benefits

In the world of herbal medicine, milk thistle stands proud, backed by solid science. Thousands of products made from it have become popular in Europe and North America. Milk thistle has many virtues, including its ability to improve various types of liver and biliary diseases including hepatitis, cirrhosis, alcohol-induced liver disease, and fatty liver. The active ingredient is silymarin, a substance extracted from the seeds, which helps protect the liver against toxic damage and, perhaps, even repair it.

Experiments confirm milk thistle improves liver function and decreases the number of deaths that occur in cirrhotic patients. Several studies also show taking milk thistle orally may improve cases of hepatitis or alcohol-induced liver damage.

More recently, milk thistle has been discussed as a possible alternative treatment for cancer. Silymarin contains a compound called silybin, which has been shown to stop cancerous tumour cells from growing.

Growing

If you have milk thistle in your garden, chances are you didn't plant it. Thistles are weeds, and most gardeners hate them. They usually tear them out, taproot and all. But I would argue milk thistle is an attractive plant when grown with purpose. Placed in the back of the garden in full sun, this drought-tolerant biennial will reseed itself year after year, offering textured foliage and bluish-purple flowers that attract bees, butterflies, and the occasional hummingbird. Plant milk thistle with caution, however, as it can be a noxious weed that must be kept in check. It may be better to simply look for it on roadsides and forest paths and in ditches.

DIFFICULTY
Easy to medium

HARDINESS
Biennial in zones 5 to 9

TIME TO PLANT
Spring

TIME TO HARVEST
Late summer to fall

LOCATION
Full sun

SOIL TYPE
Almost any, but does not do well in sandy soils

Milk thistle is a prolific producer! Each flower contains approximately 190 seeds, with an average of 6,350 seeds per plant, with over 90% being viable. That means each plant may yield about ¼ pound (120 g) of seed per season for medicinal use or to be sown again next year.

Common Varieties: There's only one species of milk thistle: *Silybum marianum*. Don't confuse this with the many unrelated plants with "thistle" in their common name, such as globe thistle (*Echinops rito*) and blessed thistle (*Cnicus benedictus*).

PLANT

You can buy milk thistle seeds, but if the weed grows in your neighbourhood you can simply collect the seeds from wild plants in late summer and fall. See my harvesting instructions below.

After the risk of frost in spring, find a sunny location, preferably away from prized garden plants. (Milk thistle is not only invasive, but it's a large plant that will easily shade others.) Directly sow the seeds in the garden at a depth of 3 mm (⅛ inch). Be generous with the seed: They sometimes have a low germination rate, so it's always better to double up on your sowing. They will take approximately 3 weeks to germinate, and you can easily thin any clumps later on when the seedlings start to mature.

Keep evenly moist until germination. As the plants mature, they will need only occasional deep watering.

GROW

Milk thistle is a weed and it grows like one! As long as the plants are in full sun and fairly good soil, they will thrive. In fact, they can be invasive and will need to be thinned. Watch out for new seedlings and remove as necessary to keep milk thistle confined to restricted areas. When removing milk thistle from the garden, pull out the entire root. And be careful not to walk around the garden holding the seed heads or you may inadvertently sow them everywhere!

Milk thistle is biennial, which means the plant takes 2 years to flower and complete its life cycle. This means that if you grow from seed, you'll probably get minimal flowers, if any, in the first year. The plant is resistant to most insects and diseases.

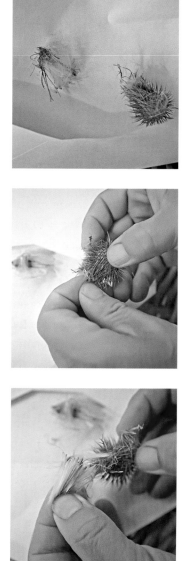

Harvesting seeds from dried milk thistle heads.

HARVEST

The biggest challenge when harvesting milk thistle is not getting stung by its prickly leaves! Wear gloves, pants, and long sleeves.

While all parts are edible, the seeds are the prized possession. Harvest spent flowers in late summer to fall: Cut the seed heads when the purple flower has dried and given way to white silky tufts. Harvest in late afternoon when all moisture has dried.

STORE

Allow seed heads to further dry by placing them in a brown paper bag in a dry location out of direct light for up to 10 days. After drying, store the seeds in an airtight container in a cool, dry place.

Put It to Work

Liver sluggish? Don't hesitate: decontaminate!
The liver is the body's central chemical dump site. It works day and night to process the air we breathe, the food we eat, and the medicines and supplements we take. The liver is capable of healing and regenerating itself, but if it is overwhelmed it can leak toxins into the bloodstream, burdening other organs and diminishing our health. You can help the liver boost productivity with milk thistle. It may even be essential to maintaining health in our pollution-filled world.

In a blender, combine 1 cup of freshly harvested milk thistle seeds with 1 cup of vodka (at least 80 proof) (1, 2) and blend on medium speed until smooth. Pour into a resealable glass jar (like a Mason jar) (3). Place wax paper over the jar and then screw the lid on tightly to seal it (4). Set aside in a cool, dark place for 4 weeks, shaking the jar vigorously every day.

After 4 weeks, using a fine-mesh sieve or coffee filter, strain the liquid into a sterile glass jar with a tight-fitting lid (5, 6). Store in a

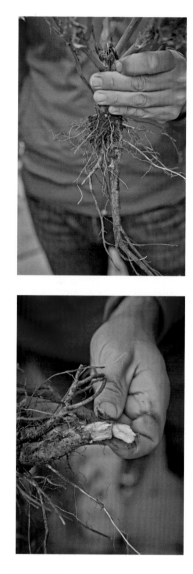

Milk thistle's tough tap root makes it a drought-resistant and resilient weed.

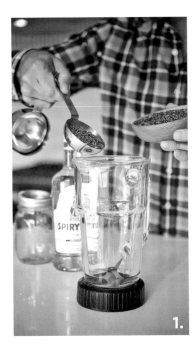

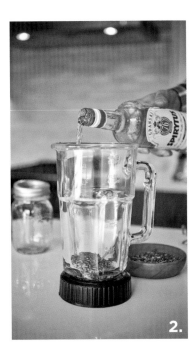

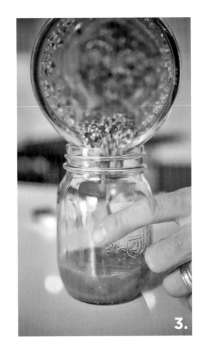

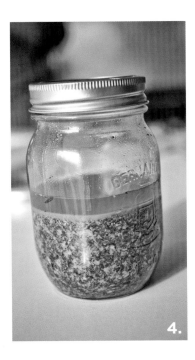

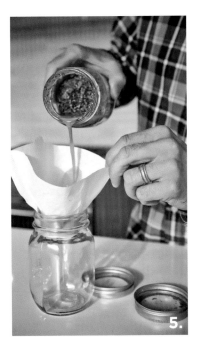

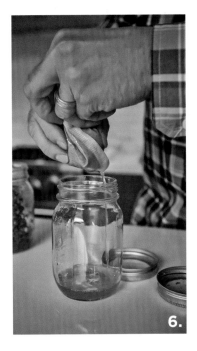

cool, dark place. Take 1 teaspoon in 2 ounces of water twice daily (between meals) for 3 months.

To help determine the success of this treatment, check your liver enzymes with your family doctor before, every 4 weeks during, and after your treatment.

Feeling toxic? How about a detox milkshake?
You can incorporate milk thistle seeds directly into your diet. The silymarin is more effective when the whole seeds are ground to a fine powder or soaked overnight. The powder has a nutty taste similar to ground flax or hemp seed. It's delicious in this milkshake, whether you prefer chocolate or vanilla.

> *1 cup milk thistle seeds*
> *1 cup filtered water*
> *2 tbsp cacao powder or 1 tsp pure vanilla*
> * extract*
> *1 tbsp pure maple syrup, agave nectar, or*
> * liquid honey*
> *½ cup ice, rice milk, or coconut milk*

In a bowl, cover milk thistle seeds with water and set aside to soak overnight.

In a blender, combine hydrated seeds with filtered water and blend on high speed until smooth. Using a fine-mesh sieve or cheesecloth, strain into a bowl (discard solids). Return the liquid to the blender. Add the cacao powder, maple syrup, and ice or milk and blend until smooth. Drink 1 cup daily to help your liver detoxify.

›› Fast Forward

Fast forward to the health food store to purchase A. Vogel's milk thistle or equivalent. Follow the instructions on the label.

! Cautions

A few people experience stomach upset, headache, and itching after consuming milk thistle; there are rarer reports of loss of appetite, heartburn, diarrhea, and joint pain. In theory, milk thistle may lower blood sugar, so those with diabetes or hypoglycemia, and those taking drugs, herbs, or supplements that affect blood sugars, should be cautious.

Avoid milk thistle if you have an allergy to any plant in the daisy family (*Asteraceae*) or to artichokes or kiwi.

Historically, milk thistle has been used to improve breast milk flow, and two studies reported no side effects in pregnant women. However, there is not enough scientific evidence to support these uses, so avoid the use of milk thistle during pregnancy or breastfeeding.

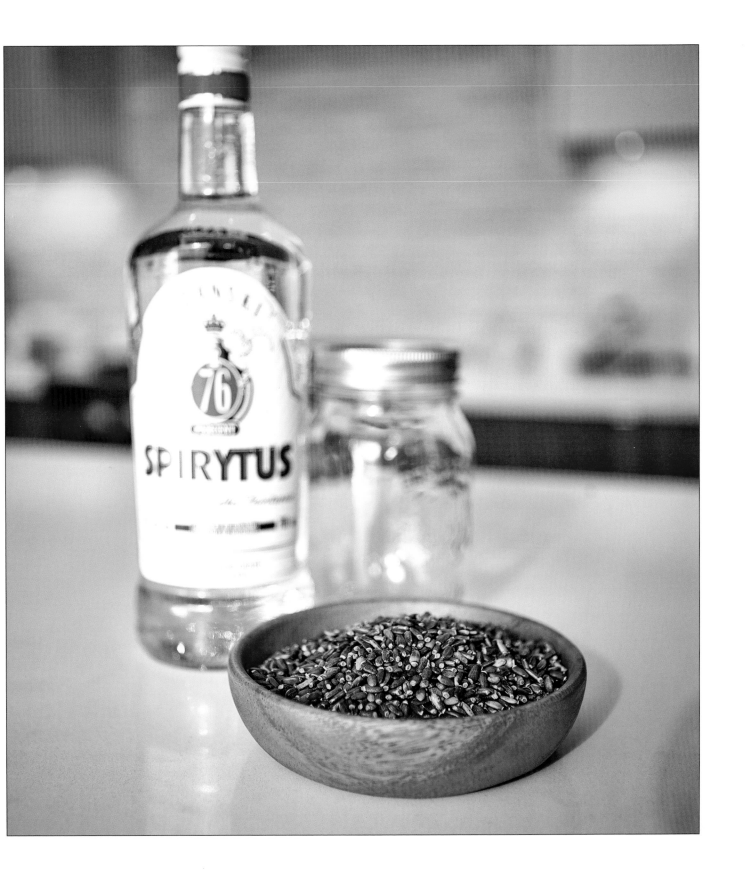

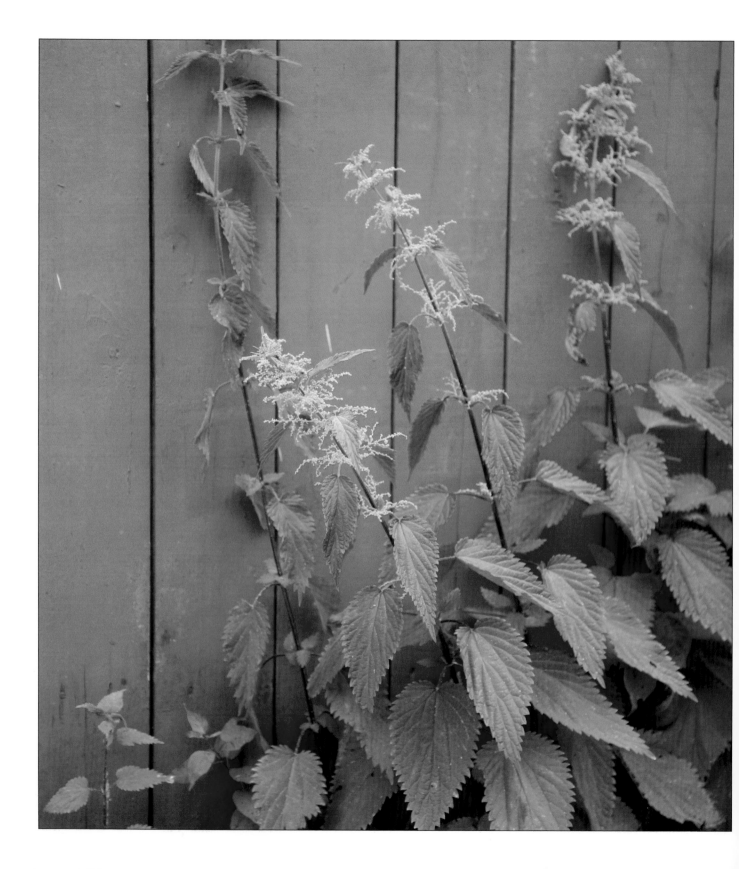

Nettle

The Latin name for this plant derives from the Latin verb *urere*, meaning "to burn."
You'll understand why if you've ever encountered nettle leaves! Sometimes you
will be walking in the country and feel like you've been stung by a wasp or a bee,
but there is no bug in sight. You may instead have been "burned" by the stinging hairs of a nettle bush. Native to Europe, Asia, and North America, the nettle
is equipped with tiny hairs filled with stinging chemicals that are released when
you touch them. Surprisingly, these compounds can actually bring relief to painful areas of the body. They have other promising medicinal uses, too, but in these
cases you'll want to cook or dry the plant to remove the sting before touching it!

Health Benefits

Nettle juice was prescribed as an external treatment for snakebites and scorpion stings some 2,000 years ago. It has also been used as a kidney tonic, for menstrual relief, as a diuretic, and as a treatment for certain respiratory disorders. Today it is generally used as a pain reliever for arthritis, for hay fever relief, and as a treatment for enlarged prostate.

A hundred or more chemicals have been identified in the nettle plant, including the neurotransmitters acetylcholine, serotonin, and histamine. If you've got arthritis, slapping your joints with these tiny needles that inject these chemicals into your skin induces a positive healing response. Nettle leaf can also relieve allergies because it contains a variety of flavonoids that have antihistamine effects.

The root of stinging nettle contains lectins and sterols, which may help with benign prostate hypertrophy (BPH). If the enlarged prostate gland presses on the tube that empties urine from the bladder (the urethra), symptoms can include reduced urinary flow, incomplete emptying of the bladder, post-urination dripping, and the constant urge to urinate. Studies have shown stinging nettle is comparable to finasteride, a medication commonly prescribed for enlarged prostate. However, scientists aren't sure why nettle root reduces symptoms, since unlike finasteride, nettle does not decrease prostate size.

Growing

Stinging nettle is an invasive weed. It's rarely planted by homeowners and usually removed when it's discovered. While nettles are useful in herbal remedies and even produce edible greens, they don't have much else going for them. They take over any

DIFFICULTY
Easy

HARDINESS
Perennial in zones 5 to 9

TIME TO PLANT
Spring

TIME TO HARVEST
Spring through first frost in fall

LOCATION
Full sun to shade

SOIL TYPE
Rich, moist

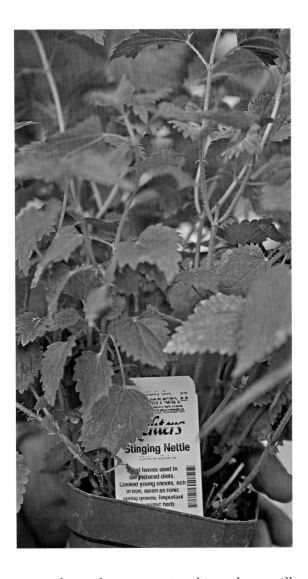

area where they grow, touching them will give you a temporary rash, and they can't be controlled by animals like rabbits or mice, as their stinging features protect them from furry friends. Even insects don't like them! I suggest you avoid planting them in the garden. Go out and steal them instead.

Common Varieties: There are several sub-species, but since you're not likely to be buying seeds or transplants, you don't need to worry about these. Just learn to identify the stinging nettle by sight.

PLANT

Always wear gloves and long sleeves when dealing with nettles. The tiny hairs are loaded with irritants that cause a burning or a sting-ing sensation that lasts for hours. Keep them away from kids!

If you ignore my advice and plant stinging nettle in the garden, divide an existing plant in spring, when the soil is workable. (Never divide a plant on a hot, dry day. The best days are overcast with a forecast of rain.) With a garden fork, remove a clump of nettles. Separate using a sharp spade or knife, ensuring sections have at least 3 to 5 eyes (sprouts). Plant the sections in a hole with good soil, making sure the fin-ished new division will be just above ground level. Water well until established and con-tinue with deep infrequent watering through the season.

GROW

Nettles don't enjoy drought and require water-ing when the sun shines for lengthy periods. As long as they have enough water, they will thrive.

I can't stress this enough: Nettles are stubborn weeds. If you choose to grow them in your garden, your biggest challenge will

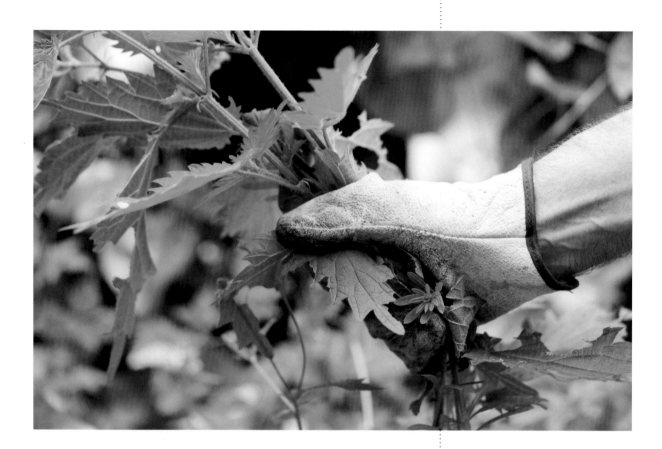

be containing them. You should remove the flower heads before they set seed, but even then you will find new nettles spreading outside your designated clump. Get rid of them immediately: Any time you find a nettle sprouting where you don't want it, tear it out, removing all the foliage and the bulk of the root system. Nettle is related to mint, and like that herb, it should be planted in a contained area of the garden, restricting roots and stems from spreading elsewhere.

HARVEST

The tender shoots of nettles can be harvested anytime during the growing season, but the best time is the spring, when growth is freshest. Harvest nettles before they set seed or flower for max-

Plants are amazing at protecting themselves! Just as nettles have a built-in mechanism (those itchy hairs!) to protect themselves against predators, other plants fight back in different ways. Roses have thorns, rhubarb has toxic leaves, and cactuses have spikes, all with the purpose of preventing the plant from getting eaten.

imum flavour. In mid-morning, when the dew has dried, cut the tender foliage (select upper leaves no wider than 5 cm/2 inches) with a sharp knife or scissors. Remember to wear gloves! Don't worry, the sting disappears once the leaves are cooked or dried.

STORE

Wrap fresh nettle leaves in paper towel, place loosely in a plastic bag, and refrigerate for up to a week. They can also be dried like many leafy herbs. You can either hang them or place them on drying trays out of direct light (see "Drying Herbs at Home" on page 365). After drying, store in airtight containers in a cool, dry place.

Put It to Work

Painful joints? Rub nettles where it hurts!

This application may sting, but that's the point! Simply rubbing nettle leaves on a painful joint can cause a numbing rash that lasts 6 to 24 hours, and should lead to less pain and reduced inflammation over time. Many people with joint pain caused by arthritis swear by it! Apply up to twice a day, morning and night.

Enlarged prostate? Take this tincture!

A few drops of this tincture may provide relief from the symptoms of an enlarged prostate.

Don a pair of gloves and fill a large resealable jar (like a Mason jar) with nettle leaf tops (this is the fresh, new growth at the top of the plant, not the large lower leaves). Still wearing gloves, rinse and, using a sharp knife, chop them into small pieces. Transfer the chopped nettle to a clean jar. Cover with at least 2.5 cm (1 inch) of vodka (at least 80 proof). Place wax paper over the jar and then screw the lid on tightly to seal it. Shake the jar well. Set aside in a cool, dark place for 1 month, shaking the jar vigorously every day.

After a month has passed, using a fine-mesh sieve or cheesecloth, strain the liquid into a sterile glass bottle with a tight-fitting lid (discard solids).

Add 1 teaspoon of the tincture to 2 ounces of water. Take 3 times daily for 3 months, and then once a day as a maintenance dose. The tincture will keep in a cool, dark place for at least a year.

Hay fever? Drink this infusion!

If you're suffering from the misery of hay fever, a nettle infusion (tea) can bring relief. Put a handful of nettle leaves (including the stems is fine) in a teapot or other container and top with boiling water. Cover and steep for 10 minutes. Strain into a cup and drink (hot or cold) 3 times daily for 2 weeks prior to and during allergy season.

Weak kidneys? Sip some nettle soup!

Nettle tops are a great spinach alternative. They can be added to soups and casseroles, or steamed on their own with a bit of butter and sea salt.

If you have been diagnosed with chronic kidney disease, your condition needs serious medical care and proper diet to avoid further damage or even total renal failure. Nettle may help! To make this dish, you'll need to pick the tender tops of the nettle plants (at a leaf intersection). They are the youngest, softest part of the plant.

This is a twist on French onion soup. It's low in sodium and very light on the cheese to keep it kidney friendly.

2 tbsp butter
2 tbsp extra virgin olive oil
3 sweet onions, sliced
Garlic powder
Freshly ground black pepper
1 tbsp pure maple syrup
4 cups fresh nettle tops
½ cup brandy or vermouth
4 cups chicken broth
½ cup grated Asiago cheese
¼ cup sliced chives

Heat the butter and oil in a large, deep skillet over medium-high heat until the butter is melted. Add the onions and season with garlic powder and pepper to taste. Cover with a lid and cook for about 10 minutes, stirring occasionally. Add the maple syrup and reduce the heat to low. Add the nettle tops, stir well, and cook for 10 to 15 minutes, until the onions have caramelized and the nettle is wilted. Add the brandy. Increase the heat to high and cook for another 5 to 10 minutes, stirring constantly, until most of the liquid evaporates. Add the chicken broth, reduce the heat to a simmer, and season with more garlic powder and pepper, if desired.

Ladle the soup into bowls. Sprinkle with cheese and garnish with sliced chives.

» Fast Forward

Fast forward to the health food store to purchase Restorative Formulations Prosta Px or equivalent. Follow the instructions on the label.

! Cautions

Fresh stinging nettle leaves can cause localized rash, itching, and stinging. This often presents like an allergic reaction, but there are no known reports of systemic allergies from this plant.

Dried or cooked nettle leaf is generally well tolerated, but the root can occasionally cause gastrointestinal complaints, sweating, and skin rash.

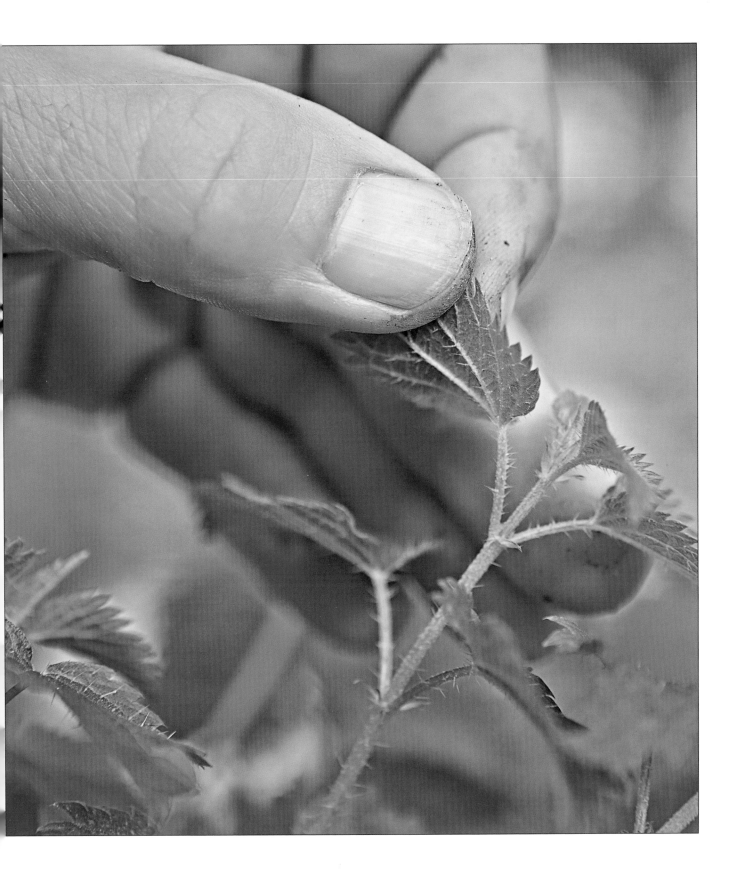

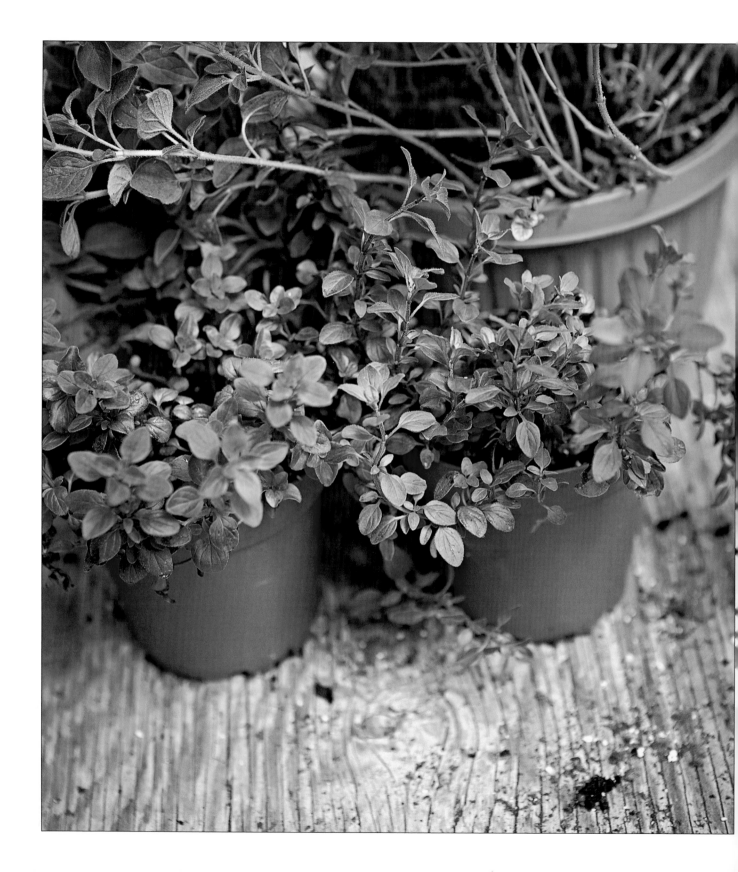

Oregano

The Greek root of the word *oregano* means "joy of the mountain." Oregano has been bringing joy since ancient times with its sweet scent, warm flavour, and healing properties. Today, oregano is best known as an herb used in pasta sauce and pizza. It is a common seasoning used in cooking and also a preservative due to its very powerful antimicrobial qualities. In fact, that is how it is used medicinally.

⊕ Health Benefits

Traditionally, oregano was used to treat respiratory, gastrointestinal, and menstrual problems. Oil of oregano was also applied to the skin for the treatment of infection. Today, it is commonly used for oral and upper respiratory infections and gastrointestinal issues, including parasites.

The leaves, stems, and flowers of oregano all contain medicinal properties, the most important of which has been identified as the volatile oil carvacrol. It also contains thymol (the main ingredient in thyme). Together, these are potent antimicrobial oils, even at low doses. The research demonstrates that oregano has antiparasitic, antifungal, antioxidant, and antibacterial properties.

Oregano oil kills germs in three important places: in the gut, in the mouth, and on the skin. But be cautious: It isn't intended for long-term use—it is very strong and can upset the essential friendly bacteria in your digestive system.

Bad bacteria in the gut are powerful. When they lurk in the grooves and crevasses of your intestines, they can be difficult

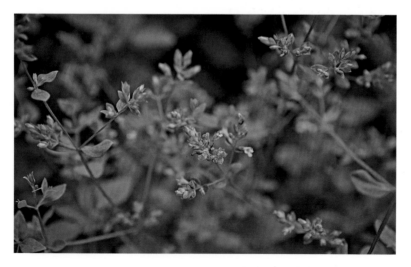

Oregano flowers. For a more productive plant, cut back before it reaches the blooming phase.

DIFFICULTY
Easy

HARDINESS
Annual (most varieties); Greek oregano is perennial in zones 5 and above

TIME TO PLANT
Spring

TIME TO HARVEST
Late spring through fall

LOCATION
Full sun

SOIL TYPE
Well-drained

for your immune cells to locate and destroy. But carvacrol helps break down the bad bacteria's defenses, making it vulnerable to your immune army.

Your mouth also contains a ton of bacteria. The good news is that carvacrol and thymol work as an antiseptic—indeed, thymol is the active ingredient in most brands of mouthwash.

Research reveals oregano oil's antibiotic ability can help eliminate the bacteria that may be responsible for a skin condition called rosacea. And unlike a prescription antibiotic, oil of oregano will fight a yeast infection instead of causing one.

Growing

Oregano is great for first-time gardeners. It's easy to grow and a great addition to any herb or kitchen garden, especially if you enjoy pasta and tomato sauce! This herb can be both an annual and a perennial, depending on the variety. A word of warning: Oregano is often confused with marjoram, a closely related herb with similar leaves. However, marjoram has a much lighter flavour.

Common Varieties: Most cultivars are annual, including compact oregano ('Compactum') and golden oregano ('Aureum'). I recommend Greek oregano (*Origanum vulgare hirtum*) for both its hardiness and its flavour.

PLANT

Oregano can be grown from seed or propagated from cuttings, and it can be transplanted easily. Sow seeds indoors 8 to 10 weeks before last frost date. When grown from cuttings, oregano will take about 4 to 6 weeks to root.

Transplants should be hardened off (see opposite) and then planted outdoors in a garden or container after the risk of frost. This plant's number-one requirement is good drainage. Water moderately until roots are established, then only when dry during

Starting seeds and cuttings indoors takes a little effort, but the feeling of growing your own is great! Before transplanting your seedlings outdoors, you need to get them adapted to light levels and temperatures. The process is called hardening off. It simply involves bringing seedlings outdoors on days when afternoon temperatures are over 15°C (59°F) and bringing them back in at night before the temperature drops. About 5 to 10 days of hardening off is recommended.

the growing season. Plant with air circulation in mind. Like most Mediterranean herbs, oregano grows best in full sun.

GROW

There is only one thing oregano hates: too much water! The main reason people fail at growing oregano is too much moisture, which causes root rot. Overwatering, high humidity, too much rain, and poor drainage can all lead to root rot and kill your oregano.

Oregano requires minimal fertilizer. When planted in the garden and amended with compost, it won't need any fertilizer at all. I do, however, recommend fertilizing containers at least once every 4 weeks during the growing season. Use a compost tea or a 20-20-20 fertilizer.

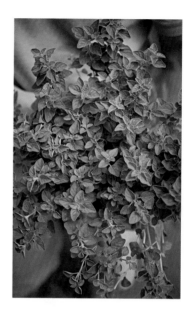

This herb is a fast grower, and to ensure a good supply of tender leaves it needs regular haircuts. Even if you don't need it, cut oregano back 10 to 15 cm (4 to 6 inches) as soon as you see flowers emerging. This will ensure healthy, fresh growth all season long. When cutting and/or pinching, remove one-third of the overall growth at a time.

Perennial varieties need to be kept in their place: Once a year, remove any section of oregano that has decided to "run." Cut and divide with a spade, ideally on an overcast day to minimize shock to the plant.

HARVEST

Oregano grows quickly and can be harvested in early spring as soon as plants measure 20 cm (8 inches) high. I recommend harvesting just before the plant blooms, as you will find the flavour most intense. Harvest mid-morning or on overcast days when foliage is completely dry.

Frequent harvests are a must; the more you cut, the busier the plant will be! Just don't cut the plant back more than 15 cm (6 inches) at a time.

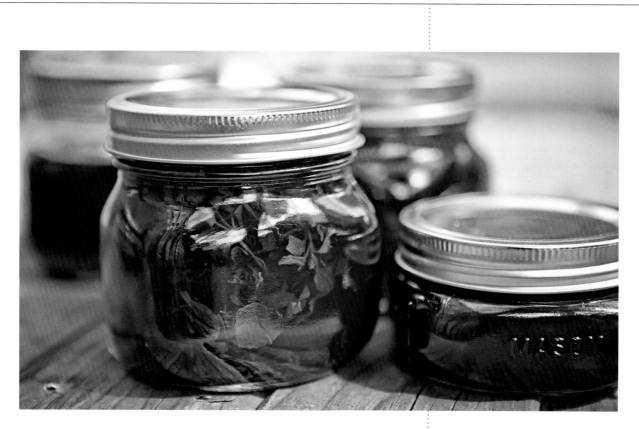

Homemade oregano tincture (left). Homemade oregano oil is an inexpensive alternative to store-bought varieties.

STORE

Oregano can be used fresh or dried. Store fresh oregano wrapped in paper towel in the refrigerator for up to a week. To dry it, hang small bunches upside down out of direct light or use drying screens (see "Drying Herbs at Home" on page 365). Once dry, the leaves will be brittle. Store the leaves (discard stems) in airtight containers in a cool, dry place.

Put It to Work

Ready to use oregano? Start by making this potent oil!

The first step in unlocking the healing properties of oregano is extracting the oil. Start with 1 cup of fresh oregano leaves, washed and patted dry. Pour into a resealable glass jar (like a Mason jar) and top the jar with 1 cup of vodka (at least 80 proof). Place wax paper over the jar and then screw the lid on tightly to seal it. Set aside in a cool, dark place for 1 week.

After a week, using a coffee filter or cheesecloth, strain the oregano mixture into a clean jar. Cover it with a clean coffee filter or cloth and set aside in a dry, warm place for at least 7 days or until the alcohol completely evaporates. What remains is pure essential oregano oil. Store in an airtight container in a cool, dark place. The oil will keep indefinitely.

Pesky parasites? Pound them with this!

First, a warning: If you're experiencing acute intestinal upset, don't simply "suspect" you have parasites. Get confirmation from a knowledgeable healthcare practitioner. Testing stool for the presence of parasites and levels of beneficial flora, imbalanced flora, pathogenic bacteria, and yeast is the best way to start. This is an ideal approach for those with sudden changes in bowel pattern, and especially for those who have been travelling abroad or camping.

Once there has been a diagnosis, treatment often requires medications such as Flagyl, Humatin, or Yodoxin, but there is compelling evidence that oregano oil can be an effective part of your recovery plan. Even chronic issues may be remedied by oregano oil. For example, it may be effective against the common protozoan parasite *Blastocystis hominis*, which lives in the gut and has been associated with irritable bowel syndrome (IBS).

Add 10 drops of oregano oil to 1 teaspoon of olive oil. Take this 3 times daily before meals.

Because oregano oil inhibits growth of Lactobacillus (good bacteria) in the gut, a course of probiotics after use is a good idea.

Faced with rosacea? Apply this oil!

Rosacea is a skin condition that typically shows up like acne on the forehead, cheeks, nose, and chin. You'll know if you've got it! It is slightly different from acne, since it presents as more of a flushing that turns into red pustules.

Excess sun exposure, alcohol, intense exercise, stress, spicy foods, and extreme hot or cold temperatures may trigger flare-ups. Often the issue is tied to "leaky gut syndrome," whereby food sensitivities are the primary trigger. Oregano oil can help.

In a sterile glass jar with a tight-fitting lid, combine 2 tablespoons of almond oil with 1 teaspoon of oregano oil. Mix well. Dip a cotton ball into the mixture and dab on the affected area every night before bed so your skin has all night to absorb it. Store at room temperature.

Gum disease? Brush with this!

If your dentist has told you that you have deep pockets, periodontitis, or halitosis (bad breath), you are overgrowing bacteria in your mouth. Recent science shows this may lead to problems elsewhere in the body, including heart disease.

To limit your chances of gum disease, place 2 drops of oregano oil on your toothbrush, top with your favourite brand of toothpaste, and brush your teeth as you normally would for 2 minutes (30 seconds in each quadrant).

» Fast Forward

Fast forward to the health food store to purchase North American Herb and Spice Oreganol or equivalent. Follow the instructions on the label.

! Cautions

Do not take oregano oil orally longer than 2 weeks unless you have been advised to by your health practitioner! It can upset the good bacteria in your gut and create a probiotic imbalance. You should also avoid oregano oil if you are pregnant or nursing.

Be cautious if you have diabetes or low blood sugar, or if you take drugs, herbs, or supplements that affect blood sugar, as the glucosides found in the oregano leaf can lower blood sugar. Oregano may also slightly increase the risk of bleeding. If you have a bleeding disorder, take drugs that may increase the risk of bleeding, or are scheduled for surgery, avoid oregano oil.

Caution is also advised in patients with low blood pressure and in those taking drugs, herbs, or supplements that lower blood pressure. Oregano oil can cause a further decrease in blood pressure.

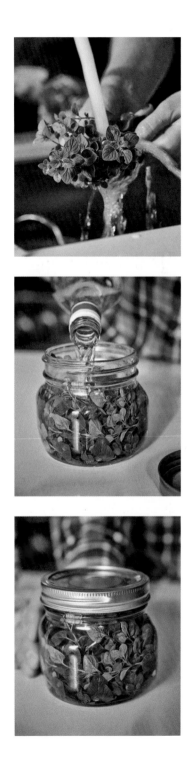

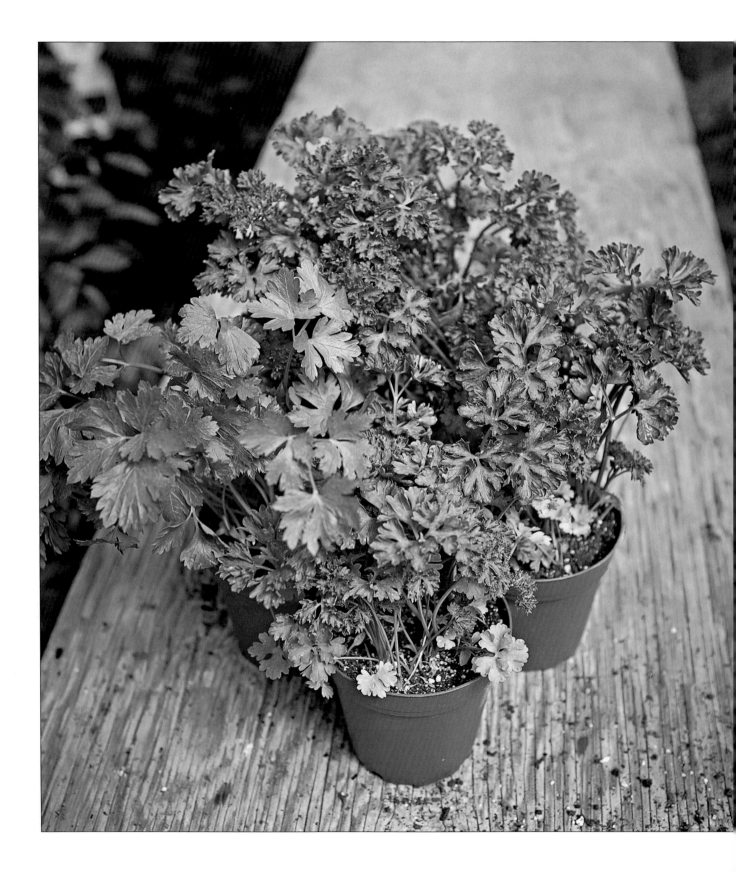

Parsley

Parsley has been part of the human diet for millennia. If you eat out you know it is arguably the most common garnish in the culinary arts. But this is no food to throw away at the end of a meal! A member of the *Apiaceae* family (which also includes carrots), it's an antioxidant-packed plant with a variety of medicinal uses. Most common forms of parsley are either of the curly-leaf or flat-leaf variety. But it doesn't matter which one you eat: they all have nearly equal health benefits.

⊕ Health Benefits

Folklore has it that ancient Greeks and Romans would feed parsley to their chariot horses to give them strength and stamina. They had it right, but parsley isn't just for garnishing or for horses: This little plant packs a wallop of energy-inducing micronutrient power.

The main indication for parsley is inflammation of the urinary tract, where it is helpful in fighting infections, expelling excess fluid, and dissolving stones and sediment from the kidneys. Parsley is also known for its ability to fight odour—it moonlights as a breath freshener. The oils found in parsley are effective in removing even onion and garlic odours. This herb also helps digestion, works as a laxative, and performs duty as a mild diuretic and as a general all-purpose health tonic.

For a green leafy plant, parsley is high in protein (coming in at 22% by weight), iron, calcium, magnesium, potassium, vitamin A, several B vitamins, and vitamin C. In fact, it has more vitamin C by volume than an orange. It also contains an antioxidant flavonoid called apiinn, which is helpful in reducing allergies, and a volatile oil called apiole, which gives the plant its diuretic and kidney-strengthening properties.

🌱 Growing

Parsley is my go-to herb! I use it all the time, in almost in every meal. I like to plant it both in the garden and in a container close to my kitchen. It's easy to grow, easy to harvest, and doesn't take a ton of space. The biggest challenge: Parsley doesn't enjoy extreme heat and it will slow down in the summer. But with the return of cooler nights—presto!—parsley will provide you with fresh taste and fantastic foliage. Parsley is a biennial, but it's treated like an annual, primarily because it goes to seed so quickly.

DIFFICULTY
Easy

HARDINESS
Perennial in zones 5 and above

TIME TO PLANT
Spring or after the threat of frost has passed. Can be sown indoors 5 to 6 weeks before last frost date. For best results, soak seeds in water for 24 hours before sowing.

TIME TO HARVEST
Spring through fall

LOCATION
Full to part sun

SOIL TYPE
Rich, moist, well-drained

Common Varieties: English or curly parsley (*Petroselinum crispum*) is the familiar type with tiny, tightly packed leaves. Italian or flat-leaf parsley (*P. neapolitanum*) is leafier. There is also a version (*P. crispum* var. *tuberosum*) grown for its carrot-like taproot.

PLANT

All parsley varieties can easily be grown from seed. Start them indoors 5 to 6 weeks before last frost date, or sow them directly in the garden as soon as the ground is workable and the risk of extreme frost has passed (temperatures below −5°C/23°F). For first-time gardeners, however, I recommend purchasing parsley plants rather than sowing seed. The plants are not costly and the experience is much easier!

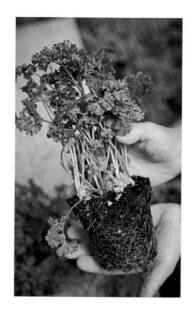

Parsley requires rich, well-drained soil, and for best results should be planted in direct sun. Amend poor soils with compost or triple mix, and avoid planting in clay or sand. For containers, use a potting mix.

If you're planting in the garden, you can locate these compact plants among flowers or in formal rows. Space them about 25 to 35 cm (10 to 14 inches) apart. Keep moist until seedlings or transplants are established.

GROW

Parsley will thrive when planted in the right soil, in the right light, and given just enough moisture. Like your lawn, it enjoys cool temperatures and moist conditions and struggles during extreme heat. In fact, parsley will go to seed during extremely hot weather, so the key for success is regular watering and ensuring the herb doesn't go through lengthy periods of drought.

When planted in nutrient-rich soil full of compost, parsley will not need fertilizer. The foliage is a good indicator of whether it's happy: Deep green foliage means you have a happy plant, while yellow or brown foliage means you have a problem. The plant may need extra fertilizer or may be suffering from not enough

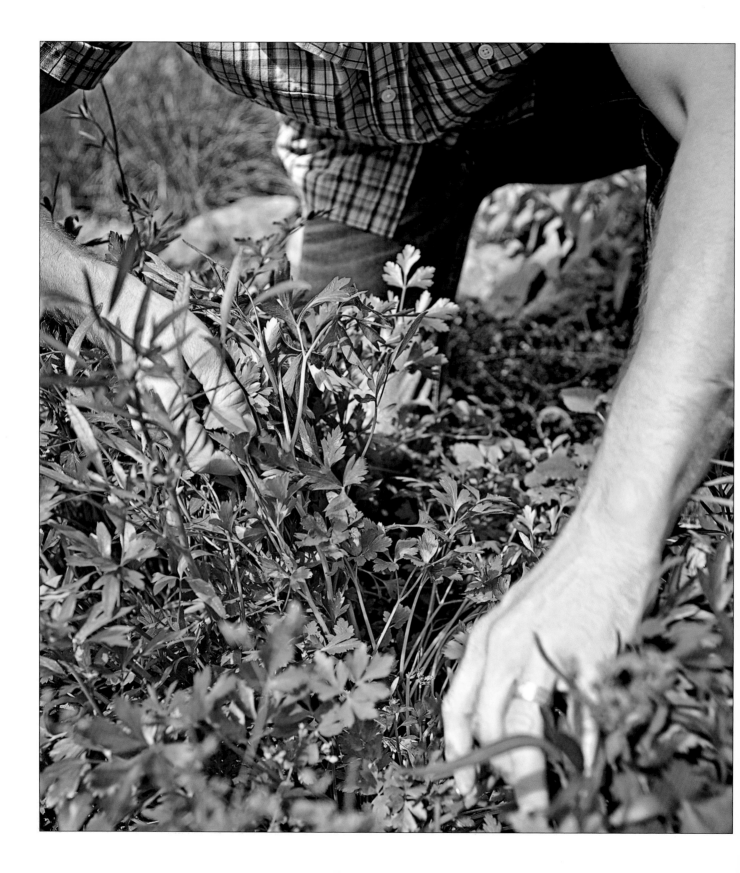

or too much water, or inadequate sun. I strongly recommend fertilizing parsley planted in pots. Use a compost tea or general-purpose garden fertilizer like 20-20-20 or 15-15-15.

Even if you don't use it, lose it! What do I mean? Parsley needs continual pruning and pinching during the growing season, so keep cutting it even if you don't need it. The key is to cut the plant back before it sets seed. Doing so will help provide you with a healthy plant and great parsley all season long.

HARVEST

Allow parsley transplants time to get established: Wait about 20 days before harvesting, or until the plant is at least 30 cm (12 inches) in height and width.

When harvesting, you can simply cut the stems and remove the uppermost tender foliage. Never remove more than one-third of the entire plant at any given time. (However, I've hacked parsley back to just 10 cm/4 inches above soil level and within 10 days it rebounded.) Harvest in the morning when plants have cooled from overnight low temperatures and the morning dew has dried.

After harvesting, tie the parsley into bunches and place the base of the stems in a pail of water or wrap with damp newspaper or paper towel.

STORE

Parsley can be used fresh, frozen, or dried. Store fresh parsley loosely wrapped in paper towel for up to 2 weeks in the refrigerator. To freeze, purée or finely chop the leaves, spoon into BPA-free ice-cube trays, and top with water. Once frozen, transfer cubes to airtight bags. Parsley can be dried by hanging or by placing on drying trays or baking sheets or using a dehydrator (see "Drying Herbs at Home" on page 365). For the freshest flavour, however, parsley is best used immediately after cutting!

Parsley plants are hosts for the caterpillars of both swallowtail and monarch butterflies. When in seed, parsley also attracts hoverflies to your garden. Some species of this insect are beneficial, as they eat pesky aphids and thrips. And—although no scientific evidence proves this—many old-time gardeners swear parsley helps repel damaging beetles!

Put It to work

Sluggish morning energy? Drink green!

Kick-start your day with this healthy green drink. It contains high levels of antioxidants, vitamins, and minerals and features parsley! This recipe makes 3 to 4 servings.

2 cups spinach

2 cups chopped cucumber

3 stalks celery

1½-inch piece gingerroot or 1 tsp ground ginger

2 bunches fresh parsley

1 green apple

Freshly squeezed juice of 1 lime

Freshly squeezed juice of ½ lemon

1 tsp psyllium fibre

In a juicer, process the spinach, cucumber, celery, ginger, parsley, and apple. Pour into a jug and stir in the lime and lemon juices and psyllium fibre. Mix well and drink.

Celiac? Make gluten-free tabbouleh!

Those who suffer from celiac disease know eating anything with barley, rye, spelt, and especially wheat (and some oats) is a major no-no. The bulgur in traditional tabbouleh is cracked wheat and therefore can't be eaten by those who are gluten-sensitive. People with a history of gluten sensitivity may also suffer from general digestive upset, something for which parsley is an excellent remedy. So, for gluten-sensitive folks—and even those who just crave better digestion—here's a tabbouleh recipe just for you.

½ cup quinoa, rinsed and drained

3 tbsp extra virgin olive oil

1 cup boiling water

½ seedless cucumber, chopped

2 cups finely chopped fresh flat-leaf parsley

½ cup finely chopped fresh mint

3 tbsp freshly squeezed lemon juice

¾ tsp sea salt

¼ tsp freshly ground black pepper

2 medium tomatoes, chopped

Combine the quinoa and 1 tablespoon of the oil in a heatproof bowl. Add the boiling water, cover bowl tightly with plastic wrap, and let stand for 15 minutes. Drain the water and transfer the quinoa to a second bowl to cool. Add the cucumber, parsley, mint, lemon juice, remaining 2 tablespoons oil, salt, and pepper and toss to combine. Gently stir in the tomatoes. Chill and serve.

Urinary tract troubles? Drink this tea!

When you combine the diuretic and antimicrobial effects of parsley with unsweetened cranberry juice, you have a powerhouse urinary tract infection cure and kidney cleanse.

Place 3 sprigs of fresh parsley in a mug. Add enough boiling water to cover the parsley.

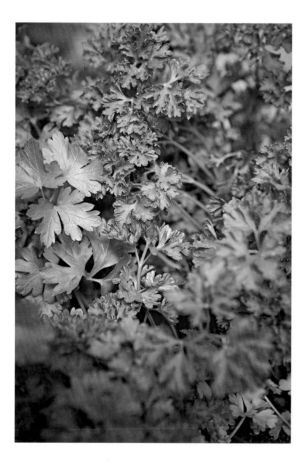

Cover and steep for 10 minutes. Strain into a clean mug. Add enough unsweetened cranberry juice to fill the mug to the top (this will also immediately cool the parsley water). Add 1 teaspoon of manuka honey (or to taste).

Drink 4 times daily to help treat a urinary tract infection.

>> Fast Forward

Fast forward to the health food store to purchase Nature's Way parsley capsules or equivalent. Follow the instructions on the label.

! Cautions

Due to its high concentration of vitamin K, use parsley with caution if you have a known bleeding disorder or take medications that may affect blood coagulation or platelet aggregation.

Consult your healthcare provider if you are diabetic, as some reports in animals suggest parsley has blood-sugar-lowering effects.

If you have low blood pressure or take blood-pressure-lowering drugs, parsley is contraindicated.

Avoid parsley if you have a known allergy or hypersensitivity to carrots, fennel, or celery, all of which are in the same botanical family (*Apiaceae*).

Pregnant women should avoid parsley seed or oil—studies show it can induce uterine contractions.

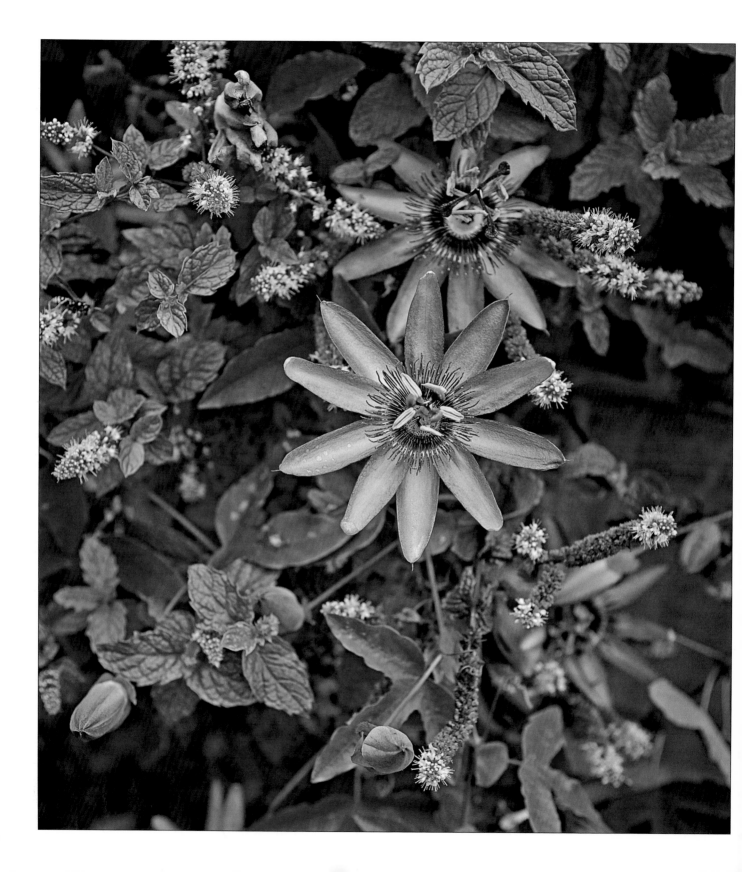

Passionflower

This incredible, eye-catching plant features a purple starburst flower that resembles a floral firework. Unfortunately, these showy flowers only last 24 hours—but the stress-busting power of passionflower extract lasts much longer. There are hundreds of *Passiflora* species, but the one most popular for medicinal use is *P. incarnata*, also called the purple passionflower, true passionflower, or maypop. While many passionflowers are tropical plants, this fast-growing vine grows wild in many parts of the southeastern United States.

Health Benefits

Passionflower is most commonly used to treat conditions associated with nervousness, restlessness, anxiety, irritability, and insomnia due to stress and tension. Many clinical trials have looked at the anti-anxiety effect of passionflower, especially when combined with other herbs with similar effects. It is known to have sedative, analgesic, and antispasmodic properties. It is particularly helpful for those who feel weak and exhausted from stress—North America's number 1 silent killer.

Passionflower is a mild sedative that doesn't cause the same "hangover" side effects most pharmaceutical drugs do. If you suffer from anxiety, doctors commonly prescribe a drug called benzodiazapine. In a study comparing the two remedies, passionflower extract seems to work at least as well and also didn't cause impairment of work like benzodiazapine did. If you regularly have trouble falling asleep—another issue that impacts workplace performance—passionflower is the herb to take before bed.

Due to its antispasmodic properties, this herb is also an excellent remedy to counter cramps, spasms, menstrual pain, PMS, and asthma. It may also help those with nerve pain as a result of shingles.

Growing

Passionflower is a sexy plant. Yes, I said it: sexy. This flowering vine grows quickly and produces unique purple blossoms. The flowers appear alien-like but extremely attractive at the same time. I call them both exotic and erotic! Passionflower grows beautifully in the garden or in a pot, and I've used it several times as a focal point and a trailer in mixed containers. Passionflower is a perennial, but it won't survive most Canadian winters, so it

DIFFICULTY
Easy to medium

HARDINESS
Perennial in zones 6 and above

TIME TO PLANT
Spring

TIME TO HARVEST
Summer

LOCATION
Full to part sun

SOIL TYPE
Moist, well-drained

should be enjoyed outdoors in the summer but brought inside before frost threatens.

Common Varieties: There are over 400 passionflower species, including some with edible fruit. *Passiflora incarnata* is the plant of choice if you're using it medicinally.

PLANT

Passionflower is easily propagated by stem cuttings and can be sown from seed, but I recommend purchasing transplants. Passionflower isn't always readily available, but you should be able to find it occasionally at larger garden centres, home improvement stores, and perhaps even flower shops.

Plant passionflower in direct sun—it thrives in locations with heat, humidity, and adequate moisture. Ensure you have rich soil that will maintain moisture but also has good drainage. I find passionflower grows best when planted in containers with potting soil.

Water often until the plant is established.

GROW

Cool summers are passionflower's biggest enemy. This plant loves the heat and likes it humid. Passionflower also enjoys moisture and requires regular watering, especially when grown in a container. Water deeply in the morning for great results, but don't overdo it. If the leaves start to yellow, allow the plant to dry out between waterings.

This fast-growing vine is self-clinging, but I recommend using a support system like a trellis, bamboo stake, obelisk, or tomato cage to guide the growth. Staking improves airflow around the plant and minimizes the chances of disease. Tie the vine with a material that will not cut into the stem, such as nylon stockings or plastic twist-ties.

Passionflower enjoys compost-rich soils and will benefit from fertilizing when planted in a container. Feed these sexy vines at least twice per month with a general-purpose fertilizer (20-20-20), compost tea, or fish emulsion.

"Vertical gardening" is about growing up instead of growing out. This style of gardening lends itself to small spaces, as its footprint is minimal. Passionflower—which is really a vine—is a perfect addition to a vertical garden, and it can provide privacy when supported by a trellis on the patio.

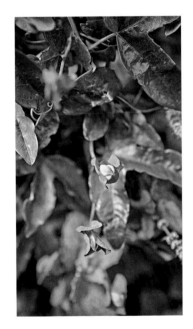

To stimulate growth and improve overall health, deadhead the spent flowers and occasionally prune or pinch back the side shoots if they appear a little out of control. Never fear, as passionflower is a tough vine and can take a good battle with the pruners!

Bugs to watch for include whiteflies, aphids, scale, and spider mites. Apply insecticidal soap every 3 weeks as a preventive.

HARVEST

The leaves, flowers, and fruits of *Passiflora incarnata* are edible. Harvest the flowers by removing them (stem included) when they're fully open mid-morning to early afternoon. Harvest the fruit in late summer. Allow it to vine-ripen, and look for full orange colour and plump appearance before you pick it. (Note that the fruits of other passionflower species may not be edible.)

STORE

Stems, leaves, and flowers should be hung to dry by placing out of direct light in a dry, warm location. Drying should take 7 to 10 days. To dry the blossoms separately, cut the flower cleanly at the base of the stem and place on a clean, dry, paper-lined surface for one week.

Fruits should be eaten fresh and can be refrigerated for up to 10 days.

Put It to Work

Problems sleeping? Drink this nightcap!
Measure 1 cup of dried passionflower blossoms and place them in a resealable glass jar (like a Mason jar). Pour vodka (at least 80 proof) into the jar until it covers the flowers by at least 2.5 cm (1 inch). Place wax paper over the jar and then screw the lid on tightly to seal it. Set aside in a cool, dark place for 1 month, shaking the jar once daily.

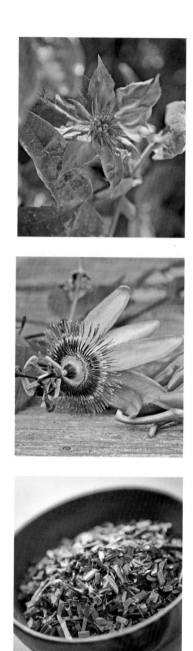

An immature passionflower bloom; full bloom; dried passionflower.

230

After a month, place cheesecloth or a swatch of linen or muslin over the mouth of a sterile jar and pour the herb-infused liquid through the cloth, straining the liquid as it enters the jar. Discard solids.

Take 1 teaspoon up to 3 times daily. The infusion will keep indefinitely stored in a cool, dark place.

Workplace stress? Drink passionflower coffee!
OK, I won't ask you to stop drinking coffee! If I did, I would be a hypocrite, since I won't give it up myself. And I'd be asking you to ignore the health virtues that come with coffee in moderation—and there are many. But coffee drinkers may experience the jitters after having more than 2 or 3 cups a day. One way to counter the effects and experience a more restful day is to power your coffee with passionflower!

Brew your coffee as you normally would, and make it extra hot. Dunk in a tablespoon of dried passionflower blooms. Cover and steep for 10 minutes. Strain out the flowers and enjoy!

Overly excitable? Try passionflower juice!
Inability to concentrate is usually related to an overly stimulated nervous system. Due to its ability to relax the nervous system, passionflower has been considered for the relief of attention deficit hyperactivity disorder (ADHD) symptoms. It's even safe for children.

To make passionflower juice, first make a passionflower infusion by placing 1 table-spoon of dried passionflower herb (leaves and flowers) in 1 cup of boiling water. Let the mixture steep for 15 minutes. Cool and add 1 cup of complementary juice, such as grape, strawberry, blueberry, or pomegranate juice. Shake well. Let us know what the teacher says about your child's behaviour after lunch!

» Fast Forward

Fast forward to the health food store to purchase St. Francis passionflower tincture or equivalent. Follow the instructions on the label.

! Cautions

Avoid driving or operating heavy machinery while taking passionflower, as it has sedative effects. You should also avoid combining passionflower with other sedatives that might increase the risk of excessive drowsiness, such as pentobarbital (Nembutal), phenobarbital (Luminal), secobarbital (Seconal), clonazepam (Klonopin), lorazepam (Ativan), and zolpidem (Ambien).

Avoid if allergic to passionflower or any of its constituents.

If you experience low blood pressure or are pregnant or breastfeeding, avoid use.

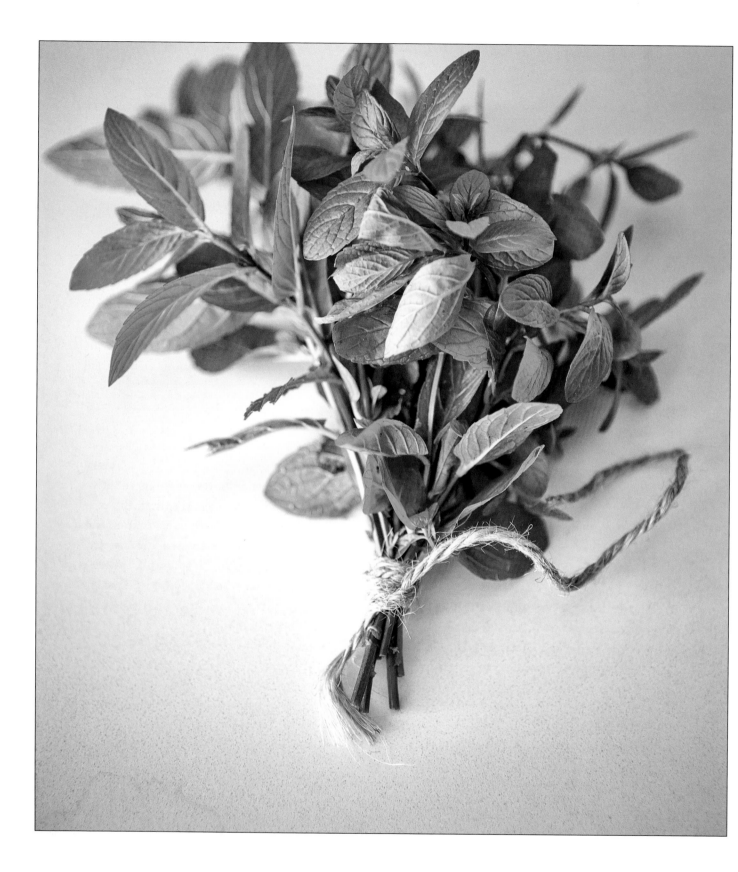

Peppermint

If you haven't tried peppermint, you've been living on some other planet. This amazing herb is renowned throughout the world. It tastes and smells great, making it everyone's favourite flavour of gum, refreshing breath candy, and herbal tea. Peppermint is a natural hybrid of two closely related species: watermint (*Mentha aquatica*) and spearmint (*M. spicata*). Like most hybrid species, it's sterile, which means it does not generally produce seeds. But its roots spread vigorously, and it's now found in the wild throughout North America and Europe.

Health Benefits

Peppermint is the richest source of menthol, the ingredient responsible for its characteristic smell and taste. Menthol has many medicinal uses. As an antispasmodic it inhibits smooth muscle contractions of the digestive system and relaxes the muscles of the esophageal sphincter. It also helps to release trapped air and reduces belching and bloating.

In one study, 79% of those who took peppermint oil experienced less pain associated with abdominal gas. Further studies show that peppermint oil relieves irritable bowel syndrome (IBS), and a double-blind study found it was more powerful than the drug cisapride, which is intended for the same symptoms.

Research shows that applying peppermint oil to the temples and forehead of a headache sufferer is just as effective as acetaminophen. It also helps to reduce symptoms of nausea when used as aromatherapy.

Growing

Peppermint is a wonderful addition to the herb and kitchen garden, and even the most incompetent gardener won't be able to kill it. All mints are extremely hardy perennials, but they're also aggressive growers that will take over if you're not careful. I call them the bullies of the garden!

Common Varieties: 'Candymint', 'Crispa', and good old traditional Peppermint.

PLANT

The easiest way to add peppermint to your garden is by getting a division from a friend—trust me, they won't mind giving you some! Divide peppermint in spring using a garden fork or sharp spade. Don't worry, you can't kill this bulletproof herb.

DIFFICULTY
Easy

HARDINESS
Perennial in zones 3 to 7

TIME TO PLANT
Spring

TIME TO HARVEST
Late spring to fall

LOCATION
Part sun (will tolerate full sun if well watered)

SOIL TYPE
Rich, well-drained (will survive in poor soils)

Now, here's where I want you to pay attention! When planting peppermint (or any mint, for that matter), keep it in a contained space. Even in the garden, I plant my peppermint in a pot and then bury the pot almost to the rim. Peppermint will send out runners, so you need to make sure these don't escape the pot.

Plant in part sun for best results, but peppermint can grow in sun to shade as long as it has adequate moisture.

GROW

Peppermint isn't threatened by bugs or disease. Its biggest struggle will come during periods of extreme heat (sometimes it doesn't enjoy direct sun).

Peppermint should be cut back often during the growing season. This herb will flower, but you should cut it back before that happens to promote vigorous growth of fresh foliage. Remember, it's the leaves you want, not the flowers! Never harvest more than one-third of the plant at any given time.

Peppermint isn't a heavy feeder, and planting in soils amended with compost is enough. For containers, I recommend fertilizing monthly with compost tea or a general-purpose fertilizer (20-20-20).

HARVEST

You can harvest peppermint leaves any time from spring through summer. Most say the volatile oils are strongest after the dew dries, so harvest mid-morning and cut the stem back to a node to get the freshest growth possible.

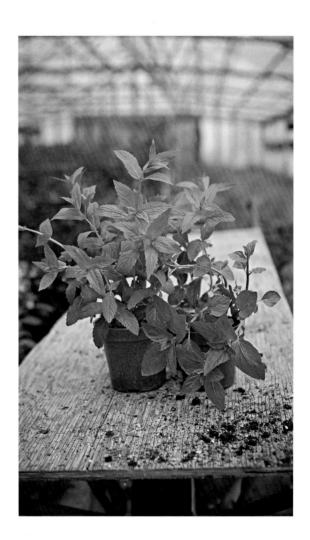

STORE

Peppermint can be used fresh, frozen, or dried. Fresh peppermint can either be wrapped in damp newspaper or paper towel or tied into a small bundle and placed in water like a bouquet and stored in the refrigerator for up to 10 days. To freeze, purée or finely chop the leaves, spoon into BPA-free ice-cube trays, and top with water. Once frozen, transfer cubes to resealable bags.

Peppermint will mould quickly, so it's best to dry it by hanging tightly tied bundles loosely covered by a paper bag or by using drying trays in a dark, dry location (see "Drying Herbs at Home" on page 365). Drying should take about 2 weeks. After drying, store the leaves in air-tight containers in a cool, dry place.

Put It to Work

Want to put peppermint to work? Make this essential oil!

To get the most potent health benefit from peppermint, you need to extract its essential oil. Among the beneficial substances found in the oil are menthol, cineole, menthone, and limonene, all of which soothe and improve intestinal function and even get rid of that pesky headache.

Wash and dry 2 cups of fresh peppermint leaves and place into a resealable bag. Press the air out and seal. Using a mallet or the butt end of a knife, gently tap the leaves inside the bag, making sure not to overly bruise them. This gentle tapping slowly releases the leaves' natural oils.

Dump the peppermint leaves into a resealable glass jar (like a Mason jar). Pour in enough vodka (at least 80 proof) to completely cover the leaves. Place wax paper over the jar and then screw the lid on tightly to seal it. Set aside in a cool, dark place for at least 4 weeks, shaking the jar once daily.

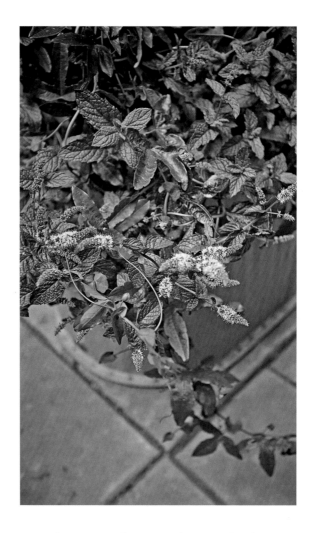

After a month, cover the mouth of the jar with a coffee filter and strain the liquid into a second jar (discard solids). Then cover it with a clean coffee filter or cheesecloth and set aside in a dry, warm place for at least 7 to 10 days or until the alcohol completely evaporates. What remains is pure essential peppermint oil.

Pour ½ cup of olive oil into the jar and shake vigorously. This will function as a

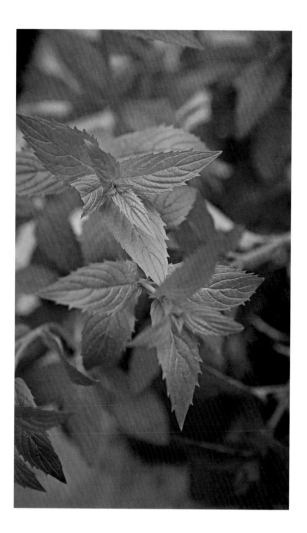

drome (IBS). It's estimated that nearly 20% of the North American population has symptoms of IBS on a regular basis. Peppermint oil can drastically improve those symptoms. Take ½ teaspoon twice daily before meals.

Bloating, gas, or distension? It's peppermint tea time!

You may not have full-blown IBS, but we all occasionally eat too much or experience an upset tummy. Peppermint tea is a godsend. In a mug, pour 1 cup of boiling water over 10 peppermint leaves, cover with a saucer, and steep for 5 to 10 minutes. Enjoy 3 to 4 cups daily between meals to relieve stomach and gastrointestinal complaints. Alternatively, add 5 drops of peppermint essential oil to a few ounces of warm water and drink as needed.

Stress headache? Rub on some relief!

Peppermint oil may help relieve a dull headache, tightness or pressure across your forehead or on the sides and back of your head, and even tenderness on your scalp, neck, and shoulder muscles. Just put a few drops of peppermint essential oil in the palm of your hand and, using your index finger, dab it on your temples. Massage the remaining oil into the muscles at the back and front of your neck.

Need a pick-me-up? Sniff it!

Smelling menthol became popular in the late 19th century after the *British Medical Journal* published an article noting the practice

"carrier oil" to dilute the very potent active ingredients. Use this peppermint oil in the preparations that follow.

Irritable bowels? Settle them with peppermint oil!

If you regularly experience indigestion that causes abdominal pressure, fullness, and gas, you may be suffering from irritable bowel syn-

relieved headaches and nerve pain. Fast forward to present day, when most scientists agree that peppermint is a strong mental and physical stimulant that can help you concentrate and stay alert.

Inhaling the aroma of peppermint oil may alleviate computer fatigue and boost your deskside energy levels. It may also help anxiety and depression. Simply dab a few drops on the back of your hand and spend 2 to 3 minutes inhaling the soothing aroma. Alternatively, burn the oil in an aromatherapy burner.

» Fast Forward

Fast forward to the health food store to purchase Nature's Way Pepogest capsules or equivalent. Follow the instructions on the label.

! Cautions

Allergic reactions to external use of peppermint oil are rare.

When you ingest a lot of peppermint oil, it is not uncommon to experience a minty-cool burning sensation in the rectum.

Peppermint tea is safe for regular consumption, but too much can cause burning and gastrointestinal upset in some people. Avoid it if you have bad heartburn, severe liver damage, inflammation of the gallbladder, or obstruction of bile ducts.

Infants and young children may choke in reaction to the strong menthol in peppermint tea, so use with caution. If you're looking to treat an infant's colic or upset stomach, go with chamomile tea cooled to room temperature, with honey added for sweetness.

Avoid applying peppermint oil near the eyes, or anywhere on the face of children.

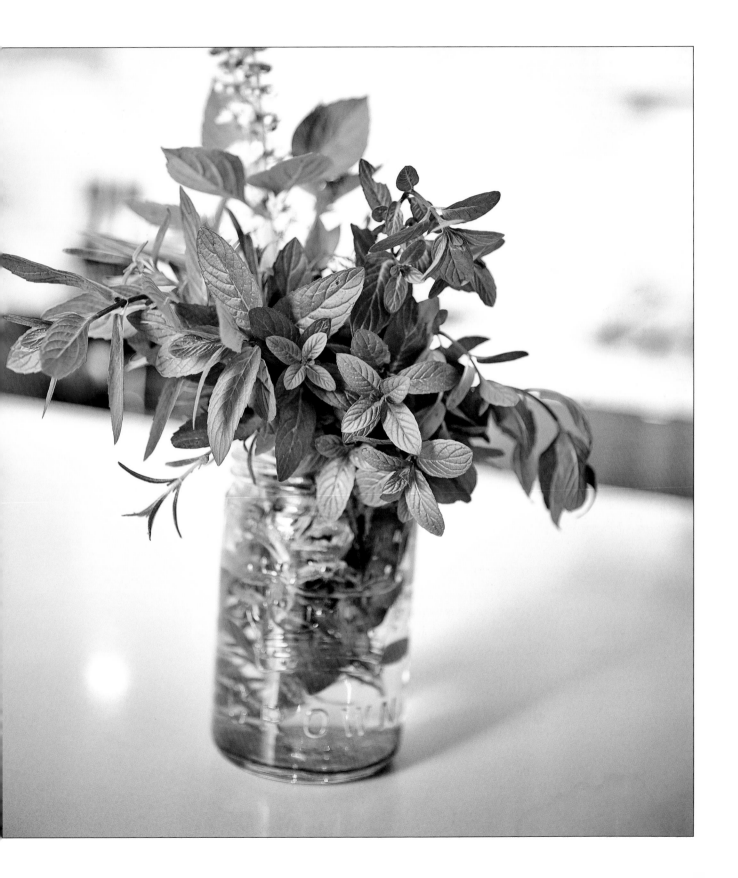

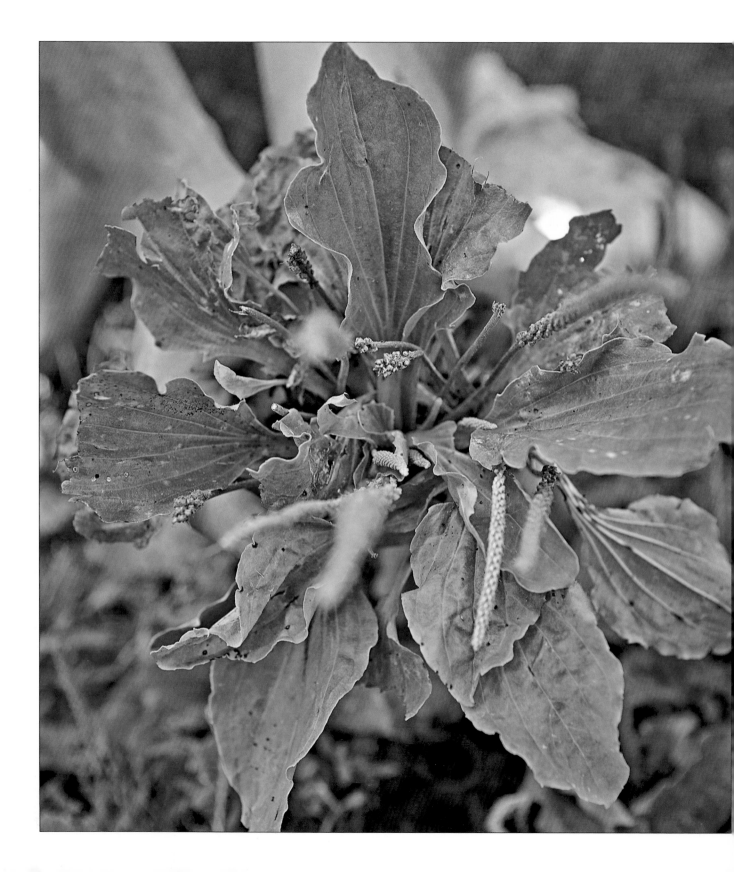

Plantain

The plantain used in herbal remedies (from the genus *Plantago*) is not to be confused with the banana-like plantain (*Musa*) found in the tropics. Other than their common name, the two plants share little in common. Plantain is a small, compact plant native to North America, Europe, and Asia that has a long history of medicinal use. The two most important species are broad-leaved plantain (*P. major*) and ribwort or buckhorn plantain (*P. lanceolata*). Plantain is found all over the world, and in many areas it has become an invasive weed.

⊕ Health Benefits

Depending on where you are in the world, plantain leaf is used to treat urogenital tract disorders, respiratory system disorders, gastrointestinal tract disorders, skin ailments, blood system disorders, nervous system disorders, cardiovascular system disorders, and rheumatism.

Recently plantain has been pegged as an herbal remedy for allergy relief, as well as for cold and flu. Germany's Commission E (a regulatory body analogous to Health Canada for herbs) approved the internal use of plantain leaf to ease coughs and irritation of the mucous membrane, which are associated with upper respiratory tract infections. It's safe for children, which is great news considering dextromethorphan (or DXM, a cough suppressant) and guaifenesin (an expectorant) have been found to be unsafe in children. Plantain may also stimulate the immune system.

Plantain is a demulcent, an agent that forms a soothing film over mucous membranes, relieving minor pain and inflammation. It also works similarly to pectin and glycerine, which are common ingredients in cough syrups and throat drops.

🌱 Growing

Plantain is a tenacious weed. You've probably got it on your lawn, gardens, patio—I've even seen plantain growing in driveways. This woody perennial has the ability to produce up to 14,000 seeds in its flowers, so once plantain gets a foothold it grows everywhere. As an avid gardener I can't in good conscience encourage you to grow it, so I'm going to recommend foraging instead!

Common Varieties: The most popular varieties for medicinal use are *P. major* and *P. lanceolata*, both of which are common weeds.

DIFFICULTY
Easy (it's a weed!)

HARDINESS
Perennial in zones 5 and above

TIME TO PLANT
Spring

TIME TO HARVEST
Spring to early summer

LOCATION
Full to part sun

SOIL TYPE
Rich, well-drained (will also grow in poor soils)

PLANT

Plantain is a perennial that spreads easily by seed. The seeds do not even require a thick covering: they just need to make contact with the soil. I will say it again: Don't plant this stuff in your garden!

So you grew it even after I told you not to, and now you want me to help you get rid of it! Plantain can be controlled early in the season by suppressing the germination of its seed. This can be done by applying corn gluten as soon as the snow disappears. Corn gluten is a natural product that reduces weeds by coating their seeds and preventing germination. Just remember you can't reseed a lawn when using corn gluten.

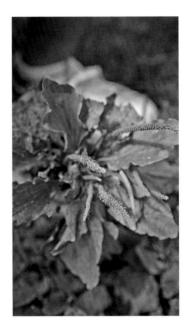

GROW

If you take my advice and avoid growing plantain from seed, I will tell you how to find it. It grows everywhere: Look in gardens, lawns, roadsides, ditches, and parks. If you're going to harvest it, look for an area where plantain is free of herbicides, pollutants, and dog urine.

Broadleaf plantain is a stout plant with broad, glossy, egg-shaped leaves and an almost leathery texture. The leaves measure about 5 to 15 cm (2 to 7 inches) long and 3 to 5 cm (1 to 2 inches) wide. Ribwort or buckhorn plantain has slightly narrower and much longer leaves: up to 30 cm (12 inches). The leaves of both varieties have parallel veins, and both produce spiky stems bearing yellow flowers that quickly turn to seed.

HARVEST

Harvest young leaves in spring, as the foliage will become tough and woody as the plant sets flowers. Harvest in the morning after the dew has dried. Remove the foliage any way you can. I wouldn't worry about harming plantain—it will grow back whether you want it to or not!

Use plantain fresh. Wash just before use. To store, wrap loosely in paper towel and refrigerate for up to a week.

⚙ Put It to Work

Stubborn cough? Drop these!

Colds and flu leave millions of people coughing every year. There are many over-the-counter remedies, but few are safe, effective, and chemical-free. Try these plantain cough drops instead. You can find gum Arabic (a natural gum used to help harden mixtures) in specialty or bulk food stores. We found that the powder doesn't work so well, so stick to the actual "rocks."

1 cup finely chopped plantain leaves

3 cups boiling water

1 cup gum Arabic, crushed

2 cups icing sugar, plus extra for dusting

In a saucepan over low heat, combine the plantain leaves with 2 cups of boiling water. Stir well and steep for 30 minutes.

In a separate saucepan over low heat, combine 1 cup of boiling water with the gum Arabic and mix until it has a goopy consistency.

Using a fine-mesh sieve, strain the steeped plantain into the gum Arabic (discard the plantain leaves). Stir in the icing sugar. Keep on low heat and stir frequently for 30 minutes.

The mixture is done when it begins to pull away from the side of the pan and form a thick ball in the centre.

Pour the mixture approximately 1 cm (½ inch) thick onto a baking sheet lined with wax paper. Let it set for about 15 minutes, until hardened. When it's fully set, break it into bite-size pieces. Dust with icing sugar to prevent the pieces from sticking together (the sugar will also absorb any residual moisture). Store the lozenges in an airtight container.

Suck 1 lozenge every 2 to 3 hours (don't exceed 6 lozenges in one day).

Stretched or scarred? Apply this salve!

When you're pregnant or nursing you have every reason to be cautious about what you apply to your skin. This cream has wondrous healing powers, and it can help reduce stretch marks from pregnancy or scars from an injury. The ingredients are natural and chemical-free, and therefore safe even for people with skin sensitivities.

1 cup plantain leaves

½ cup olive oil

½ cup coconut oil

2 oz beeswax

1 tbsp vitamin E oil

In a blender, combine the plantain leaves and olive oil and blend on high speed until smooth. Using a fine-mesh strainer, coffee filter, or cheesecloth, strain the plantain oil into

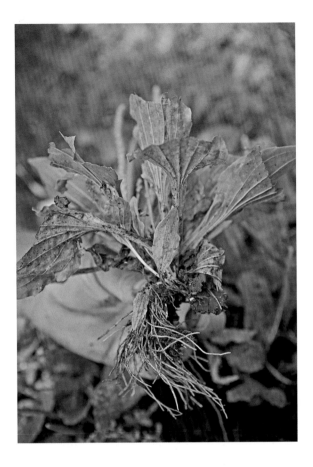

a heatproof glass bowl (discard solids). Place the bowl over a small pot of boiling water (acting as a double boiler) and warm—but do not overheat—the oil. Add the coconut oil and beeswax and mix continuously. (Do not cover, as condensation will ruin the salve.) Once all the ingredients have melted, add the vitamin E oil and stir vigorously. Pour into small glass containers (do not cover) and let them sit overnight. The next morning the cream will be ready to use. Apply liberally to the affected areas twice daily, morning and before bed.

» Fast Forward

Fast forward to the health food store to purchase Clef des Champs plantain syrup or equivalent. Follow the instructions on the label.

! Cautions

Since demulcents can cause more mucus production in the lungs, they are best used to relieve dry, stubborn coughs.

Plantain has no known side effects and is thought to be safe for children. There is no information available about its use by pregnant or nursing women, though topical application appears to be safe.

There have been rare reports of plantain supplements being adulterated with digitalis, a potentially toxic plant. Be sure to purchase herbs from reputable companies.

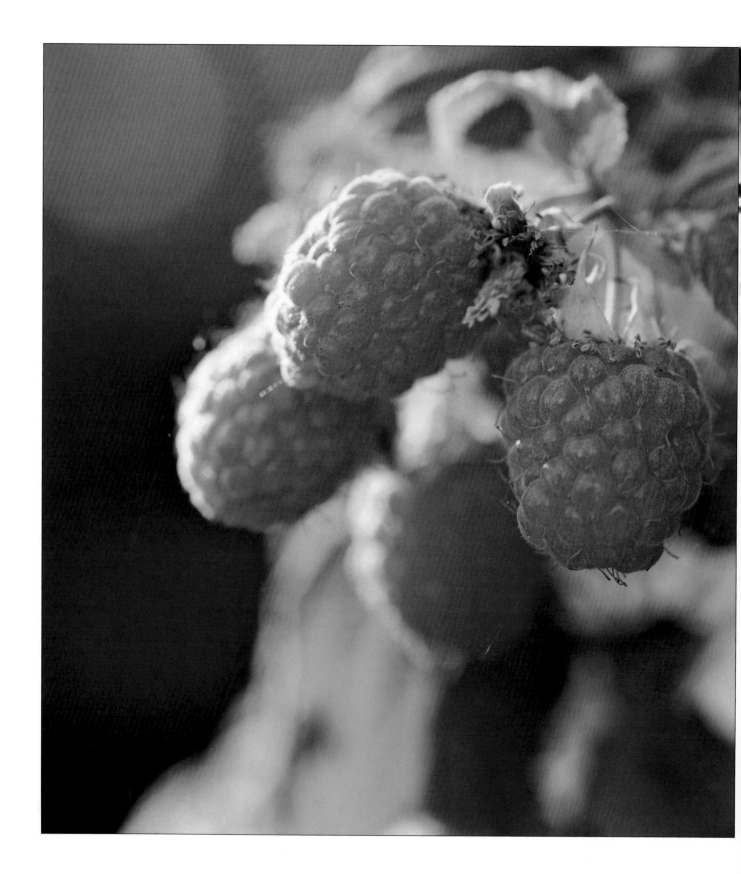

Raspberry

When you eat a raspberry it's hard not to marvel at its delicate architecture—each raspberry has about a hundred little "drupelets," or self-contained fleshy lobes with tiny seeds perfectly sized to get stuck in your teeth! Their mouth-watering sweet-tart taste isn't quite as popular in jams and jellies as some other berries, but they are enjoyed around the world. Raspberries (there are many species in the genus *Rubus*) are genetically related to roses, which won't come as a surprise to anyone who has brushed up against their prickly, woody canes. The most popular varieties are red, although black, golden, and even white (albino) berries are available.

⊕ Health Benefits

Raspberries have historically been used to treat inflammation of the digestive tract, gum disease, anemia, stomach ache, and fever. Tea made from the leaves has been used for centuries as a folk medicine to treat wounds, diarrhea, colic, and respiratory diseases.

Traditionally, midwives use raspberry to address menstrual concerns and to reduce the pain of labour. It alleviates morning sickness, may prevent miscarriage, and decreases postpartum bleeding. An early study shows that raspberry leaf may be safe for both mother and child. It is thought to tone the muscles of the uterus to help it function better during labour. (These effects take several weeks to accumulate in your body, so it won't work to bring on labour if you are overdue.)

Labour and giving birth are a tremendous feat of endurance. What the body goes through during the hours it takes to bring a new life into the world is nothing short of a miracle. The physical stress and strain endured by the female body includes free radical damage (inflammation from oxidative stress in the muscle tissue). The powerful antioxidants in raspberries can help.

New evidence in the world of sports medicine suggests that endurance athletes—who face physical demands much like the marathon that mothers go through during labour—require significant antioxidant support after exercise. Raspberry extract can help meet that demand, too.

🌱 Growing

Raspberries are delicious, and growing them in your garden sounds like a good idea. They're fairly easy to grow, your kids love picking them, and you all love eating them. But there's a big but! They take a lot of space, some varieties can be invasive,

---

DIFFICULTY
Medium

HARDINESS
Perennial in zones 2 to 7
(depends on variety)

TIME TO PLANT
Spring

TIME TO HARVEST
Summer through early fall
(depends on variety)

LOCATION
Full sun

SOIL TYPE
Rich, well-drained

and they may require time-consuming pruning. Before you plant them, look for any patches of wild raspberries on fence rows, ditches, and vacant lots in your area. You may be able to harvest them for free!

Common Varieties: There are two main types of raspberries, summer-bearing and everbearing. Summer-bearing raspberries—as you probably figured out—yield their fruit in early summer only. Everbearing raspberries give you a crop in the summer and another in the fall. There are many cultivars of each type, with berries of various colours and sizes. I like the following:

- Summer-bearing red raspberry varieties: 'Prelude', 'Boyne', 'Nova', 'Titan', 'Glen Ample'
- Everbearing red rasberry varieties: 'Autumn Bliss', 'Caroline', 'Josephine', 'Polka'
- Black and purple raspberry varieties: 'Jewel', 'Royalty'
- Yellow raspberry variety: 'Fall Gold'

PLANT

Plant raspberries in spring—that's when you'll find the best selection at garden centres. (You can also plant them in early fall.) Look for large pots with several canes, and pay attention to whether the variety you are purchasing is summer-bearing or everbearing. This will not only tell you the time to harvest and the type of fruit, it will also guide your pruning practices.

Locate the plants in full sun, in well-drained soil rich in organic matter or compost.

GROW

Raspberries are not maintenance-free. They need regular weeding, occasional watering (at least 25 mm/1 inch per week), annual fertilizing, mulching, and inspection for bugs and disease. But the critical—and time-consuming—task is pruning. When and how to prune is determined by the type of raspberries you grow and the wood on which they produce their fruit.

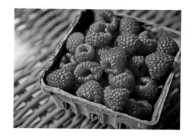

Do you have a friend with raspberry plants? If you do, they will definitely have some to share! Raspberries tend to spread and should be divided annually to keep them in check. This is best done in early spring when the ground is workable and the plants are dormant. Divide using a sharp spade. Never fear; it's hard to hurt a raspberry. Wrap root divisions in damp newspaper and plant where desired. Voilà, free raspberry plants!

Summer-bearing raspberries need to be pruned twice each year. In early spring the goal is to remove all weak canes (anything thinner than a pencil) and cut back any others damaged by heavy snow or that appear too tall or out of control (over 2 metres/6 feet). The second pruning happens after the harvest. Now the goal is to remove any canes that produced fruits this season, because summer-bearing raspberries produce fruit on old wood, or last year's growth. The canes are biennial, so they will die off after bearing fruit.

Everbearing raspberries produce berries on new wood, so they require only one pruning per year. In late fall or late winter, just mow your everbearing raspberries to the ground! Since new wood is what you want, you can remove any and all old wood from last season.

Always remove any diseased canes and those growing in unwanted places or directions.

Finally, raspberries should be staked, since the canes grow tall and fast. When growing them in rows, support can be as easy as placing stakes and stringing lines outside of rows to keep the canes contained.

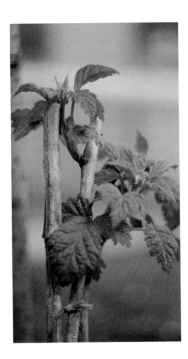

Freshly pruned summer-bearing raspberry canes in the spring.

HARVEST

It takes almost two growing seasons to get good raspberry yields. Harvest the berries immediately when they're ripe: They will appear plump and come off canes easily. Berries that squish or fall from canes are overripe and will lack flavour.

Put on a pair of gloves and harvest berries after the morning dew has dried and the fruit is still cool from overnight temperatures. Never pick raspberries in the rain unless you want to eat them immediately!

The flowers can be harvested in mid-spring to early summer. For maximum potency, harvest raspberry leaves in spring or early summer, preferably in mid-morning after the dew has dried. Don't defoliate entire canes: just remove leaves sporadically.

STORE

Wash raspberries only before eating. Store them in an airtight container in the refrigerator for up to 7 days. Remove rotten berries as soon as you see them. I say "eat 'em while they're fresh," but raspberries can also be frozen (place in a single layer on a baking tray, freeze, then transfer to resealable bags), preserved into jams or jellies, or made into wine.

The flowers should be used fresh. The leaves can be used fresh or dried on drying trays in a dry, warm location out of direct light (see "Drying Herbs at Home" on page 365).

 # Put It to Work

Hemorrhoids? Raspberry flower power!
Hemorrhoidal veins in the rectum are similar to varicose veins in the legs. When there is a long history of constipation, the pressure from bearing down fills the veins beyond their normal capacity, stretching them like overinflated balloons. Over time they become permanently dilated and can even hang out of the rectum and bleed, a chronic and often painful or itchy condition. There is a solution, however: raspberry flower paste.

1 cup freshly cut raspberry flowers (prior to fruit harvest)
½ cup olive oil
1 cup petroleum jelly
¼ cup shaved beeswax

Wash and strain the flower tops. Put them in a blender with the oil and blend on medium-low speed for 1 minute or until smooth. Pour into a resealable glass jar (like a Mason jar). Place wax paper over the jar and then tightly screw the lid on the jar to seal it. Set aside in a cool, dark place for 1 week.

After a week, cover the mouth of the jar with a coffee filter or cheesecloth and strain the liquid into a bowl (discard solids). This is your raspberry flower oil.

In a small heatproof bowl over a pot of boiling water (acting as a double boiler), melt the petroleum jelly. Add the flower oil and stir well. Add the beeswax and stir until combined.

Pour the mixture into a sterile glass jar with a tight-fitting lid and refrigerate. When the paste has cooled and hardened, use a tissue to apply it liberally to the affected area twice daily (in the morning and before bed). Store in a cool, dark place for up to 3 months.

Recovering after baby? Raspberry leaf tea!
You don't need to be postpartum to enjoy the amazing health benefits of raspberry leaf tea. But if you are, this simple recipe is ideal! Raspberry leaves are high in tannins, which are water-soluble antioxidants that help protect your body from inflammation.

Place 1 teaspoon of chopped dried raspberry leaves or 3 teaspoons of chopped fresh raspberry leaves in a mug and add 1 cup of boiling water. Cover and steep for 2 hours for

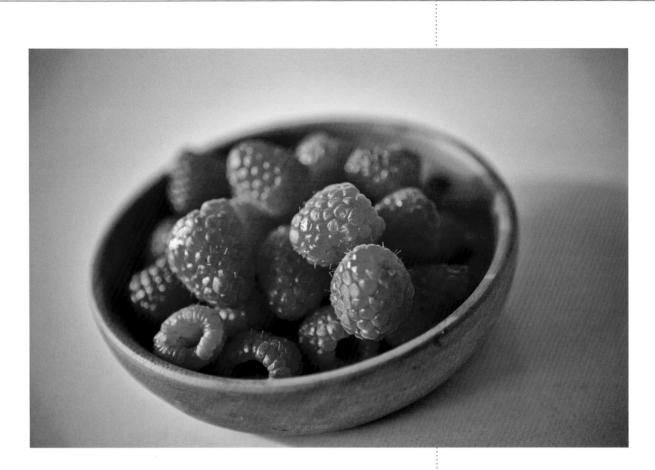

a full and robust infusion, then strain the tea into another mug.

You can drink 2 cups a day during the last two months of pregnancy—but don't use this tea earlier in pregnancy (it could cause early contractions). Always check with your healthcare provider before taking raspberry tea during pregnancy, as you may experience complications.

Endurance training? Use raspberry syrup sport gel!

Nearly every sweet sport gel these days is made up of artificial colour and flavour, but not homemade raspberry syrup sport gel. This one is 100% natural and delicious. And it isn't just pretty-looking; it's packed with a huge antioxidant punch. You can find the capsules and tablets needed in this recipe in health food stores or specialty pharmacies.

2 lb fresh raspberries

4 cups water

2 cups granulated sugar

1 tsp sea salt

3 100-mg magnesium bisglycinate
  capsules

3 99-mg potassium tablets

¼ cup gum Arabic

In a medium saucepan over high heat, combine the raspberries and the water and bring to a boil. Reduce the heat to low and simmer for 30 minutes. Using a spoon or ladle, skim the foam that rises to the top, but be careful not to crush the raspberries. After 30 minutes, the raspberries will have lost most of their colour, but the water should be deep pinkish-red.

Using a fine-mesh sieve, strain the raspberry liquid into another saucepan, being careful not to compress the remaining berries (if you attempt to extract more juice, your raspberry sport gel will be cloudy and may not set); discard the berry solids.

Add the sugar, salt, and the contents of the magnesium capsules to the raspberry juice. Using the back of a spoon or a mortar and pestle, crush the potassium tablets and add them to the pan, too. Add the gum Arabic and stir. Bring the mixture back to a boil, reduce the heat, and simmer, stirring frequently, for 10 minutes or until everything is completely dissolved and the mixture has thickened to a semi-thick gel. Cool completely.

This recipe makes enough for about 28 "gel packs" (in small resealable bags). Spoon about 3 tablespoons of the gel into each bag. Press out the air and seal. The packs should stay fresh in the refrigerator for about 2 weeks or in the freezer for 6 months.

When you're out on a run or heading to the gym, take one with you and eat it mid-workout to supply your body with the natural nutrients it needs to get through the intense training.

» Fast Forward

Fast forward to the health food store to purchase Traditional Medicinals red raspberry leaf tea or equivalent. Follow the instructions on the label.

! Cautions

Raspberries are considered very safe. Any adverse effects generally arise from contaminated fruits, which can cause gastrointestinal upset, vomiting, diarrhea, weight loss, fatigue, and fever. Always thoroughly wash raspberries as they may carry Norwalk-like viruses.

Avoid if you have an allergy to raspberries or other plants in the rose family (*Rosaceae*).

Don't consume high amounts of raspberries if you are in early pregnancy. It's a uterotonic; i.e., it will induce uterine contractions.

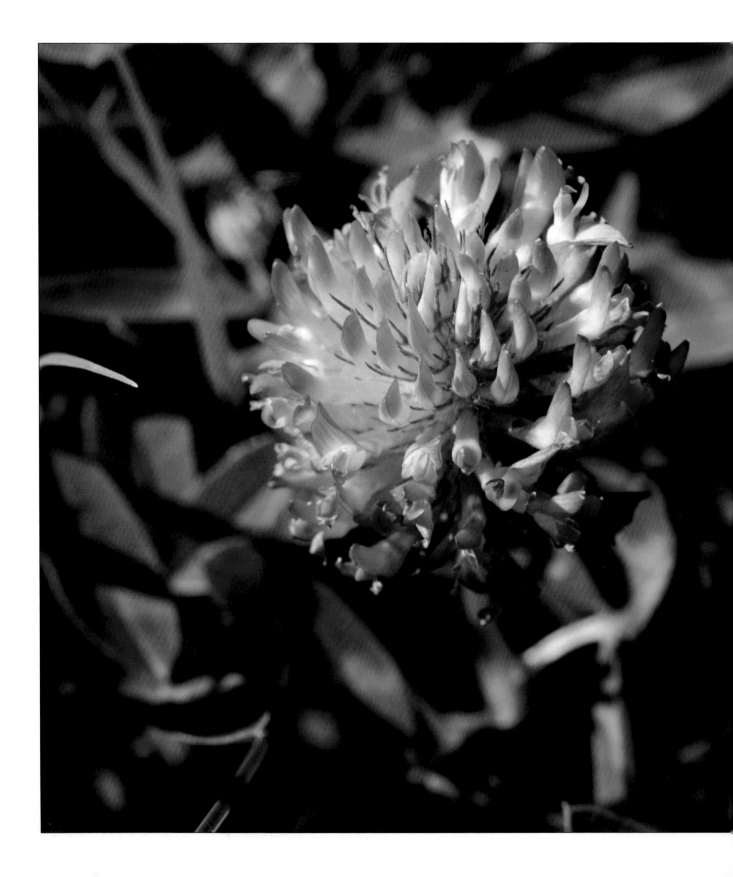

Red Clover

Red clover is—perhaps surprisingly—a legume from the same family as peas and beans (*Fabaceae*). It's a popular ground cover with trifoliate leaves and a reddish-pink globe-shaped flower. Traditionally, red clover leaves are eaten as salad greens, and the flowers are dried for use in teas. It's also the source of a tasty treat: Red clover nectar is a favourite of bees, who turn it into a delicious variety of honey.

⊕ Health Benefits

The Chinese traditionally used an infusion of red clover flowers as an expectorant. Europeans used it for liver and digestive ailments, and Native American peoples used the plant to treat cough, fevers, and menopause symptoms.

Red clover has become a popular over-the-counter treatment for the symptoms associated with menopause. It contains plant hormones called phytoestrogens (specifically, isoflavones), which are similar in chemical structure to the body's own estrogen. Isoflavones can help women over 45 when levels of hormones are naturally declining. They are effective at reducing menopausal hot flashes and slowing bone loss (osteoporosis) in postmenopausal women.

Red clover isoflavones have also been shown to have a positive effect on blood pressure and cholesterol. They maintain arterial wall elasticity, preserve the feel and appearance of the skin, regulate mood and emotions, and improve the ability to concentrate.

🌱 Growing

Red clover isn't a popular plant in the world of gardening, but it's gold in the agriculture business. It's commonly grown for livestock feed and planted as a "green manure." Farmers plant it to add nutrients to the soil before they grow other crops. Red clover is extremely good at fixing nitrogen from the air, suppressing weed growth, reducing erosion, and improving soil structure. It can perform those roles in your garden, too. If you grow vegetables organically, a cover crop of red clover may be the best way to feed the soil naturally!

Common Varieties: There are dozens of varieties, but red clover is so hard to find that I recommend whichever variety you can get your hands on!

DIFFICULTY
Easy

HARDINESS
Perennial in zones 4 and above

TIME TO PLANT
Early spring or late fall

TIME TO HARVEST
Late spring and summer

LOCATION
Full sun

SOIL TYPE
Well-drained

PLANT

This is a really easy plant to grow, but the seed isn't readily available at garden centres. You'll have to make a special request or try a farm supply store. Purchase seeds that have been inoculated with a bacterium called *Rhizobium trifolii*, which helps them grow.

Red clover is a fast-germinating seed and should be sown in early spring as soon as soil is workable, or in late fall before extremely cold temperatures set in—it will germinate before the snow flies. If you're using the plant for weed suppression, soil improvement, and erosion control, then broadcast the seeds by hand to cover the whole area. If you are growing it for medicinal purposes in a smaller area, sow in rows. Red clover is a small seed that requires only a light covering or contact with the soil.

The greater frequency of rain in early spring and fall will usually be sufficient for germination, but water during dry periods.

GROW

Red clover lives fast and dies hard! Although it's a perennial, it will usually last only 2 to 4 years. It can die in hot, dry conditions, and it suffers from insects that prey on its roots. Keep your plants alive with deep, infrequent waterings.

The upside is that red clover isn't typically an invasive plant. While you will occasionally have to remove it from unwanted spaces, it doesn't travel too much, and if it does it won't last long!

HARVEST

Harvest red clover during its early bloom stage by removing flowers just below the first cluster of leaves. The flowers can be harvested 3 to 5 times during the growing season. I suggest collecting them during dry weather and preferably on an overcast day. Hot, humid weather isn't ideal, as red clover blossoms will rot quickly.

STORE

Dry the flowers on drying trays, spacing them so the blooms do not touch, for 10 to 14 days. Place the trays out of direct light in a dry

No space and no time? Red clover can easily be found growing in lawns, on roadsides, and in farmer's fields. If you go looking for it, red clover is best identified by its pinkish-red flowers and its characteristic "clover-like" oblong leaves, which are variegated with a white arrowhead-shaped mark.

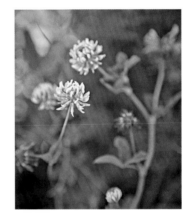

Don't be fooled by white clover! Red clover bears red to purple flowers, whereas white clover bears white to pink blooms, like the ones here. If that isn't clear enough, look at the plant's growth habits: Red clover is taller and more upright, while white clover is short and grows laterally.

location. To dry the leaves, hang bunches in a cool, dark, and dry location. (See "Drying Herbs at Home" on page 365.) Store the flowers and leaves separately in airtight containers.

Put It to Work

Need a refresher? Sip a red clover watermelonade!
Enjoy the health benefits of red clover in this fruit-packed beverage.

> *3 cups water*
> *1 cup freshly cut red clover blooms*
> *2 cups fresh watermelon juice*
> *6 strawberries, blended*
> *Freshly squeezed juice of 2 limes*
> *2 tbsp liquid honey*

In a saucepan, bring the water to a boil. Add the red clover blooms and boil for 5 minutes. Using a fine-mesh sieve lined with cheesecloth or a coffee filter, strain into a jug or pitcher (discard solids). Cool and add watermelon juice, strawberries, lime juice, and honey. Stir well and chill. Serve with ice.

Hot flashes? Iced tea!
Traditionally, red clover tea is taken hot, but here's an iced version to cool those hot flashes! Collect a few cups of clover blossoms. Put the blooms between two paper towels and set aside in a warm, dry location for 2 to 3 days to dry out. (You can speed up the process by spreading them over a baking sheet and baking in the oven on low heat, checking them frequently until they are totally dry.) Once the blossoms are dry, remove the petals and dispose of the thick stalks.

Place the petals into a mug and pour boiling water over them. (You can add a few mint leaves if you desire.) Cover with a saucer and steep for 15 minutes. Add honey to taste. Chill and serve over ice.

Menopause? Red clover tincture!
Whether you're experiencing hot flashes, worried about bone loss, or simply feeling that your hormones are out of whack, red clover can help. The most concentrated form you can make on your own is an alcohol tincture.

Fill a resealable glass jar (like a Mason jar) with red clover flowers. Pour vodka (at least 80 proof) into the jar, filling it right up to the top. Press the flower tops down with a fork to displace any air and then top up with additional vodka to cover the plant material. Place wax paper over the jar and then tightly screw the lid on to seal it. Shake well. Set aside in a cool, dark place for at least 4 weeks, shaking the jar once daily.

After a month, cover the mouth of the jar with a coffee filter or cheesecloth and strain the liquid into a sterile jar (discard solids).

Take 1 teaspoon twice daily with meals. The tincture will keep for up to 5 years stored in a cool, dark place.

Seeking optimum health? Get your daily dose! Honey is a preservative, and when it's mixed with the edible flower blossoms of red clover it will capture the flavour of the plant from which it is often derived.

In a resealable glass jar (like a Mason jar), combine 2 cups of freshly cut clover blossoms with 1 cup of liquid honey. Set aside for 3 days, stirring vigorously every 24 hours. That's it—it's ready to eat! If the blossoms were properly dried, the clover-infused honey should last a long time.

» Fast Forward

Fast forward to the health food store to purchase Novogen Promensil capsules or equivalent. Follow the instructions on the label.

! Cautions

Studies show virtually no side effects from red clover extracts after 1 year of treatment. Theoretically, based on the estrogen-like action of red clover seen in laboratory studies, side effects could include weight gain or breast tenderness, but these effects have not been documented.

If you are taking hormone replacement therapy (HRT) or birth control pills, you should only use red clover with the strict supervision of your healthcare provider.

If you have low blood pressure, or if you are taking medications that lower your blood pressure or thin your blood, avoid using red clover.

Red clover is not recommended during pregnancy and breastfeeding due to its estrogen-like activity. Women who have had breast cancer should not use red clover.

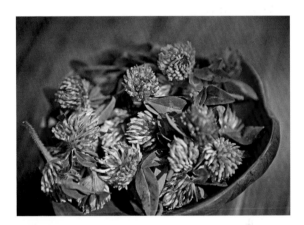

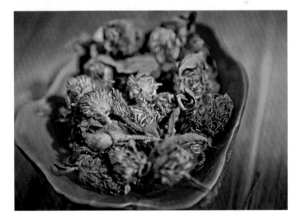

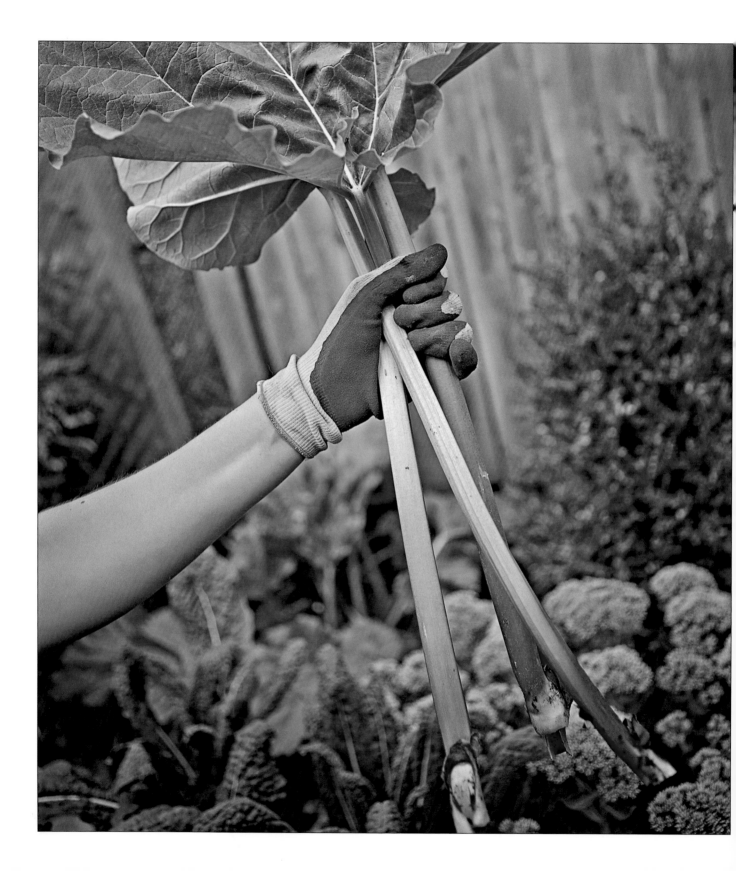

Rhubarb

Rhubarb has been used in traditional Chinese and Tibetan medicine for more than 5,000 years, and it gradually spread to India, Russia, Europe, and eventually North America. Rhubarb belongs to the same family as buckwheat and sorrel (*Polygonaceae*). It produces huge leaves on reddish celery-like stalks. These stalks have a distinctly tart taste, but when sweetened with sugar they make a popular food. Both the stalks and the root of the plant are used to make medicines. The leaves, however, contain highly toxic oxalic acid and should never be consumed.

⊕ Health Benefits

Herbalists have traditionally used rhubarb as a laxative, as a diuretic, and to treat kidney stones, gout, and liver diseases. It is also used externally to heal skin sores and scabs. In traditional Chinese medicine, rhubarb is used as an ulcer remedy and to "clear heat" from the liver, stomach, and blood. It is also used for de-worming, fever, toothache, and headache.

"Swedish bitters" is a popular tonic, especially in Europe, and it includes rhubarb as one of its active ingredients, along with aloe and senna. But frequent use of this tonic is not recommended due to the risk of bowel dependence.

Research has identified several active compounds in rhubarb that may act to fight cancer, reduce inflammation, and lower cholesterol, as well as protect the eyes and brain. These compounds are strong antioxidants called anthraquinones. One of these, emodin, is found in high concentrations in rhubarb, and promising new research suggests it might inhibit cell proliferation, induce cell death in cancer cells, and prevent cancer from spreading.

Rhubarb also contains anthocyanins (the type of pigment also found in blueberries), lutein, and zeaxanthin, as well as significant amounts of vitamins (C, K, B-complex) and the essential minerals calcium, potassium, and manganese.

🌱 Growing

There is nothing like the taste of strawberry rhubarb pie to say spring! Rhubarb is one of the few perennial vegetables that will grow in Canada and other cold climates. It's a massive plant—about 90 x 150 cm (3 x 5 feet) wide—that requires a lot of space, but it makes an excellent addition to both the perennial and veg-

DIFFICULTY
Easy

HARDINESS
Perennial in zones 3 to 8

TIME TO PLANT
Spring

TIME TO HARVEST
Spring

LOCATION
Full to part sun

SOIL TYPE
Rich, moist, well-drained

Rhubarb stalks are tasty, but their leaves can be deadly! The foliage of rhubarb is toxic: Not only should it never be eaten, but you shouldn't even throw the leaves in the composter.

etable garden. In addition to its valuable stalks and roots, rhubarb also makes a scene with its dramatic foliage, and its seed heads offer ornamental interest, too.

Common Varieties: My favourites include 'Victoria', 'Timperley Early', 'Hawke's Champagne', 'Crimson Red', 'Canada Red', and 'Strawberry'.

PLANT

Rhubarb grows from "crowns," or segments of rhizome (root) removed from parent plants. Each crown should be firm and have one to three eyes, or reddish buds.

Plant the crowns in spring as soon as the ground is workable. Dig a hole 30 to 60 cm (1 to 2 feet) deep and 60 cm (2 feet) in diameter. Add composted manure to the bottom of the planting hole. Backfill with more compost and soil, placing the crown in the centre of the hole, covering the buds with 2 to 3 cm (¾ to 1 ¼ inches) of soil. Water deeply and infrequently until established. Soil should be kept moist.

Do not plant rhubarb in containers.

GROW

Rhubarb is disease- and insect-resistant, requiring only occasional watering and fertilizing. Feed the plant in midsummer by adding a layer of composted manure around the crowns.

Remove the flower stalks as they appear, and in late summer keep the plants clean by removing dead leaves and any surrounding weeds.

Monitor regularly for yellowing or dead leaves and remove them as they appear. If the entire plant shows signs of wilting or yellowing, remove and destroy the crown—this is called crown rot. Don't plant rhubarb in this location for several years.

Divide or trim rhubarb every 3 to 5 years or when the foliage appears to weaken. Segments can be removed from the parent using a sharp knife or spade and planted elsewhere.

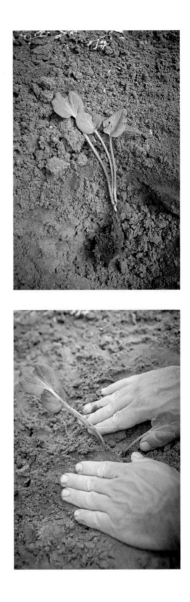

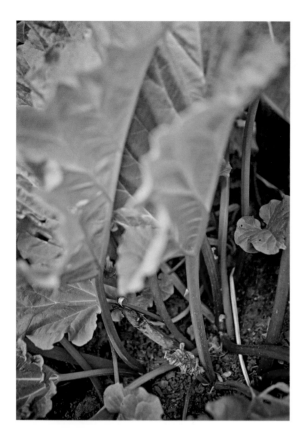

HARVEST

Do not harvest rhubarb stalks in the first year: The foliage will help support the roots, producing increased yields for future years.

In subsequent years, once stalks measure 30 cm (1 foot) they are ready for harvest, in mid- to late spring. Slide your thumb down the inner groove of the stalk as far as it will go toward the ground. Grasp, twist, and tug upward. The stalk will separate from the crown. Do not overharvest: Take only one-third of the stalks per harvest.

STORE

Rhubarb can be used fresh or frozen. Store fresh rhubarb with the base wrapped in aluminum foil in the refrigerator for up to 2 weeks. To freeze, chop the stalks, arrange the pieces in a single layer on a baking sheet lined with wax paper, and freeze. Once frozen, transfer the pieces to a resealable bag. Rhubarb will keep in the freezer for up to 9 months. You can also preserve rhubarb in jams.

Put It to Work

Sluggish digestion? Try cinnamon rhubarb compote!
This delicious compote is the perfect complement to yogurt, cereal, or pancakes.

> *4 cups chopped fresh rhubarb*
> *¼ cup water*
> *½ cup liquid honey*
> *½ cup golden raisins*
> *½ cup granulated sugar*
> *1 tbsp finely chopped gingerroot*
> *¼ tsp ground cinnamon*

Combine all of the ingredients in a saucepan and simmer for 10 to 15 minutes or until the rhubarb is soft. Let cool. Store in an airtight container in the refrigerator for up to 2 weeks.

Bloated? Try this safe laxative!
Rhubarb tea has many health-promoting ben-

efits, but above all it's a seriously powerful laxative. It will also act as a diuretic, so it can strengthen the kidneys. However, you should not use this tea for longer than 2 weeks at a time because you can develop dependence.

4 stalks rhubarb
2 cups boiling water
¼ cup psyllium husk
1 tbsp blackstrap molasses
1 cup cold water

In a blender, combine the rhubarb and boiling water and blend on medium-low speed until smooth. Add the psyllium husk, blackstrap molasses, and cold water. Pulse for 15 to 30 seconds to combine. Drink immediately. Do not exceed 2 drinks daily.

Gingivitis? Rinse with rhubarb!
If you suffer from inflamed gums, the answer to your problems might be to rinse nightly with rhubarb. Rhubarb contains powerful astringents and antioxidants that can strengthen your gums and reduce inflammation.

Place 4 cups of chopped rhubarb in a resealable glass jar (like a Mason jar). Pour in enough vodka or brandy (at least 80 proof) to cover the rhubarb completely. Place wax paper over the jar and then tightly screw the lid on to seal it. Shake well. Set aside in a cool, dark place for 2 weeks.

After 2 weeks, cover the mouth of the jar with a coffee filter or cheesecloth and strain the liquid into a sterile jar with a tight-fitting lid (discard solids).

Swish ½ ounce in your mouth for 1 minute every night before bed after brushing your teeth and flossing your gums. The infusion will keep in a cool, dark place for up to 4 months.

» Fast Forward

Fast forward to the health food store to purchase Herb Pharm's rhubarb tincture or equivalent. Follow the instructions on the label.

! Cautions

Remember, the leaves of rhubarb are toxic and must be avoided.

Occasionally, ingesting rhubarb can cause severe abdominal cramping, but this can often be alleviated by reducing the dose.

Rhubarb is a diuretic and can cause potassium loss, so it should not be taken in combination with cardiac medications, cathartics, steroids, or other diuretics or laxatives. Although it was formerly indicated for kidney stones, those with a history of this condition should actually avoid it because its oxalic acid may in fact cause kidney stones.

Avoid during pregnancy (it's a uterine stimulant).

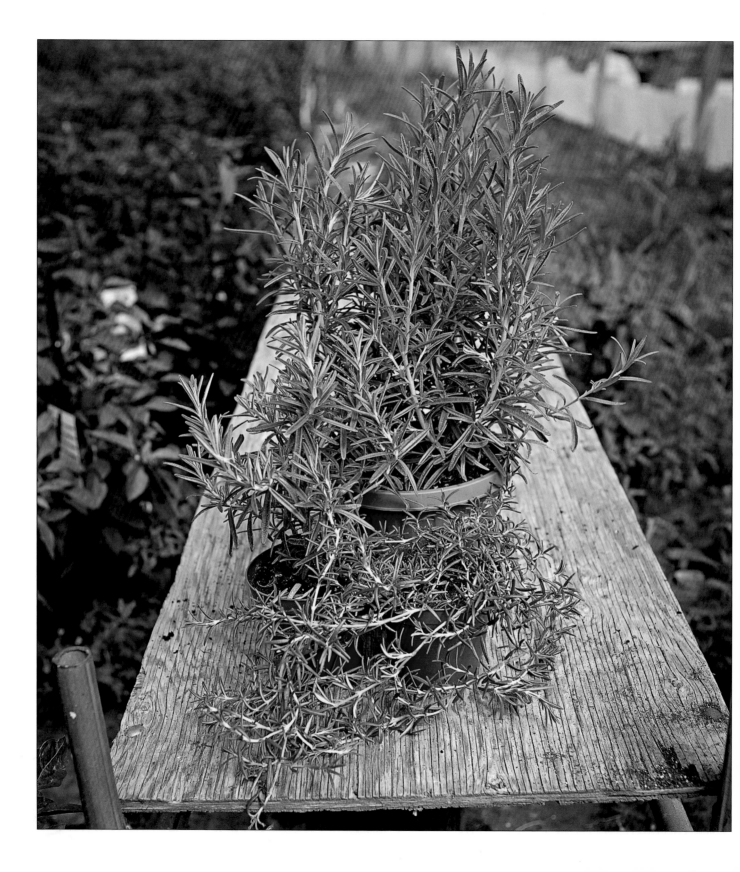

Rosemary

Rosemary is part of the mint family (*Lamiaceae*) and is native to the Mediterranean region, where it is popular as a spice for meats such as lamb and chicken. Its aroma is potent and unmistakeable: a mix of eucalyptus and pine trees on a rainy morning with a juniper finish. Rosemary is known as a powerful antioxidant, and it is used today by the food industry not only as a flavouring, but also as a preservative.

Health Benefits

Rosemary is a versatile plant in botanical medicine. Historically it was known as the "herb of remembrance" for its ability to help with memory. It has also been used to treat kidney stones and painful menstruation, to relieve symptoms caused by respiratory disorders, and even to stimulate the growth of hair. Extracts of rosemary are also used in aromatherapy to treat anxiety-related conditions and increase alertness.

Rosemary has a number of beneficial compounds, including eucalyptol (also called cineole), which is considered to have potent antibacterial effects and may relax smooth muscles in the lungs. Another ingredient of rosemary, known as carnosol, has been shown to inhibit cancer in some animal studies. These compounds have powerful antioxidant properties and are under investigation as potential therapies for liver toxicity, inflammatory conditions, and cancer.

The herb can even be used to help prevent cancer by adding it to your meat and veggies before you grill them. Consuming anything charred (especially meat grilled on the barbecue) can contribute to colon cancer because polycyclic aromatic hydrocarbons (PAHs) are produced from the combustion of organic material. However, studies show that if you first spice up your meat with rosemary, the antioxidants in the herb can help neutralize the PAHs.

Growing

The grey-green foliage of rosemary makes it attractive and fragrant in the herb garden—and best of all, it's great with chicken! Skilled gardeners can even shape some varieties of rosemary into attractive topiaries and hedges. Rosemary is not a particu-

DIFFICULTY
Medium

HARDINESS
Treat as annual (perennial in zones 7 to 10)

TIME TO PLANT
Spring

TIME TO HARVEST
Late spring through early fall

LOCATION
Full sun

SOIL TYPE
Well-drained

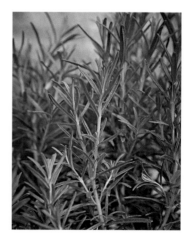

larly easy herb to grow in some climates, however; it won't survive frost, it does poorly if you bring it indoors in winter, and it's vulnerable to mildew.

Common Varieties: There are many cultivars of *Rosmarinus officinalis*. One of the hardiest is 'Arp', which is also excellent for cooking. 'Spice Islands' is a tasty variety that can be trained into a topiary. 'Prostratus' is a creeping variety. Other popular cultivars include 'Miss Jessopp's Upright', 'Tuscan Blue', 'Albus' (white rosemary), and 'Majorca Pink'.

PLANT

Rosemary can be grown from seed or stem cuttings, but I wouldn't recommend either. The best way to add rosemary to your herb garden is to purchase a transplant in spring from a garden centre or even a grocery store. Look for healthy plants that are free of mould, with lush greyish-green foliage. If any leaf drop is visible, do not purchase.

For best results, plant in full sun in spring after all risk of frost has passed. You can grow rosemary in the garden or in containers, but it tends to do poorly indoors. Rosemary will grow in most soils as long as there is good drainage. It can thrive even in poor, rocky soils, but it hates clay. If you plant it in containers, use a potting soil or a soilless mix.

GROW

The number 1 killer of any rosemary plant is overwatering. Only water when the soil is completely dry.

The other key to growing rosemary successfully is pinching. It needs to be regularly pruned or the result is a thin, sad-looking herb. Regularly pinch off the new growth tips, removing up to 5 cm (2 inches) at a time to promote happy, healthy, and busy rosemary!

Rosemary's biggest threat is mildew, which is often the result of several days of rain. Once mildew takes hold of rosemary, your

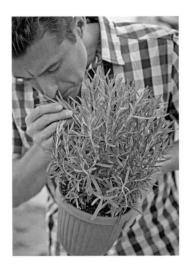

Rosemary trees have become a popular gift at Christmas. Rosemary is an evergreen that can be easily shaped, and it looks great with holiday decorations. But a rosemary tree will only be happy indoors for about 10 to 14 days before it begins to yellow, and it will usually die within 30 days. The reason for its short life is the dryness of our homes. Rosemary is a Mediterranean plant that likes "dry feet," but it also enjoys the humidity it would get from the ocean in its natural setting. Adding a humidifier will help, but don't water the tree unless it is completely dry.

chances of bringing it back are slim. As soon as you see stems with a white substance on them, remove and discard them. Before touching the remaining plant, wash your hands and wipe your scissors or pruners with bleach. You can help prevent mildew by improving the air circulation around the plants: Keep the surrounding garden weed-free and do not overplant.

HARVEST

You can harvest rosemary plants the day you buy them—indeed, the newest growth often gives the best flavour.

Never overharvest: Don't remove more than one-third of the plant at any given time. Harvest after the morning dew has evaporated, and choose a dry day. Just clip what you need using scissors or shears. I recommend wearing gloves, because the leaves have a sappy residue that will stick to your hands when collecting larger batches.

STORE

Rosemary is best used fresh and can last a long time after being pinched from the plant. I recommend storing it with the cut stems in a glass of water on the counter (only the stems should be in the water, not the leaves). Rosemary can also be dried by hanging small bundles in a dark, dry, warm place or by using drying trays (see "Drying Herbs at Home" on page 365). Rosemary is dry when both the stems and leaves are brittle. Store dried rosemary in airtight containers.

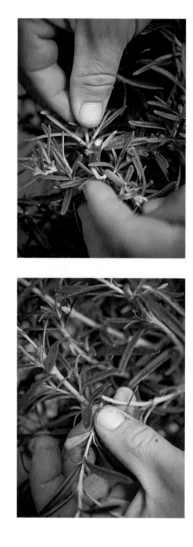

🛠 Put It to Work

Exam time? Have a rosemary bath!
The ancient Greeks swore by the power of rosemary as a memory aid. The sharp, camphorous odour of rosemary can make for a soothing bath the night before a big exam. Finely chop 4 to 5

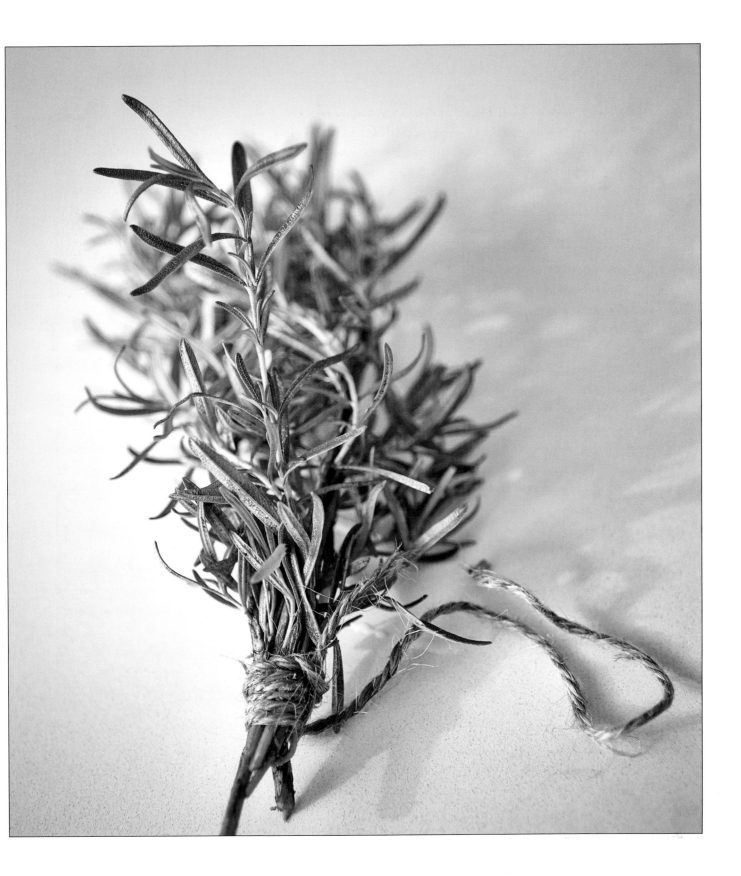

sprigs of rosemary, tie up in cheesecloth (to make a kind of tea bag), and add to a hot bath with 1 cup of Epsom salts (if you have them). Don't get your cheat sheets wet while you study them once more by candlelight. Good luck!

Thinning hair? Rub on the rosemary oil!

Theoretically, rosemary oil may help promote hair growth by promoting cell division, dilating blood vessels, and stimulating hair follicles. There are few known balding remedies that actually work, but rosemary may at least improve circulation in the head and nourish hair follicles. In a blender, blend 3 sprigs of fresh rosemary leaves with ½ cup of olive oil until well combined. Strain using a coffee filter or fine-mesh sieve into a sterile glass jar with a tight-fitting lid (discard solids). Apply immediately to thinning hair and leave in for 1 hour before using a natural tea tree shampoo to rinse off.

Poor circulation in the feet? Wear rosemary to bed!

Rub rosemary oil (recipe above) into your feet 20 minutes before bed. Cover with a pair of wool socks. The phytochemicals and antioxidants in the rosemary oil will increase circulation to your feet and also deal with any fungus that lurks between your toes!

Menstrual headache? Switch out aspirin for rosemary tea!

Headaches during the menstrual cycle can be overwhelming, so you'll need more than just your average tea. This calls for every bit of rosemary's medicinal power!

Place dried rosemary in a mortar and pestle and grind it into a powder. (You can also use a clean coffee or spice grinder.) In a mug, combine 1 tablespoon of the powdered rosemary with 1 cup of boiling water, whisk, cover, and steep for 30 minutes. Strain using a fine-mesh sieve. Drink every 2 to 3 hours as needed. People around you may ask where the lamb and potatoes are roasting, but at least you won't have a headache!

» Fast Forward

Fast forward to the health food store to purchase Genestra's Rosemary Young Shoot Liquid or equivalent. Follow the instructions on the label.

! Cautions

Avoid if you have a known allergy to rosemary or other plants in the mint family (*Lamiaceae*).

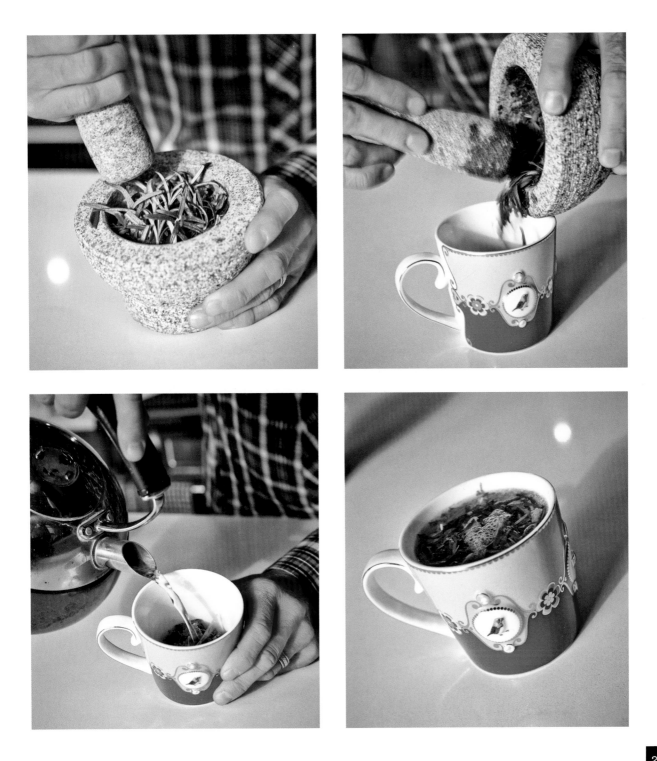

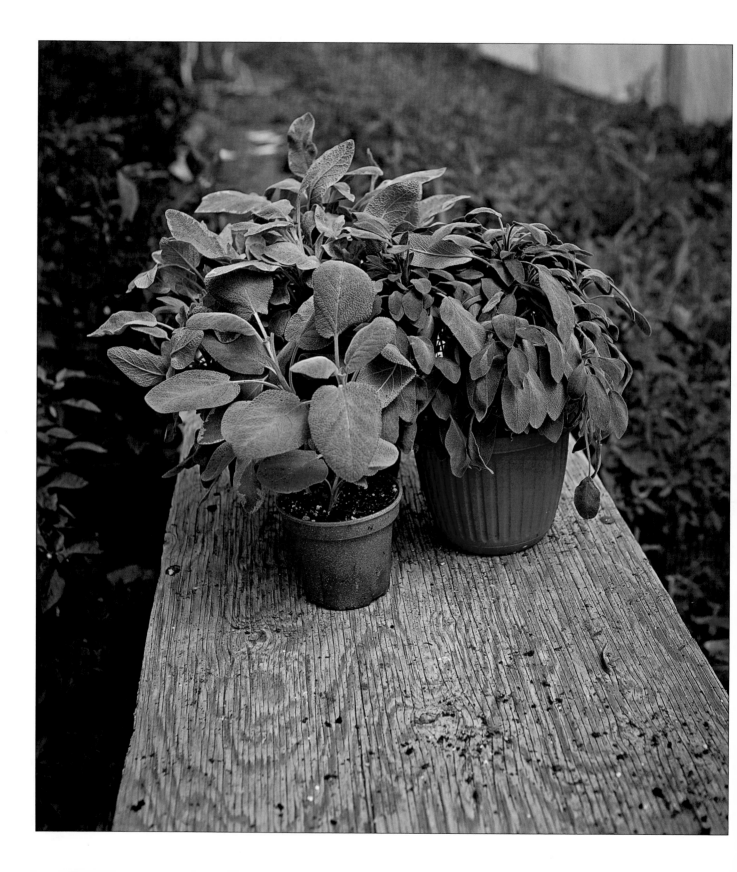

Sage

If you're going to Scarborough Fair, sage is right there alongside parsley, rosemary, and thyme. In fact, these four herbs are the most popular on your typical spice rack. They have stood the test of time not only because of their flavours, but also due to their anti-inflammatory, antioxidant, and anti-cancer properties. If you're looking for some sage advice: Grow and consume this herb! Sage is one of the many medicinal *Salvias* that belong to the mint family (*Lamiaceae*). Common sage (*S. officinalis*) bears pretty blue-purple flowers and aromatic leaves. If you're having a hard time placing its taste or smell, think of the dominant flavour of Thanksgiving turkey stuffing.

⊕ Health Benefits

Many people make their own echinacea extract (see page 108) when they feel a cold coming on. If you're coming down with a sore throat, the first thing to do right after you've taken your echinacea is to chew some tender sage leaves for their juice, which will numb the soreness of your throat and speed healing.

Sage is also used in reducing excessive perspiration, including sweat caused by menopausal hot flashes.

The plant has also been used for centuries with the intention of improving memory, and more recently it has garnered interest as a possible treatment for Alzheimer's disease. In a recent study, 30 people with moderate Alzheimer's took sage or a placebo over 4 months. In the end, those who took sage improved significantly. Sage may help prevent the breakdown of acetylcholine, a neurotransmitter that plays a role in the disease.

🌱 Growing

Sage has become one of my favourite plants in the garden. I don't just love it for its flavour and its medicinal benefits: I love sage for its foliage. Whether in the garden or in pots, this large leafy herb offers all-season interest. Sages are one of the showiest of all herbs, with vibrant flowers of various colours (usually purple or blue). This perennial evergreen herb is adored not only by gardeners but also by bees, butterflies, and hummingbirds.

Common Varieties: There are countless *Salvia* species, but most are ornamental; for culinary and medicinal use, look for *S. officinalis*. One of my favourite varieties is 'Tricolor', which has silver-green leaves trimmed in white and tinted with purple. 'Purpurascens', or purple sage, is not as hardy and not as useful as a spice, but looks great in the garden.

DIFFICULTY
Easy

HARDINESS
Perennial in zones 5 to 9

TIME TO PLANT
Spring

TIME TO HARVEST
Late spring through fall

LOCATION
Full sun

SOIL TYPE
Moist, well-drained

PLANT

Sage can be started from seed or grown from cuttings that take 4 to 6 weeks to root. But for those looking for an easy growing experience, I recommend transplants. The range of leaf colours available increases every year, and you may be tempted to try something exotic, but good old common sage still rules. It's available everywhere, and it's the easiest to grow.

Plant sage in full sun, either in a container or in the garden: Just make sure drainage is good. Use potting soil in a container, and in a garden use good compost or triple mix. If your soil is rich, sage rarely requires fertilizer. I recommend feeding only if plants appear weak or lacking in vibrant leaf colour. In a pot, sage should be fertilized once or twice a month using compost tea, fish emulsion, or a general-purpose fertilizer (20-20-20).

Sage is a good companion to many vegetables. Planting it close to carrots, cabbage, strawberries, and tomatoes may help to improve their overall growth.

GROW

If you can't grow sage you might want to give up on gardening! If you forget a watering, it will forgive you. If you forget to fertilize, it will forgive you. If you forget to pinch it, you can just do it later and your sage will bounce back.

Sage will suffer in wet soils and eventually get root rot, so do not overwater. The plant will become woody over time, and it does benefit from aggressive cutting back and dividing. Perennial sages should be divided every 2 to 4 years or when plants appear weak.

To promote overall health, pinch it back during the growing season, even if you don't need the herb. The plant will improve every "pinch" of the way!

Insects to watch out for include aphids, whiteflies, and thrips; control using insecticidal soaps.

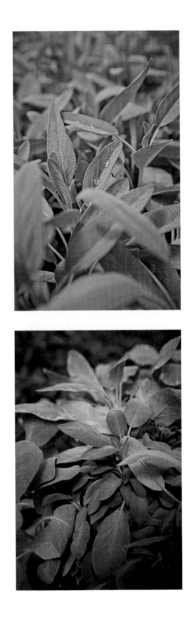

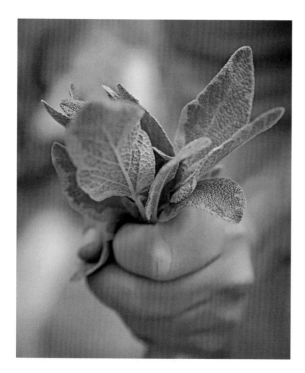

HARVEST

Sage can be harvested during the entire growing season. Cut the tender new foliage first (the newest leaves will be lighter in colour). Clip the leaves during mid-morning after heavy dew has dried. Do not cut the woody stem, as new leaves will grow on it. And be careful not to impact the main stem of the plant, known as the crown.

During the fall you can aggressively remove most of the plant, but never harvest more than one-third of the plant on any given day. The goal is to allow your sage to rebound with more growth and more leaves for future harvests.

STORE

Sage can be used fresh or dried. I recommend storing fresh sage with the cut stems in a glass of water on the counter (only the stems should be in the water, not the leaves); it will keep for up to 10 days. To dry your sage, tie it in small, loose bundles. Cover with a paper bag with some slits cut in the sides for improved airflow. Hang the bags in a dark, dry, warm location for up to 2 weeks or until the leaves become brittle. Once they're dry, remove the leaves and discard the stems. Store the leaves in an airtight container in a cool, dry place. (See "Drying Herbs at Home" on page 365.)

Put It to Work

Hot flashes or excessive perspiration?
Salvia salvation!

Menopause is not a disease and cannot be prevented, but many of its symptoms—which are related to hormonal changes—can be mitigated. Hot flashes and night sweats can both be reduced with sage.

In a teapot, combine 2 cups of dried sage leaves with boiling water. Cover and steep for 30 minutes (to make it very strong). Pour into a BPA-free ice-cube tray and freeze. Add 2 to 3 ice cubes to your lemonade, water, or even beer before bed. You'll be feeling better in minutes and experience fewer night sweats.

If you are an excessive sweater (a condition called hyperhidrosis), consuming 6 to 8

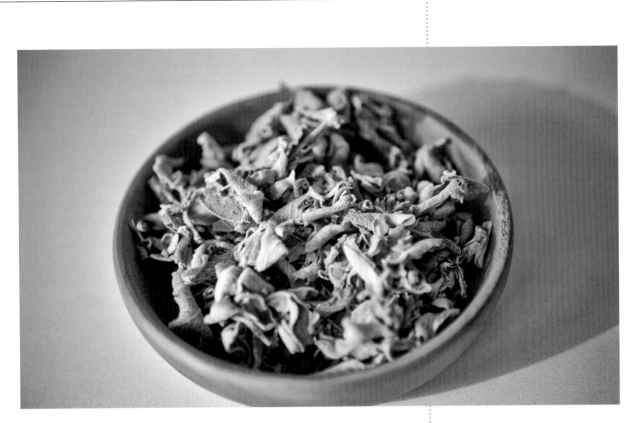
Dried sage leaves.

ice cubes per day in several doses can reduce the amount of perspiration you produce.

Alzheimer's prevention? A sage infusion!
Historically, a sage infusion was thought to help with memory loss. Now researchers are proving it. Alzheimer's prevention seems to be strongly linked to a diet high in antioxidants, including herbs, spices, fruits, and veggies that manage inflammation. Sage and these other foods may guard against low levels of the neurotransmitter acetylcholine, which is related to the loss of brain function in someone with Alzheimer's.

Perhaps you're already taking fish oil for cognitive enhancement, or just because you know how amazing it is in the prevention of many diseases. But there is something even better: You can supplement with sage-infused squid oil!

Squid oil is high in DHA, the omega-3 essential fatty acid most important in cognitive support. Wild squid is one of the richest sources of this compound—it contains 35% more omega-3 than wild salmon. This super-sustainable source of omega-3s is the way to go for Alzheimer's prevention and support.

Pick ½ cup of sage leaves from the garden. Wash and lay out on paper towel to dry overnight. The following morning, combine the contents of a 200 mL bottle of squid oil (I recommend Ascenta DHA oil) with the sage leaves in a blender. Blend on high speed until smooth. Pour into a resealable glass jar (like a Mason jar). Refrigerate for 1 week. Using a funnel lined with a coffee filter, strain the mixture into a sterile bottle with a tight-fitting lid (discard solids).

Take 1 teaspoon twice daily. The infusion will keep in the refrigerator for up to 1 month.

Sore throat? Spray sage!

Sage is excellent for a sore throat for many reasons: It can help numb the inflamed area, and it also has antiviral properties. You can gargle with a sage tincture or, even better, spray it at the back of your throat at the first sign of a cold.

Collect a few handfuls of sage leaves from your garden. Wash, pat dry, and lay out to dry overnight. The following morning, roughly chop the leaves (1) and place in a resealable glass jar (like a Mason jar) (2). Pour vodka (at least 80 proof) into the jar until it covers the sage (3, 4, 5). Place wax paper over the jar and then screw the lid on tightly to seal it. Set aside in a cool, dark place for 2 weeks, shaking the jar vigorously once daily to mix the ingredients (6).

After 2 weeks, cover the mouth of the jar with a coffee filter or cheesecloth and strain the liquid into a clean glass container (discard solids). Use a funnel to transfer the tincture into small sterile bottles equipped with a spray pump.

At the first sign of a sore throat, spray 3 to 4 pumps into the back of your throat. The tincture will keep for up to 3 years stored in a cool, dry place.

» Fast Forward

Fast forward to the health food store to purchase A. Vogel's sage tablets or equivalent. Follow the instructions on the label.

! Cautions

Do not use sage if you are pregnant or breastfeeding. Thujone, one of its active ingredients, can stimulate the uterus in pregnant women, as well as dry up milk supply in nursing mothers.

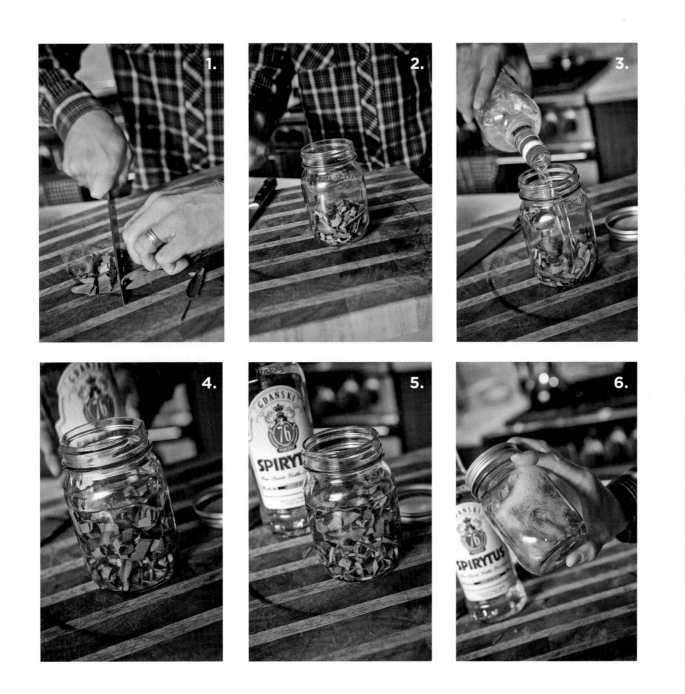

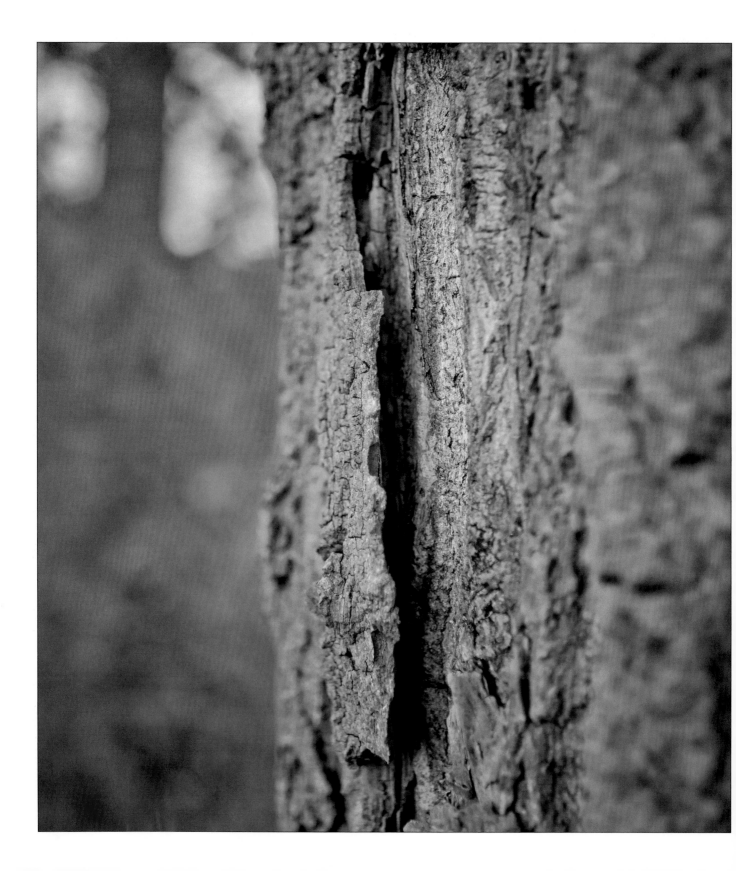

Slippery Elm

Slippery elm is a tall tree native to eastern North America; it can grow up to 18 metres (60 feet) tall. It gets its name from the thick "mucilage" of its inner bark, which can be made into a porridge—in fact, George Washington's soldiers apparently lived off the stuff for 12 days during a bitter winter in the American Revolutionary War. The inner bark has also been used as an herbal medicine for centuries by Native American healers. Also known as red elm, this species is less prone to Dutch elm disease than its larger cousin, the American elm (*Ulmus americana*), but it's not immune. It also contends with other pests that make it a rather challenging tree to grow.

Health Benefits

The inner bark of slippery elm has been used to treat a multitude of ailments, including skin abrasions, ulcers, eye injuries, and coughs, as well as to manage inflammation of the urinary tract, digestive system, skin, and mucous membranes. Poultices made from slippery elm bark can be applied to bruises and black eyes, and are often recommended to treat minor burns and abrasions.

Research on slippery elm's active constituents suggests it contains antioxidants that reduce inflammation in the digestive tract as well as immune-boosting properties. It isn't digested by the body, but the mucilage works by coating and soothing the digestive tract, absorbing toxins, softening waste, and supporting the growth of friendly bacteria in the gut.

Until the 1960s, elm bark was commonly used in mainstream medicine as a demulcent (a product used to soothe mucous membranes), an emollient (a skin softener), and a cough suppressant. Today the bark is powdered and included in herbal teas, throat lozenges, and poultices and taken in capsules and tablets. It is also one of the four ingredients in the popular herbal formula "Essiac" (see page 56).

Growing

Slippery elm is a large and attractive shade tree that can have a dramatic impact on a landscape. But while I love all elms, I recommend investigating Dutch elm disease in your area before planting one. Even if the disease isn't a problem in your area, you'll find slippery elm to be a high-maintenance tree. If you already have one on your property, cherish it and fight for it!

Common Varieties: Slippery elm, or red elm, is usually iden-

DIFFICULTY
Medium to hard

HARDINESS
Perennial in zones 3 and above

TIME TO PLANT
Spring or early fall

TIME TO HARVEST
Early spring

LOCATION
Full sun

SOIL TYPE
Moist, well-drained

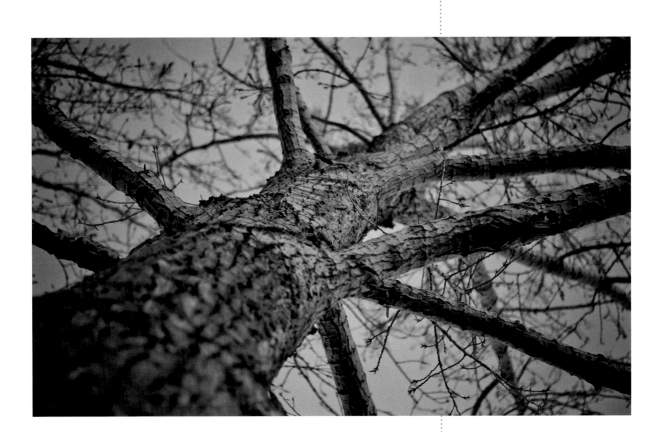

tified by the Latin name *Ulmus rubra*. However, in the context of herbal medicine slippery elm is sometimes called *U. fulva*. This is a synonym for the same species.

PLANT

If you choose to plant a slippery elm, remember it will eventually take up a huge amount of space: When mature it can reach 18 metres (60 feet) high and 12 metres (40 feet) wide.

Purchase healthy trees from a reputable nursery and ask about Dutch elm disease. Most nurseries will offer a 1-year guarantee.

Plant in spring or in early fall when the ground is workable. Choose a location with well-drained soil and full sun. Water deeply and frequently until established, then reduce watering. Some nurseries recommend using transplant fertilizer or root

When growing a vulnerable tree like slippery elm, enlist the help of an arborist, or tree doctor. Through careful pruning, feeding, and pest management, an arborist can help your tree stay healthy and prolong its life. An arborist will also inspect trees for dangers such as rubbing branches or rotted stems that can lead to property damage or injury.

stimulant to reduce shock and speed root establishment.

After you plant your new elm, stake it to prevent it from being uprooted during windstorms. Use two stakes (one on each side of the tree), and never secure the tree with material that can cut into the bark. Stiff wire shielded with a section of old rubber hose will work well.

GROW

While slippery elm is less susceptible to Dutch elm disease than American elm, it can be devoured by the elm leaf beetle. This insect (the larvae do the most damage) has few natural enemies and insecticides may not be effective against it. Your best bet is to wait out the infestation and minimize shock to the tree by continuing to water it regularly. Remove weeds or turf from the base so they won't compete with the tree for moisture.

Slippery elm requires occasional pruning, ideally in early spring: Just remove broken or dead stems, crossing branches, and any branches growing toward the centre of the tree.

HARVEST

When you prune your elm in the spring, that's the perfect time to harvest the inner bark. When pruning, use a sharp tool and ensure your cuts are clean. Pruning paste or pruning tape is not required, as the tree will heal itself.

Use a sharp knife to peel the bark away from the branches and cut deep enough to remove the green "slippery" substance along with it. That's the medicine!

STORE

Use sharp scissors or pruning shears to cut the bark into small pieces. Put the pieces on a drying tray in a cool, well-ventilated room for 2 to 3 weeks or until they're brittle. (Putting a fan on them speeds up the drying process.) You can also dry slippery elm with a food dehydrator. When the bark is dry, put the pieces in a clean coffee or spice grinder and grind them into a fine powder. Store the powder in an airtight container.

Put It to Work

Dealing with diaper rash? Bottoms up!

Diaper rash is most often caused by a yeast that loves a warm, moist environment. One of the best things you can do is ensure the child's bum gets ample air. Slippery elm can help, too. Simply mix three parts of your favourite diaper cream with 1 part slippery elm powder in a small glass container. Apply liberal amounts to the affected area, or on healthy skin to prevent rash.

Upset tummy? Soothe it with a smoothie!

Do you have diarrhea, cramping, or upset stomach? More than half of the world's population is lactose intolerant, so the last thing I'd suggest is conventional dairy ice cream. Try this instead: In a blender, combine 1 cup of rice ice cream, 1 banana, and 2 tablespoons of slippery elm powder and blend on high speed until smooth. Sip slowly. (If you have

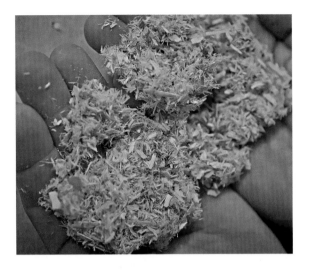
Dried bark ready to be ground into slippery elm powder.

very loose stools, consider the BRAT diet for 24 hours: bananas, rice, applesauce, toast. This smoothie qualifies as part of that diet.) If making for a child, halve the ingredients.

Battered and bruised? Try this poultice!
Whether you're banged, bumped, or bruised, this poultice can bring relief! In a bowl, mix 3 teaspoons of slippery elm powder with 1 ounce of boiling water. Let it cool. Spoon onto a piece of gauze, fold the gauze over, and apply to the affected area for 30 to 60 minutes. (Just one or two applications should help.) Never apply slippery elm to an open wound.

» Fast Forward

Fast forward to the health food store to purchase Mediherb's slippery elm capsules or equivalent. Follow the instructions on the label.

! Cautions

The Food and Drug Administration (FDA) in the United States recognizes slippery elm for its safety and efficacy. There have been no reports of serious side effects.

Topically, slippery elm extracts may cause dermatitis in some people who are allergic. However, usually the pollen, not the bark, is the allergen.

Slippery elm has been deemed safe even for use during pregnancy or breastfeeding, but always check with your doctor or healthcare specialist before using it.

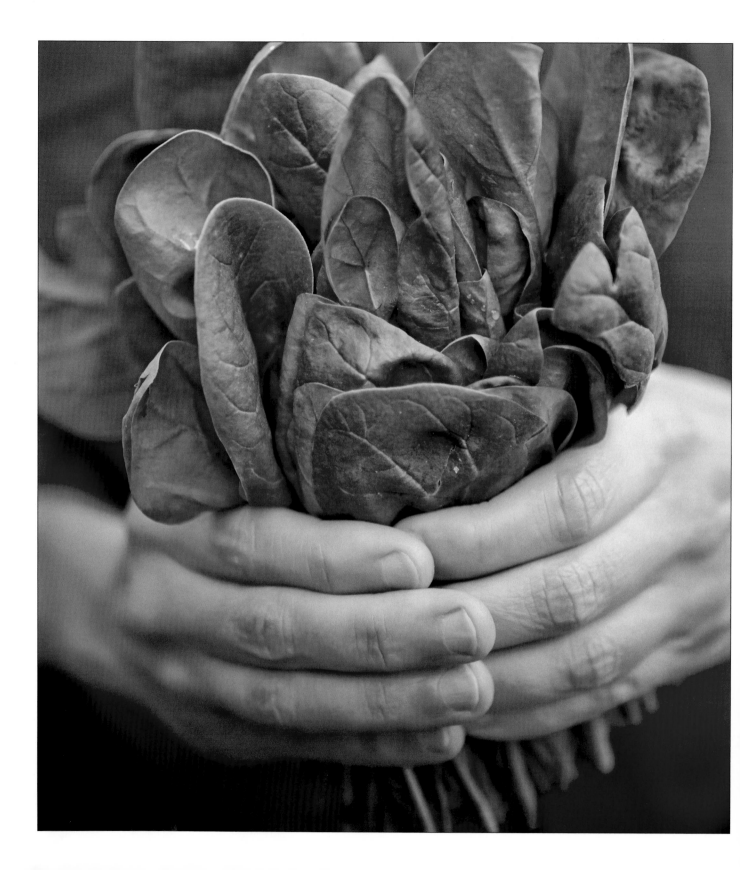

Spinach

Most of us remember the pleas from our parents and grandparents to "eat your spinach so you'll grow big and tall." They weren't far off. Spinach is one of the world's healthiest vegetables: It's packed with vitamins, minerals (especially iron and calcium), carotenoids (beta carotene, lutein, and zeaxanthin), fibre, and a host of other phytonutrients. Spinach is thought to have originated in ancient Persia and later been introduced to India and China. It probably made it to Europe sometime in the Middle Ages. By the 16th century, it reached the taste buds of Catherine de Medici, who left her home in Florence to marry the king of France. She supposedly was so addicted to spinach that she brought along her own cooks to prepare it. Ever since, anything prepared on a bed of spinach is referred to as " à la Florentine."

⊕ Health Benefits

Good food is medicine, and spinach is the perfect example. Studies suggest this leafy green vegetable has anti-cancer, antioxidant, and anti-inflammatory properties. Spinach may also reduce your chance of cataracts and loss of eyesight as you age.

Popeye maintained his strength eating spinach (and spitting out the can), but what the cartoon didn't show you was that he was also protecting himself against inflammation, oxidative stress-related problems, heart disease, bone problems, and cancers at the same time!

🌱 Growing

Spinach is a sure sign of spring! Fast to germinate from seed, it's one of the first crops ready for harvest in the vegetable garden. The only difficulty is that spinach doesn't enjoy extreme heat: It's a crop that loves short days and cool temperatures. But plan your planting carefully and you'll be able to enjoy spinach for much of the growing season.

Common Varieties: Spinach varieties fall into three categories: smooth leaf, savoy (which have crinkly leaves), and semi-savoy. My favourites include 'Giant Nobel' and 'Olympia' (both smooth-leaf varieties), 'Bloomsdale' (a savoy), and 'Melody' (a semi-savoy).

PLANT

Spinach should only be grown from seed. For the best selection, purchase the seeds in late winter. Sow them as soon as the soil is workable in early spring: Use 12 to 15 seeds per 30 cm (1 foot) of row, and plant rows 30 to 60 cm (1 to 2 feet) apart. Lightly cover with soil. When the plants are 3 to 5 cm (1¼ to 2 inches) tall, thin

DIFFICULTY
Easy

HARDINESS
Annual

TIME TO PLANT
Early spring and late summer (use succession planting)

TIME TO HARVEST
Spring, early summer, fall

LOCATION
Full to part sun

SOIL TYPE
Rich, moist, well-drained

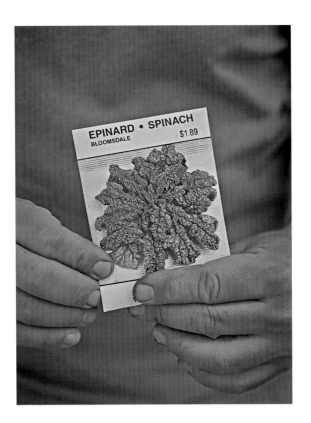

Bloomsdale is an easy-to-find spinach variety—and one of my favourites.

For small spaces, spinach can be grown in containers when temperatures are cool in early spring and early fall.

Heat accelerates the life cycle of spinach, causing it to bolt. That's another way of saying it will go to seed. You can't prevent this from happening, but if you live in warmer climates you can purchase hybrid spinach varieties that are slow to bolt, such as 'Olympia'. These varieties are also good if you want to try for a summer harvest.

GROW

Spinach likes cool nights, warm days, and adequate rain, so it's easy to grow in spring. The difficulty begins when evening temperatures go on the rise and rain is minimal. During dry periods, water spinach deeply in the morning.

Spinach enjoys rich soil, so if plants appear light green and are growing slowly, you need to fertilize with compost tea, fish emulsion, or general-purpose garden fertilizer (10-10-10).

Fungal diseases and blight are common with some varieties of spinach, especially during lengthy periods of wet or humid weather. Look for spinach varieties resistant to mould, and make sure the soil is well drained.

Spinach is loved by furry friends like groundhogs, rabbits, and mice. You can discourage them with a plastic owl, cayenne pepper, or dog hair. The key is to figure out what the animal doesn't like to see, smell, hear, touch, or taste. In extreme cases, you may need

them so the remaining plants are 5 to 10 cm (2 to 4 inches) apart. (If you don't thin them, don't worry. You'll still be okay!) Make sure the plants get plenty of sun and rich, moist soil. Add some composted manure if necessary.

Spinach is a fast grower: From sowing to harvest takes only about 40 days. To get multiple harvests, plan on succession planting (planting small batches at 14-day intervals). Since spinach hates the heat, it's best to halt sowing in late spring and then start again in late summer for a fantastic fall harvest.

a fence. If the problem is rabbits, the fence needs to be buried at least 40 cm (16 inches) deep—rabbits dig!

Spinach rarely needs to be weeded. In fact, because of its shallow roots, any heavy cultivation should be avoided.

HARVEST

Timing is key when harvesting spinach: If you wait too long, the plant will bolt or the leaves will have a bitter taste. Harvest spinach as soon as its rosettes have 5 or 6 leaves. (Spinach harvested before this is known as baby spinach, and it has a sweeter flavour.)

You have two options: For a continual harvest, use a pair of scissors to cut the outer, older leaves first, allowing inner leaves to mature. For a full harvest, cut the whole plant off at the base. Often this will stimulate more growth and lead to another harvest in the future.

The best time for harvesting spinach is mid-morning or late afternoon.

STORE

Spinach will keep in the refrigerator for up to 10 days. Loosely bundle stems together, wrap with a paper towel, and place in a resealable bag. Handle it gently and do not store anything on top of it—spinach bruises easily.

To freeze spinach, steam or sauté it first, then chop it and store in airtight containers in the freezer.

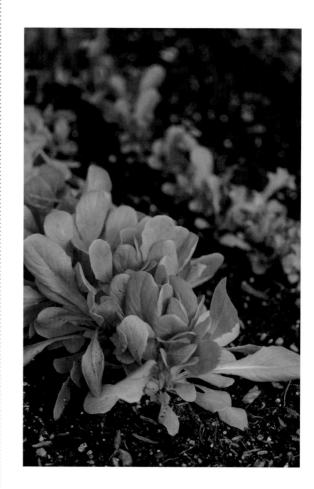

Put It to Work

Want to lock in the goodness? Boil it!

It turns out Popeye's habit of eating cooked spinach was actually healthier than eating it raw. There's nothing wrong with a baby spinach salad, but steaming or boiling spinach is even better. This vegetable contains a high concentration of oxalic acid, which can leach minerals from your body. Even "flash-boiling"

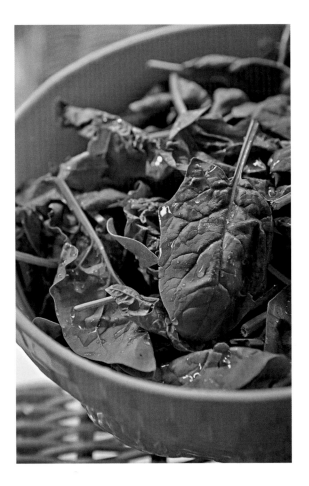

Weak bones? Spinach sauté!

Spinach is an excellent source of vitamin K, magnesium, manganese, and calcium, all of which are extremely good for bone health. It is also an excellent vegetarian source of muscle-building protein, energy-producing phosphorus, and vitamin B1. Here's a simple way to go green.

2 large bunches spinach
2 tbsp extra virgin olive oil
3 cloves garlic, chopped
Sea salt

In a skillet over medium heat, heat the oil. Add the garlic and sauté for about 1 minute, until lightly browned. Add the spinach and stir to coat well. Cover the skillet and cook for 1 minute. Uncover and turn the spinach. Cover and cook for an additional minute. Season with salt to taste. Serve immediately.

Low energy? Spinach smoothie!

Spinach packs a heart-healthy punch of potassium, folate, and other B vitamins. And it doesn't stop there: It has a ton of energy-producing iron and the antioxidants lutein and zeaxanthin, as well as beta carotene, vitamin C, and vitamin E.

Dark green veggies are the most important item in your diet, and they provide you with energy to boot. But it can be a challenge to get Health Canada's recommended 4 servings every day. A smoothie is the perfect way

will help remove the oxalic acid while minimizing nutrient loss and preserving the flavour.

By quickly boiling spinach in large amounts of water (the same way you would pasta) you may reduce the oxalic acid by as much as 50%. Just bring a large pot of water to a rapid boil, add the spinach, and boil for 1 minute. Do not cover the pot (you'll release more of the acids with the rising steam). Drain and enjoy.

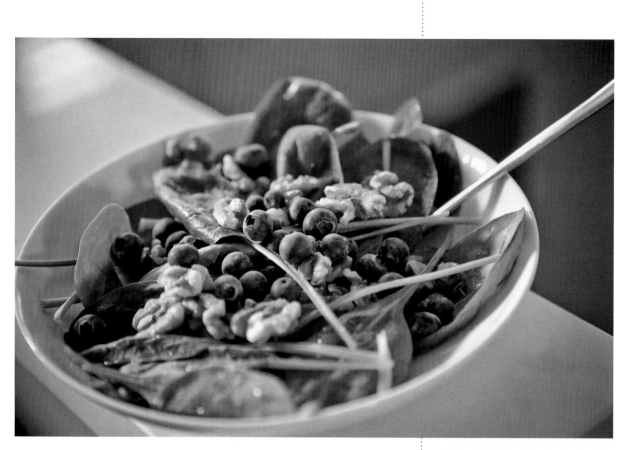

A simple baby spinach salad with blueberries and walnuts is another quick and easy way to add more healthy leafy greens to your diet.

to get a few servings into you. This isn't too different from a regular berry smoothie, so don't worry about the taste. Here's a tip: If you want to flash-boil your spinach for this smoothie, do a large amount ahead of time and then freeze it in BPA-free ice-cube trays.

1 cup spinach (fresh or flash-boiled)
1 cup blueberries (fresh or frozen)
½ cup raspberries (fresh or frozen)
½ cup blackberries (fresh or frozen)
½ cup freshly squeezed orange juice
1 tbsp plain low-fat yogurt

Combine all of the ingredients in a blender, add ice if desired, and blend on high speed until smooth. Makes 2 servings.

Aging too quickly? Antioxify!

"Antioxify" isn't a real word, of course, but it may as well be! There are countless creams, sunblocks, and makeup products claiming to rustproof and protect your skin from aging. But antioxidants work best from the inside out. That means eating spinach will do a lot more to prevent wrinkles than any cream you might put on your face. Spinach and many of its green allies will add years to your life! Enjoy this simple spinach soup.

3 cups vegetable broth
5 cups spinach
1 cup broccoli
1 cup green peas
1 sweet onion, quartered
3 cloves garlic
1 tbsp minced gingerroot
1 tsp ground turmeric
1 tsp ground coriander
1 tsp ground cumin
¼ tsp cayenne pepper (or to taste)
½ cup chopped fresh coriander leaves
2 tbsp extra virgin olive oil

In a high-speed blender or food processor, purée all of the ingredients. Pour into a saucepan over low heat and bring to a simmer. Serve hot.

» Fast Forward

Fast forward to the health food store to purchase Jarrow CarotenALL capsules or equivalent. Follow the instructions on the label.

! Cautions

Spinach is much loved by pests, so commercially grown crops may get a heavy spray of pesticide in the field. You will minimize health risks by avoiding store-bought spinach (or buying organic) and growing your own.

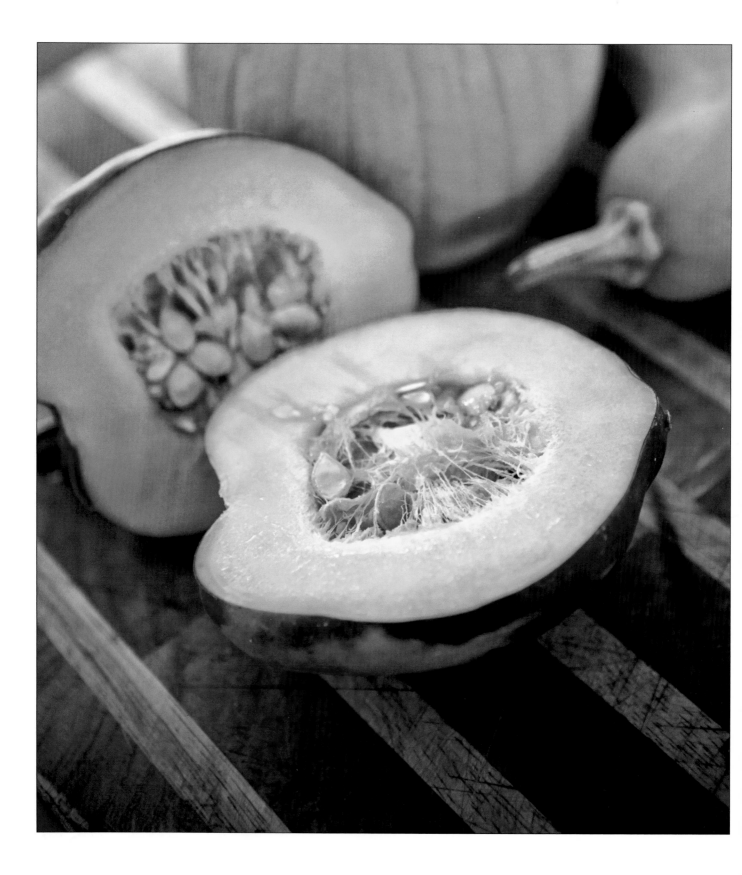

Squash

Squashes are a group of vegetables with an extraordinary variety of shapes, colours, textures, and tastes. You probably didn't know that orange pumpkins, green zucchini, and yellow spaghetti squash are all varieties of the same species: *Cucurbita pepo*. Other *Cucurbita* species give us butternut squash, Hubbard squash, and countless other cultivars. Summer squashes are delicious in soups or on the grill, while fall varieties are more likely to end up as ornamentals—either as Halloween jack-o-lanterns or in Thanksgiving pies. But you can enjoy their health benefits year-round.

Health Benefits

A simple way to determine the powerful health benefits of a squash is by the colour of its interior flesh. The darker and richer the colour, the higher the flesh will be in vitamin A, beta carotene, lutein, zeaxanthin, and other antioxidants. So choose butternut squash over zucchini.

Squash is particularly high in beta carotene, which is important for your eyes, lungs, heart, and immune system. Beta carotene is considered a provitamin because it can be converted to active vitamin A. Vitamin A deficiency leads to eye problems, abnormal bone development, disorders of the reproductive system, and untimely death. In just 1 cup of butternut squash, you're getting more than the recommended daily allowance of vitamin A!

New research also reveals that a type of carbohydrate found in squash is unusually high in pectin, which is linked to protection against diabetes, better balancing of blood sugar, and weight loss.

Growing

Squash is easy to grow. Given enough light and heat, one plant will produce a ton! The limiting factor is space; some varieties can take up entire backyards. So ask yourself two things: Do I have enough space? Do I need so many squash? I've seen a lot of friends bringing zucchini loaf to work—a sure sign of one too many plants!

Common Varieties: There are two main groupings: summer squash and winter squash. Summer squash (zucchini is the most popular example) grows on bush-type plants and is harvested before the rind hardens and the fruit matures. These should be

DIFFICULTY
Easy (if you have the space!)

HARDINESS
Annual

TIME TO PLANT
Spring

TIME TO HARVEST
Summer or fall (depends on variety)

LOCATION
Full sun

SOIL TYPE
Rich, moist, well-drained

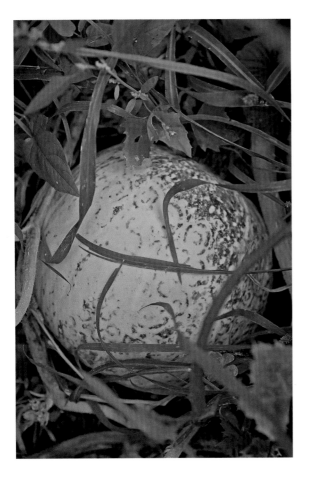

Squash needs space—especially between squash varieties. This picture is an example of what happens when you plant zucchini too close to pumpkins. Maybe we should call it a pumpkini?

eaten fresh. Winter squash (including butternut, acorn, spaghetti, and pumpkin) tend to grow on vine-like plants. They have tougher rinds and can generally be stored for several months.

PLANT

Both summer and winter squash can easily be grown from seed. If you start them indoors, sow them in pots using a seed-starting mix. Don't be too anxious: The seeds germinate very quickly (4 to 8 days), so approximately 2 to 3 weeks before last frost date is early enough. Alternatively, sow the seeds directly in the garden after the risk of frost.

If you're using transplants, remember squash despise the cold. Plant outdoors only after threat of frost has passed, and cover them on cold nights.

Squash love sun and heat, so plant in direct sun, protected from wind. The plants are heavy feeders, so I recommend amending the soil with manure before planting.

Follow seed packs for specific directions, but in general summer squash should be spaced 45 to 60 cm (18 to 24 inches) apart in rows 1 metre (3 feet) apart, with an average space of 0.8 square metres (9 square feet) per plant. Space winter squash 60 to 90 cm (24 to 36 inches) in rows 1 to 1.5 m (3 to 5 feet) apart, or with an average space of 1.4 to 1.8 square metres (15 to 20 square feet) per plant.

GROW

Help your squash grow with regular watering and occasional fertilizing. Only water the roots and avoid getting water on the foliage to minimize the risk of disease. Another way to avoid diseases like powdery mildew is to avoid handling squash when wet. Mulching helps, too, by maintaining moisture and preventing soil pathogens from splashing up on the foliage during heavy rain.

Not all insects in the garden are bad. In fact, squashes produce both male and female flowers and need bees to pollinate them. You can also hand-pollinate a squash bloom by taking a small brush and lightly moving from flower to flower.

After the blooms fall off, the plant will need a lot of nutrients. If your soil is poor, apply a compost tea or topdress with manure. Once the fruit has set (the blooms appear to fall off) and squash begin to form, remove any new blooms to focus energy on fruit production. (When winter squash vines measure 1.5 metre/5 feet, pinch off the leading tip to promote fruit-producing side shoots.) To avoid rot, place larger winter squash and pumpkins on a board, a flat rock, or some mulch.

Monitor often for the bad bugs, including squash vine borers, cucumber beetles, and whiteflies. You can help with an occasional spray of insecticidal soap. Another trick is to plant nasturtiums nearby: Insects will be kept busy eating them instead of your squash!

If some squash plants show signs of disease such as wilt, yellowing, and white powder on leaves, discard them to minimize the spread of disease.

HARVEST

Summer squashes like zucchini can be ready in as little as 40 to 50 days. Don't wait for them to grow too big; harvest while they are tender. The ideal length is about 15 to 20 cm (6 to 8 inches) with a diameter of 10 to 15 cm (4 to 6 inches). Harvesting before the fruit is fully mature will stimulate additional flower buds, leading to more harvests in the coming weeks.

Winter squash (such as acorn and butternut) must be fully vine-ripened before harvest. This takes almost double the time: An average of 80 to 100 days. Harvest in late summer or early fall when the vines start to yellow and die back. Choose a dry day and use a knife to remove the fruit from the vine. Set your harvested squash in the sun to help dry the stems. Be careful when handling squash to avoid bruising.

STORE

Summer squash is best enjoyed fresh (I love grilling it on the barbecue). It will keep in the refrigerator for up to 10 days. Squash can be preserved by freezing, drying, canning, pickling, or turning it into relish. For best results, blanch summer squash before drying or freezing. When freezing, slice squash into equal portions, arrange in a single layer on baking sheets, and freeze. Once frozen, transfer to resealable bags. To dry, use a dehydrator.

Do not wash winter squash if you're going to cold-store it! After the stems have turned grey in the sun, place the squash in a dry location with temperatures of 5° to 10°C (40° to 50°F), such as a cold room. It will keep for up to 5 months.

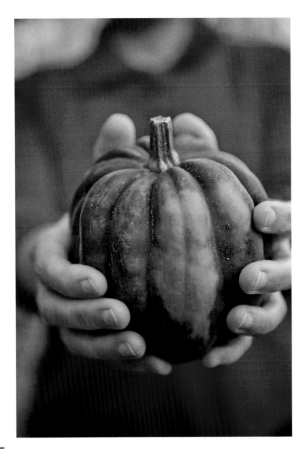

Put It to Work

Want an ACE up your sleeve? Deal with this squash soup!

You often hear about the virtues of vitamins C and D when it comes to your immune system. They are very important antioxidants and can help you thwart the next virus or bacterium that comes your way. But if you're "holding the ACEs," you stand an even better chance. That means getting a good level of vitamins A, C, and E from squash soup!

1 medium butternut squash or acorn
   squash or pumpkin
1 sweet onion
1 orange bell pepper
2 tbsp extra virgin olive oil
½ cup pure maple syrup
1 tsp sea salt
½ tsp freshly ground black pepper
¼ tsp ground cinnamon
¼ tsp ground nutmeg
2 cups boiling water
1 cube vegetable bouillon
Dollop low-fat sour cream
Chopped fresh parsley

Peel the squash, remove and discard the seeds, and chop into 2 cm cubes. Cut the onion and orange pepper into small pieces (about the same size as the squash). Arrange the vegetables in a single layer on a baking sheet.

In a small bowl, combine the oil, maple syrup, salt, pepper, cinnamon, and nutmeg. Drizzle evenly over the vegetables and toss to coat well. Bake, uncovered, in a preheated 200°C (400°F) oven for 20 minutes. Flip the vegetables, increase the temperature to 230°C (450°F), and bake for an additional 10 minutes or until dark golden brown.

Transfer the cooked vegetables to a blender, add the boiling water and stock cube, and blend on high speed until smooth. Pour into bowls while hot. Top with a dollop of low-fat sour cream and garnish with chopped fresh parsley, if desired.

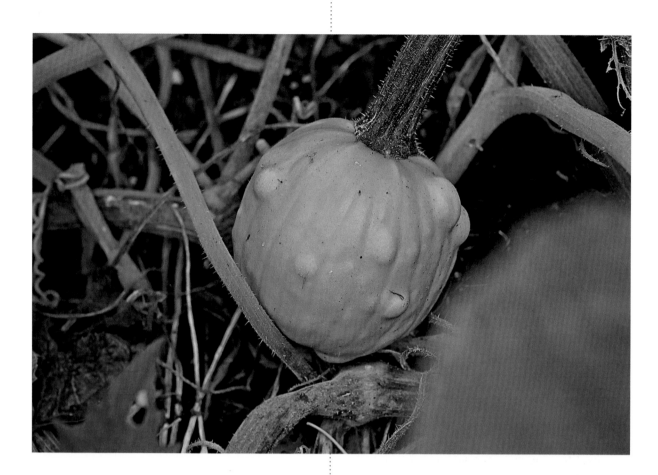

Looking for a healthy snack?
Try a squashsicle!

One of the best ways to sneak nutrients into a kid (or yourself!) is through a frozen treat. The cold on the tongue actually numbs the taste buds and decreases the odds that your olfactory bulb—responsible for so much of the taste experience—figures out that you're trying to sneak in some healthy vegetables! Try this orange and mango "squashsicle" instead of ice cream.

1 medium butternut squash, peeled, seeded, and cubed
2 cups freshly squeezed orange juice
2 cups mango purée
Freshly squeezed juice of 2 lemons
1 cup granulated sugar

In a saucepan of boiling water, cook squash for 20 minutes or until soft (a fork or knife should easily poke through). Strain and transfer the squash to a blender. Add the orange juice, mango, lemon juice, and sugar and blend on high speed until smooth. Pour into ice pop moulds and freeze.

High cholesterol? Try spaghetti squash and Brussels balls!

One thing we know for sure: A plant-based diet will lower your cholesterol and add years to your life! Instead of your typical refined white-flour pasta, why not try a baked spaghetti squash? And to replace your usual saturated-fat-laden meatballs, how about some garlic-roasted Brussels sprouts?

1 spaghetti squash
15 Brussels sprouts
¼ cup extra virgin olive oil
Sea salt and freshly ground black pepper
3 cloves garlic, minced
¼ cup slivered almonds
Grated Parmesan cheese

Cut the spaghetti squash in half. Using a spoon, scoop out the seeds and discard. Place the squash face down on a lightly oiled baking sheet. Place the Brussels sprouts on a separate baking sheet, drizzle with the oil, and season with salt and pepper to taste. Place both trays in a preheated 175°C (350°F) oven.

After 20 minutes, sprinkle the Brussels sprouts with the minced garlic and almond slivers, and roast for another 5 minutes. Remove from the oven, cover, and keep warm.

After 40 minutes, remove the squash from the oven and let it cool for 15 minutes. Using a fork, gently scoop out the squash strands, leaving as much intact as possible, and evenly divide among plates. Top with the Brussels sprouts, drizzle with olive oil, season with salt and pepper, and sprinkle with Parmesan. Enjoy immediately.

» Fast Forward

Fast forward to the health food store to purchase Natural Factors beta-carotene capsules or equivalent. Follow the instructions on the label.

! Cautions

You can enjoy squash with no concern about side effects or interactions.

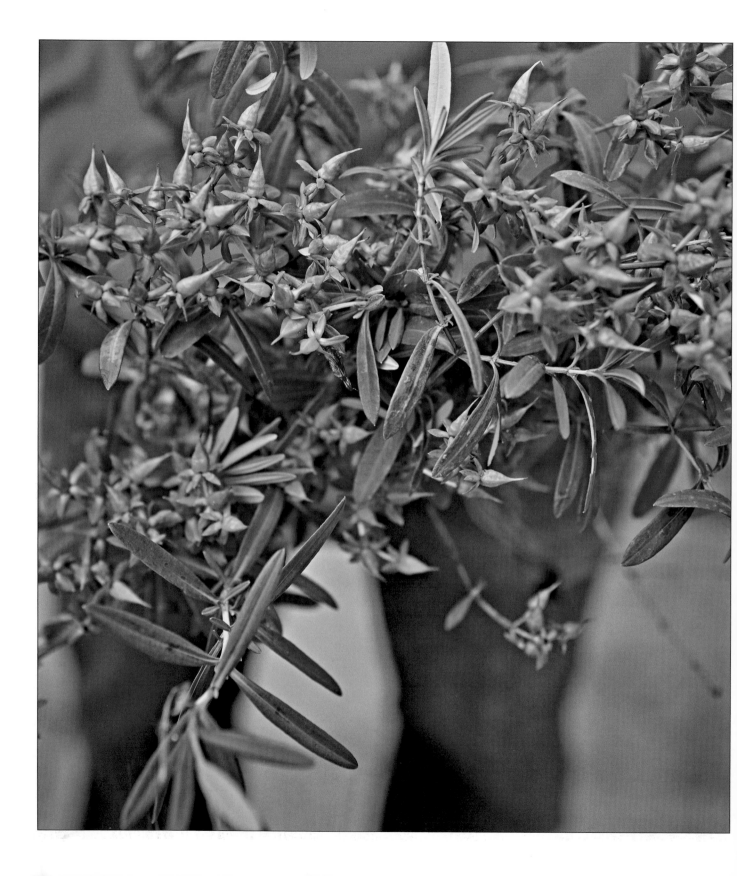

St. John's Wort

The five-petal yellow flower of St. John's wort may have become the unofficial icon of natural medicine. The herb has attracted a lot of attention since the 1990s, when the public caught wind of studies that found it could be used to treat mild depression without the side effects of drugs such as Prozac. This plant is native to Europe and Asia but now grows all over North America, and in many Canadian provinces it's a nuisance because it can be toxic to livestock. It can also cause foraging animals to become sun-sensitive, a side effect that's shared by humans. We're not sure whether the plant also makes cows happier and less depressed going into middle age!

⊕ Health Benefits

Since ancient Greece, St. John's wort has been hailed as a remedy for wounds, sores, burns, bruises, sprains, inflammation, and nerve pain. It was used for coughs, nervous exhaustion, epilepsy, depression, and even psychosis.

Today, St. John's wort is most commonly used to relieve anxiety, nervousness, seasonal affective disorder (SAD), and depression. It's not clear exactly which compounds in the plant have antidepressant properties. Some research suggests St. John's wort extract increases production of feel-good chemicals in the brain—namely the neurotransmitters serotonin, norepinephrine, and dopamine.

St. John's wort works well both internally and externally. However, sensitivity will vary from person to person, so if you're making your own herbal remedies you may need to experiment to find the appropriate dose for you.

🌱 Growing

St. John's wort is a relatively low-maintenance deciduous shrub that is both functional and beautiful. It produces flowers in summer on multiple stems measuring 1 to 1.5 m (3 to 5 feet), displaying vibrant yellow blooms that attract a host of pollinators including bees and butterflies. St. John's wort can be enjoyed as a cut flower, in mass landscape plantings and containers, as a ground cover, and in woodland gardens and cottage gardens alike. The plant isn't a heavy feeder, and it can survive without water for lengthy periods.

Common Varieties: There are hundreds of species of *Hypericum*, including annuals, perennials, shrubs, and even trees. For medicinal use, *H. perforatum* is the species of choice. For ornamental use in the garden, however, you can substitute *H. kalmia-*

DIFFICULTY
Easy to medium

HARDINESS
Perennial in zones 4 to 9

TIME TO PLANT
Spring

TIME TO HARVEST
Summer

LOCATION
Full to part sun

SOIL TYPE
Rich, well-drained (will also tolerate poor soils)

num (varieties include 'Ames' and 'Kalm's') or *H. androsaemum* ('Albury Purple').

PLANT

St. John's wort can be propagated from seed or stem cuttings, but it's easiest just to buy a transplant. A 2-gallon container is the perfect size to give you a head start.

Plant in spring in a location with full to partial sun and rich, well-drained soil. While St. John's wort will survive in poor soils, it will thrive if there's more organic matter. St. John's wort does not enjoy wet feet, so drainage is very important. Do not plant in clay soils.

Score the roots before planting to loosen the compacted fibres. Then dig a hole twice the width of the container and one-and-a-half times the depth. Ensure the root ball is slightly above ground level, firmly tamp soil, and keep evenly moist until established. Within 4 to 6 weeks the shrub will start to root in.

GROW

A general rule for flowering shrubs is "prune only after bloom." This holds true for St. John's wort. You can prune this shrub when you harvest the flowers: Just make sure not to remove more than one-third of the plant.

St. John's wort is disease- and insect-resistant, as well as drought-tolerant, so it pretty much takes care of itself. It will benefit from mulching and occasional weeding.

Some varieties of St. John's wort spread by sending roots underground, making this an ideal ground cover. But in some areas the plant will require thinning and some removal to prevent it from overtaking the entire garden.

HARVEST

Harvest whenever the flowers appear in midsummer. Wait until the dew has dried but the air is still cool. Use sharp shears and never harvest more than one-third of the plant at a time.

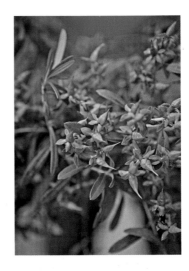

One key to gardening success is purchasing healthy plants. When you visit the garden centre look for rich, green foliage that's free of any damage or sign of disease (such as holes or spots). The roots should not be growing out of the bottom of the pot, and when you slide the plant out of the pot they should appear white and firm (black and soft roots are a sign of root rot). Stems should be firm and strong. I also recommend not purchasing plants that are already flowering: It's better to buy them when they're budding.

STORE

St. John's wort flowers can be used fresh or you can dry them by hanging bunches in a cool, dry, dark place for 7 to 10 days (see "Drying Herbs at Home" on page 365). Other drying options include using a dehydrator or baking on a baking sheet at low temperature until the leaves have curled, but air-drying works best. Store the dried flowers in an airtight container out of direct light.

Put It to Work

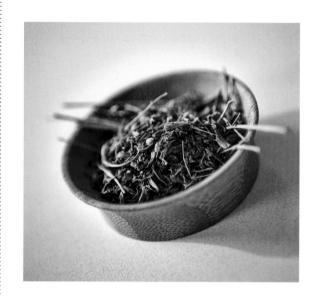

Mild depression? Try this tincture!

Depression is a serious condition, so don't self-diagnose. Get evaluated by a doctor who will determine whether your case is truly mild. If you don't need more conventional medication, this tincture can help. It's very potent stuff, so use it sparingly and cautiously!

Collect a resealable glass jar (like a Mason jar) full of flower tops from your St. John's wort plants. (Your fingers will turn red as you pick them—don't worry, it's normal.) Fill the jar to the brim with vodka (at least 80 proof). Place wax paper over the mouth of the jar and then screw the lid on tightly to seal it. Within minutes you should see the flowers turning red as they release their active ingredients into the tincture. Set aside in a cool, dark place for 4 weeks, shaking the jar once daily to release the oil.

After 4 weeks, cover the mouth of the jar with a coffee filter or cheesecloth and strain the liquid into a sterile dark-coloured jar with a tight-fitting lid (discard solids).

To aid with mild depression, take 1 teaspoon twice daily with food. The tincture will keep indefinitely stored in a cool, dark place.

Crush a finger or toe? Go, pain, go!

Ever slam a finger in a door, stub your toe on a chair leg, or smack your head on a wall? We've all done it, and it hurts so badly! If you can get to the St. John's wort oil in time, however, you'll be amazed at how quickly you can find relief.

Combine ¼ cup freshly cut St. John's wort flower heads and 1 cup of almond oil in a resealable glass jar (like a Mason jar) and seal tightly. Set aside at room temperature for 6 weeks, shaking frequently. Cover the mouth of the jar with a coffee filter and strain the liquid into a sterile dark-coloured glass bottle with a tight-fitting lid.

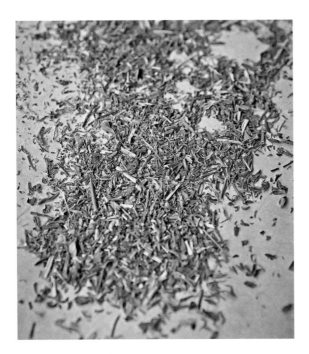

For crushing nerve pain or trauma, rub liberally onto the affected area. The infusion will keep in the refrigerator for up to 3 months.

Feeling gloomy or moody? Drink this tea daily!
If you're feeling low or moody, St. John's wort tea can provide the benefits of the herb at a very mild dose. It has a slightly woody and bitter taste, but this can be balanced with the addition of honey and peppermint.

Collect ¼ cup of St. John's wort flower heads in a mug. Pour boiling water over top, cover with a saucer, and steep for 10 minutes. Add 2 to 3 peppermint leaves and 1 teaspoon honey. Drink it daily as a nerve tonic, and as a nightcap to calm the mind and the bladder.

 # Fast Forward

Fast forward to the health food store to purchase Genestra St. Johnswort tincture or equivalent. Follow the instructions on the label.

! Cautions

St. John's wort may interact with medications used to treat depression or other mood disorders, including tricyclic antidepressants, selective serotonin reuptake inhibitors (SSRIs), and monoamine oxidase inhibitors (MAOIs). Taking St. John's wort with these medications could lead to a dangerous condition called serotonin syndrome.

Because it's processed by the same enzyme in the liver that metabolizes many drugs, St. John's wort can potentially cause drug interactions that have not yet been reported.

Adverse effects such as stomach upset, fatigue, itching, sleep disturbance, and skin rash have been reported.

St. John's wort can make the skin much more sensitive to sunlight.

People with a history of manic-depressive illness (bipolar disorder), or a less severe condition known as hypomania, should avoid St. John's wort as it may trigger a manic episode.

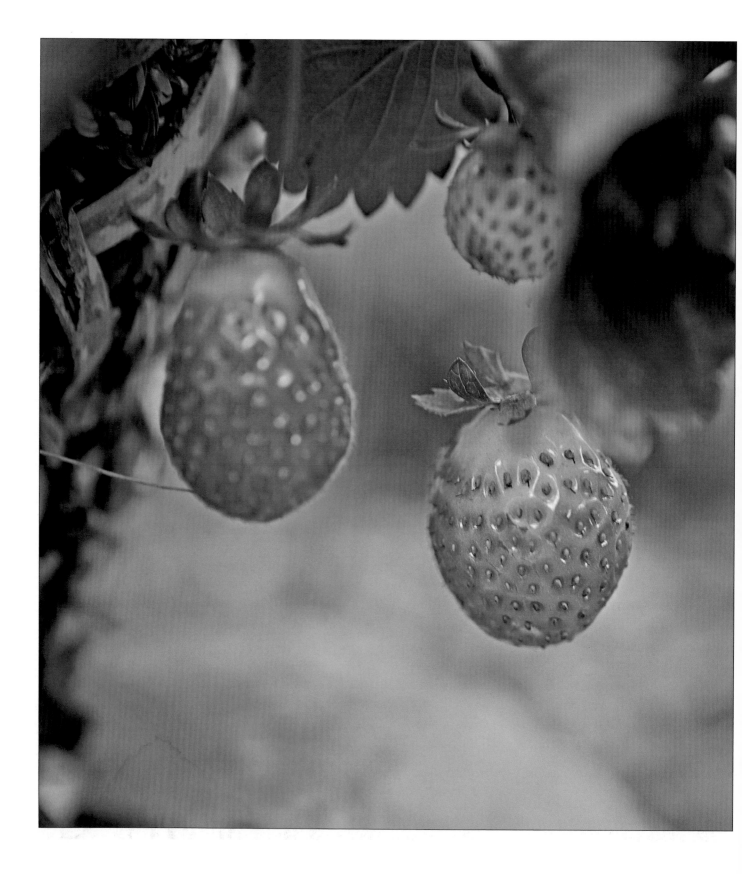

Strawberry

The strawberry belongs to the same family as the rose (*Rosaceae*) and is one of nature's most succulent, sweet, and healthy fruits. It may be the third most popular ice-cream flavour (trailing chocolate and vanilla), but it's second to none when it comes to producing fresh berries. Technically it's not a true berry, because its dry, yellow seeds are on the outside. True berries, such as blueberries and cranberries, have seeds on the inside. Wild strawberries have been eaten and used in medicines since antiquity, but the hybrid species we enjoy today was cultivated in France in the 18th century.

Health Benefits

Fresh strawberries are particularly high in soluble fibre, which is the type that dissolves in water. Most of us are familiar with psyllium husk, which is an insoluble fibre. Insoluble fibres are important because they add bulk to the diet and help prevent constipation, but they pass through the gastrointestinal tract in their original form. By contrast, soluble fibres attract water and form a gel, which slows down digestion and delays the emptying of your stomach. That makes you feel full and helps control your appetite, and therefore your weight. When your stomach empties more slowly, your blood sugar levels are lower, too. Soluble fibre can even help lower LDL (bad) cholesterol.

Strawberries are high in vitamin C, folic acid, potassium, and many powerful antioxidants. They have anti-inflammatory properties (providing you're not allergic) and may also help iron absorption.

Studies show that regular consumption of strawberries may even reduce the risk of colorectal cancer, thanks to the anthocyanins, ellagic acid, and other polyphenols they contain. These same compounds might also slow the effects of aging on the nervous system and help protect against the damage typical of Alzheimer's and other neurodegenerative diseases.

Growing

There is nothing like a fresh strawberry to celebrate the start of the edible growing season. One of the first berries in spring, strawberries are a versatile crop that can be planted in rows in formal vegetable gardens, used among perennials in flower gardens, or even grown in pots. Some even offer attractive flowers as well as edible berries. They're relatively easy to grow, and within

DIFFICULTY
Easy to medium

HARDINESS
Perennial in zones 3 and above

TIME TO PLANT
Spring

TIME TO HARVEST
Late spring to summer

LOCATION
Full sun

SOIL TYPE
Rich, moist, well-drained

one year of planting a row of 25 tiny transplants can yield over 22 kg (50 lb) of fruit!

Common Varieties: There are countless varieties of strawberries in three broad categories: June-bearers, everbearing, and day-neutrals.

June-bearers (including 'Honeoye', 'Guardian', 'Kent', 'Redchief', 'Delite', and 'Jewel') have the largest and most flavourful fruit. The downside is that they produce "runners" (see opposite), which means they need ample space, require a little more work, and will not produce a good yield in their first year.

Everbearing varieties ('Quinalt', 'Ogallala', 'Fort Laramie') produce one crop in spring and the other in fall, but the fruit itself is smaller and generally less flavourful.

Day-neutrals ('Tribute', 'Tristar', 'Fern') produce berries all summer long. They have few runners, so they require less work, and they will produce fruit in their first year. However, the yields are smaller and later than June-bearing varieties and the plants are more susceptible to disease.

PLANT

Plant in spring after the risk of hard frost and when the ground is workable. All varieties need full sun and moist soil that is rich in organic matter, so amend with manure just before planting. Look for a location with good air circulation but protected from northwest winds. Airflow will help reduce the chance of disease.

Plant June-bearing strawberries in "matted rows" with the plants flush to the ground and surrounded by straw. Space them 40 to 60 cm (16 to 24 inches) apart in rows separated by 90 to 120 cm (3 to 4 feet).

Plant everbearing varieties using the "hill system." Dig out a trench and mound up the soil you remove. Place your plants in these mounds, setting them 25 cm (10 inches) apart in two or three rows. Leave a walkway about 1 metre (3 feet) wide between the hills.

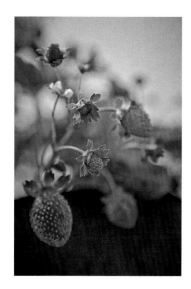

"Runners" will run away with your yield! Runners are the side shoots that grow out of the crown of a strawberry plant. They are energy suckers that detract from future fruit production. If you've grown strawberries but have never enjoyed good yields, I'll bet you didn't pinch away the runners. Removing them takes a little extra effort, but it pays back in baskets of berries!

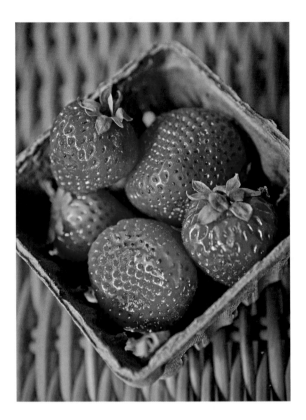

Plant day-neutrals in pots or gardens, in groups or on their own. Space them 25 cm (10 inches) apart.

In all cases, plant so the crown (the base of the stem) is level with surrounding soil. Mulch with clean straw or alternative (do not use stone), making sure the mulch does not cover the crowns. Water deeply and infrequently until established.

GROW

The first rule when growing June-bearing and everbearing strawberries is to remove the flowers in the first season. This will allow the plant to get established and will create healthier plants and greater yields in the second season.

The second rule is to remove runners during and after harvest when they appear between the rows. Runners filling spaces within the rows can be left alone.

Water deeply and infrequently, and do your best to avoid watering foliage, flowers, or fruits. Remove diseased and overripe fruit throughout the harvest season. Monitor for disease and insects and treat accordingly. Common problems include powdery mildew, spider mites, slugs, and beetles. If birds become a problem, place netting over the plants. Weed frequently. Use a hoe between rows, but hand-weed in among plants, especially during the first growing season, to prevent damage.

After the growing season has finished and a few hard frosts have occurred, mow the foliage and cover the rows with straw or leaf mulch to a depth of 10 cm (4 inches). The following spring, just after leaves start to emerge on deciduous trees, remove the covering and dress with composted manure.

In future seasons, thin plants and rotate patches to new areas every 3 to 5 years to ensure good health.

HARVEST

Within 3 to 6 weeks after the first flowers appear, your strawberries will begin to ripen. Strawberries are most flavourful when left on the vine to fully ripen, but they can be harvested when over 60% of the red colouring has appeared. Harvest mid-morning after the dew has dried. You can collect fresh berries every couple of days. Remove the stem and a few leaves along with the berry.

STORE

Wash strawberries just before use. Store at room temperature if you're using them immediately. Refrigerating will extend their life, but the flavour will diminish. For best results when refrigerating, store in an open container. To freeze, remove leaves and stems, wash, slice in half, and place in resealable bags. You can also purée strawberries, spoon into BPA-free ice-cube trays, and freeze. Preserve by making into jams or jellies.

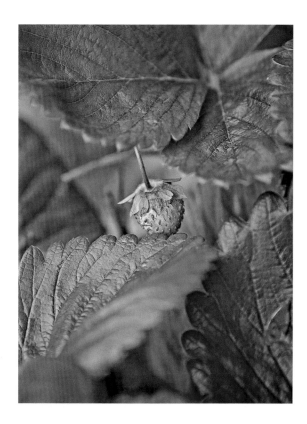

 # Put It to Work

Yellow teeth? Try a strawberry whitener!
Yellow or stained teeth are not necessarily unhealthy, but they can make some people self-conscious. Strawberries, believe it or not, can serve as a natural whitening agent.

In a blender, combine 1 tablespoon of baking soda, the juice of half a lemon, and 6 large strawberries and blend on high speed until smooth. Wipe saliva from your teeth using a clean cloth or paper towel. Use a cotton swab to apply the mixture liberally, but avoid your gums. Leave the mixture on your teeth for up to 3 minutes before gently brushing it off with a toothbrush. (Leaving it on your teeth for longer could cause the tooth enamel to erode.)

Low iron? Try this salad!
About 80% of menstruating women are clinically anemic. The best way to treat anemia from a dietary perspective is to eat steak (providing you're not vegetarian) and spinach. Adding strawberries provides a crucial punch of vitamin C, which allows the iron to be absorbed into your body. Here's the meal that will do it for you!

4 oz steak, grilled and sliced
2 cups baby spinach
½ cup cherry tomatoes
½ cup sliced strawberries
¼ cup slivered almonds
¼ cup poppyseed dressing

Combine all of the ingredients in a large bowl and toss gently to mix. Enjoy!

Insatiable craving? Smother it with a strawberry smoothie!
The main reason you crave unhealthy foods is that you've gone too long without eating and your blood sugar has dropped too low. To bump it back up, you need a sugar fix—often salty-sweet or fatty-sweet.

Plan your meals so they are never more than 4 hours apart. Between meals, strawberries are the ideal snack. If you're just sitting at your desk, 4 or 5 of them will do just fine.

For a more substantial alternative to that unhealthy snack you crave at night, try this strawberry smoothie. It has flavour to satiate, soluble fibre to aid in weight loss, and tons of antioxidants to support you until the morning.

½ cup plain Balkan or Greek yogurt
1 cup strawberries
½ cup mango purée
½ cup coconut milk
1 tbsp coconut sugar crystals
5 ice cubes

In a blender, combine all of the ingredients and blend on high speed until smooth. (Add more ice cubes to suit your taste.) Enjoy!

» Fast Forward

Fast forward to the grocery or health food store to purchase organic strawberry spread or equivalent.

! Cautions

Strawberries are a common allergen. Avoid them if you have any known allergy or hypersensitivity to the fruit or any members of the rose family (*Rosaceae*).

Eat organic strawberries only. Conventionally grown fresh strawberries and premade commercial strawberry salads have been found to contain high pesticide levels as well as bacterial and viral contamination. If you can't get organic varieties, consider washing your strawberries with a solution of 1 part vinegar to 9 parts water.

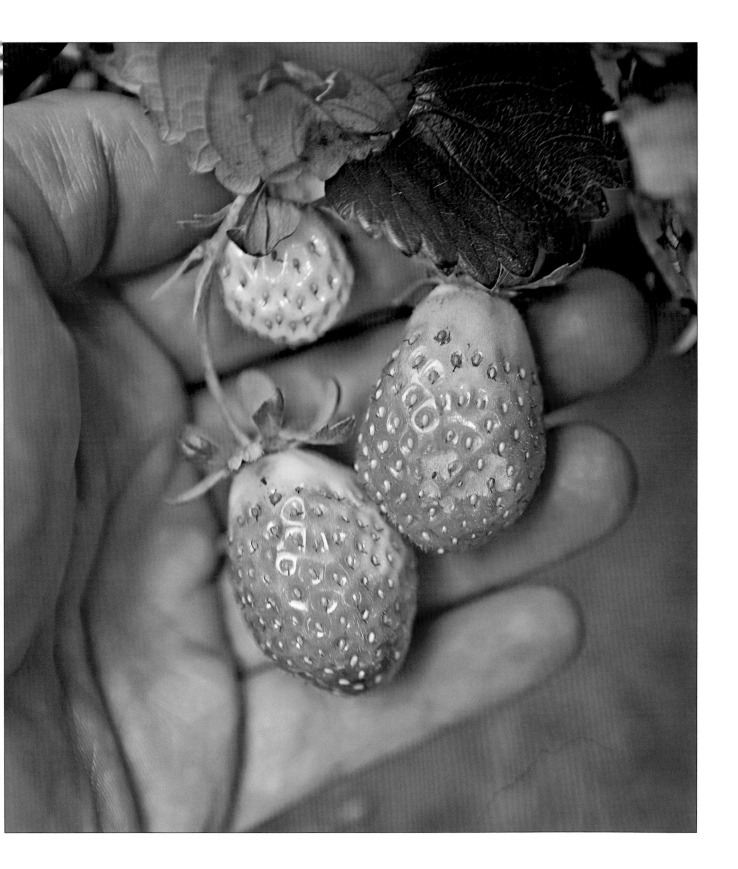

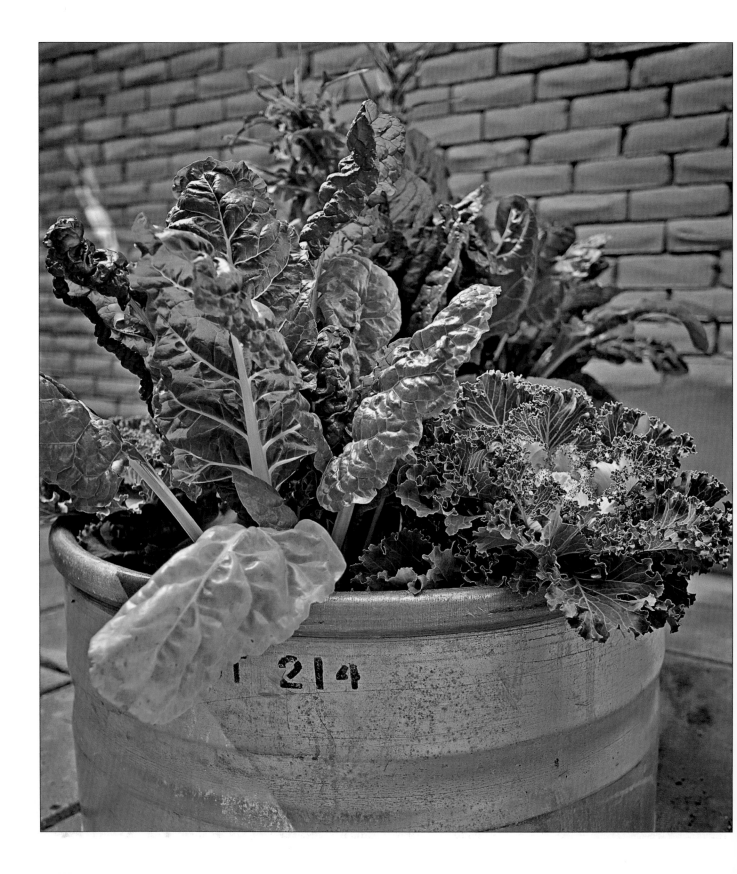

Swiss Chard

Despite its name, Swiss chard doesn't originate in Switzerland; it's native to the Mediterranean region. This leafy vegetable looks a little like spinach, but its ribs are a beautiful red, pink, or yellow. If the red-ribbed variety reminds you of beet tops, that's not a coincidence. Swiss chard and beets are actually cultivars of the same species (*Beta vulgaris*). If you mixed the nutritional virtues of spinach and beets, you'd get Swiss chard. It's one of the healthiest vegetables available: It's loaded with vitamins, essential minerals, fibre, and an army of antioxidants.

✚ Health Benefits

Swiss chard has not been studied as extensively as beets and spinach, but it has a valuable role to play in health. Like beets, Swiss chard contains plant compounds called betalains. These are the pigments that give the colour to the stalk and veins of the chard leaves, and they deliver powerful antioxidant, anti-inflammatory, and liver-detoxification support. They help the liver make more of the most powerful antioxidant in the body, known as glutathione.

The leaves also contain an antioxidant called kaempferol, which offers potent heart protection, and syringic acid, which balances blood sugar and supports the production of insulin.

The antioxidants in chard act as anti-inflammatory agents that decrease the risk of obesity, atherosclerosis, type 2 diabetes, high blood pressure, and several forms of arthritis.

Besides being an antioxidant powerhouse, chard is no slouch when it comes to conventional vitamins and minerals. It contains vitamin K levels that make it third only to kale and spinach. Though most of the attention focuses on calcium, magnesium, and vitamin D, vitamin K helps prevent bone loss. And friendly bacteria in the intestines convert vitamin K1 into vitamin K2, which activates osteocalcin, a protein whose job is to anchor calcium molecules inside the bone.

🌱 Growing

Swiss chard in the landscape is a triple treat: It's edible, it's incredibly healthy, and above all, it's sexy! Okay, ornamental at least. This low-maintenance vegetable is the crop that keeps on giving: It continues to grow for a second, third, fourth, and even fifth harvest. Swiss chard comes in a rainbow of stem colours,

DIFFICULTY
Easy

HARDINESS
Annual

TIME TO PLANT
Spring

TIME TO HARVEST
Summer through fall

LOCATION
Full to part sun

SOIL TYPE
Rich, well-drained, slightly acidic

from white, to yellow, to red, adding flair to any garden it graces. It's a cool-season plant that can take light frost and will fill both containers and gardens well into the fall.

Common Varieties: My favourite varieties include 'Rhubarb', 'Ruby', 'Bright Lights', 'Lucullus', 'Rainbow', and 'Fordhook Giant'.

PLANT

Swiss chard is one of the few plants that novice gardeners can grow from seed sown directly in the garden. As soon as the ground is workable in spring, plant the seeds 1 cm (½ inch) deep in soil that's rich in organic matter. Space the seeds 1 to 3 cm (1 to 1¼ inches) apart in rows 20 cm (8 inches) apart. Keep well watered and the seeds will germinate in 7 to 14 days. Thin seedlings to the spacing recommended on the seed packet as soon as chard has developed 3 to 5 leaves.

When growing from transplants, space them 15 to 25 cm (6 to 10 inches) apart in the garden. If you're planting Swiss chard in containers, ensure the pots have adequate drainage and use potting soil.

You can sow Swiss chard in the garden again in late summer for an additional fall harvest!

Make sure you fertilize at the right time. Water-soluble fertilizers such as compost teas, fish emulsions, and synthetics like 20-20-20 are best applied after rain or watering. When the soil is moist, the roots can absorb the nutrients more easily.

GROW

The two Ws are a must with Swiss chard: weeding and watering. Weeds will constantly compete for moisture and nutrients and attract unwanted pests, so remove them weekly. To minimize weed growth and maximize moisture retention, use mulch to a depth of 5 to 10 cm (2 to 4 inches).

Ideally, your crop should get 20 to 30 mm (1 to 2 inches) of water per week, but once the plants are established you can get away with occasional deep soaking during periods with no rain. Swiss chard may "burn up" during lengthy periods of heat, especially if it's not watered. If this happens, salvage what you can and re-sow in late summer for a fall harvest.

Swiss chard grown in containers must be fertilized. I recommend at least twice per month using a fish emulsion or water-soluble 20-20-20 fertilizer.

This vegetable may be the target of furry friends, including deer and rabbits, and may be enjoyed by slugs, snails, aphids, and even cutworms. But with minimal care (slug baits are a good idea), you should not have much trouble with these pests. Other ways to reduce the risk of infestation include avoiding planting near beets or spinach and rotating crops annually to ensure Swiss chard is not planted in the same location in successive years.

HARVEST

With Swiss chard you can go big or small. You can remove just a few leaves by breaking them

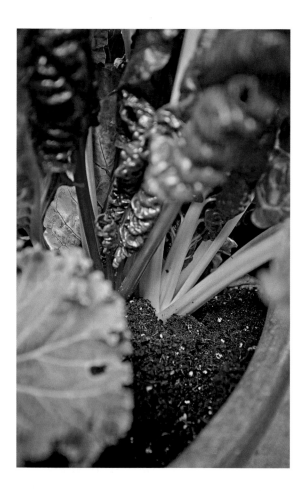

off (harvest the large outer leaves only, allowing smaller ones to mature) or cut a whole bunch with a sharp knife. Harvest in early to mid-morning, just before the dew dries. Cut the stalks 5 to 10 cm (2 to 4 inches) from the base. Bundle and wrap the ends in damp newspaper or place them in water.

Within 3 to 5 days, chard will start to regrow from the base, allowing for additional harvests if there's enough growing time left in the season!

STORE

Wash Swiss chard just before use. Swiss chard can be stored for up to 10 days in resealable bags in the refrigerator. Another option is to blanch the leaves in boiling water for 1 to 2 minutes, drain, cool, and freeze in airtight containers.

Put It to Work

Need to drop weight fast? Try the Swiss chard shredder!

You've probably heard of miracle diets that promise you'll lose 10 pounds or more in a week. Well, guess what: This one works! If your doctor gives you the go-ahead, this 4-week diet will help you lose weight fast without any rebound if you stick to a healthy lifestyle thereafter.

The "chard cleanse" helps detoxify the liver, balance blood sugar, regulate your bowels, clear your skin, strengthen your bones, and help you shed pounds! Aim to do this twice annually (4 weeks each time). Caution: Do not proceed if you are pregnant or have diabetes.

The 7-day chard juice primer: During this primer, don't eat or drink anything but what is recommended each day. Drink about 6 ounces at a time, 7 to 10 times daily. The limits on solid foods are described below. There is no limit on your consumption of pure water.

Juice the following each day (enough to make 42 ounces of juice), storing it in individual 6-ounce serving sizes for convenience.

Keep refrigerated or in an insulated lunch bag and shake before drinking. Be warned: I never said this would taste like a milkshake!

> *2 lb Swiss chard*
> *½ cup ground turmeric (reduces and clears any lingering inflammation)*
> *2 pineapples or 4 cups fresh pineapple chunks (the bromelain enzyme will cleanse the small intestine)*
> *Freshly squeezed juice of 3 lemons (acidifies, detoxifies, and cleanses the liver)*

Limit yourself to the following solid foods each day for 7 days:

- 2 servings of berries (½ cup per serving)
- 4 cups of lightly steamed vegetables
- ½ cup of whole grain (quinoa, kasha, and buckwheat are all good choices) mixed with ½ cup of any bean or legume, seasoned with fresh herbs from your garden
- ½ cup of plain low-fat unsweetened yogurt

A day in your life while on the 7-day primer looks something like this:
- Morning (on waking): 6 ounces of Swiss chard juice
- Breakfast: ½ cup of whole-grain and bean mixture accompanied by ½ cup plain low-fat yogurt and 1 serving of berries
- Mid-morning: 6 ounces of Swiss chard juice
- Half an hour before lunch: 6 ounces of Swiss chard juice

- Lunch: 2 cups of lightly steamed vegetables
- An hour after lunch: 6 ounces of Swiss chard juice
- Mid-afternoon: 6 ounces of Swiss chard juice
- Dinner: 2 cups of lightly steamed vegetables and ½ cup of whole-grain and bean mixture
- An hour after dinner: 6 ounces of Swiss chard juice
- Snack: 1 serving of berries
- Before bed: 6 ounces of Swiss chard juice

You might experience common detoxification symptoms such as mild nausea, loose bowels, headaches, muscular aches and pains, and skin rashes. Don't be alarmed by these symptoms. Consult with your doctor if any symptoms persist after the week you are on this primer, to make sure they are not caused by an illness or infection.

The 21-day brown rice cleansing diet: On day 8, you're ready to move on to the brown rice diet for the next 3 weeks. You'll receive all the nutrition your body needs while you're on this diet. You don't have to go hungry, and you don't have to count calories or weigh food. You are allowed to eat when you're hungry, but stop before you're overly full. Try the Japanese practice of *hara hachi bu*, which means eating until you are 80% full. It's better to eat several small meals a day rather than three large ones.

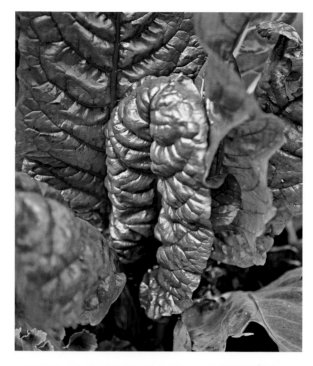

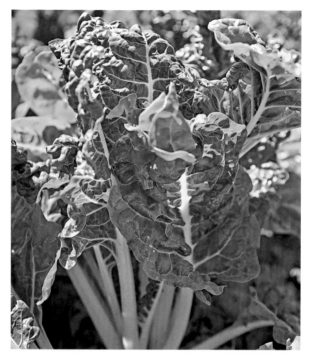

Swiss chard is both edible and ornamental, offering colour through its foliage in gardens and in containers. It boasts a range of stem colours, from ruby red through to hot pink, white through to golden yellow. Pictured here are 'Ruby Red', 'Large White Ribbed', and 'Rhubarb'.

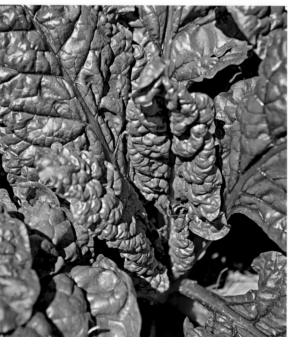

Here's what's allowed on the diet:

- Protein: lentils, rice cakes, sesame seeds, ocean fish, organic free-range chicken, hummus, tofu, and tempeh
- Carbohydrate: organic brown rice (no more than 1 cup twice daily)
- Vegetables: Focus on Swiss chard every day. Add other veggies you like, lightly steamed. Onions are especially good for cleansing and are very sweet and tasty when steamed. Try a plate full of carrots or broccoli with fresh garlic.
- Fruits: any kind except oranges (including orange juice), bananas, and dried fruits. It's best to consume only organic produce whenever possible. However, as this is not always possible, buy locally grown seasonal fruits and vegetables and wash them thoroughly before eating.
- Seasonings: cayenne pepper and a no-salt herbal seasoning; lots of fresh garlic and gingerroot
- Drinks: Water is always best. Use vegetable or fruit juice minimally (it's best if fresh-pressed from a juicer). Otherwise use juices with no additives, sugar, or chemicals, and little or no salt (a good variety can be found in health food stores).

» Fast Forward

Fast forward to the health food store to purchase Natural Factors L-Glutathione Reduced Form or equivalent. Follow the instructions on the label.

! Cautions

Swiss chard is perfectly safe when eaten in normal quantities. The leaves contain oxalic acid, which may be problematic for people with urinary tract stones. The vegetable also has a high vitamin K content and should be avoided by those taking anticoagulants such as warfarin.

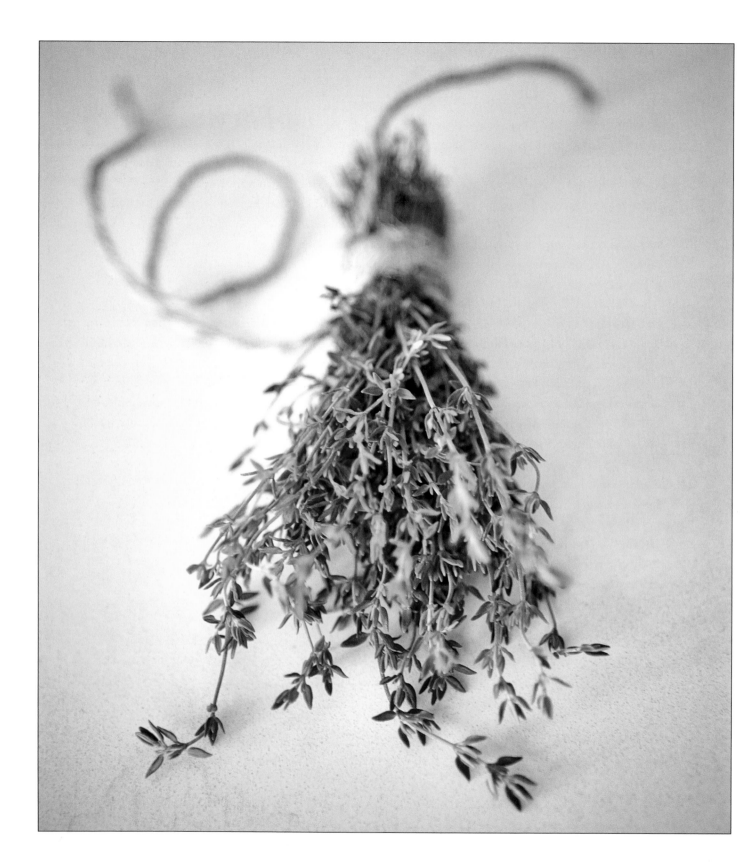

Thyme

Everyone could use a little more time and a lot more thyme! This familiar herb is a member of the mint family (*Lamiaceae*), and its savoury leaves have been used in cooking and in medicine for centuries. An old adage in culinary circles is "When in doubt, use thyme." The preservative properties of thyme were discovered by the ancient Egyptians, who used it to embalm the dead. Later the Greeks burned it in temples to disseminate an aroma they believed would deliver strength and courage to soldiers. Today it's on every cook's top 10 list and remains popular as a natural remedy.

⊕ Health Benefits

Thyme has been used medicinally for thousands of years. It was recognized for its antiseptic properties long before science understood what really caused infections. It was also used as a treatment for coughs and spasms, though these uses are less common today.

The plant's most important ingredient is thymol, a compound that has a powerful ability to kill germs such as bacteria and fungi. Thymol is found in other herbs, such as basil and oregano, but no plant has higher concentrations than thyme.

Thymol is a popular ingredient in antiseptic mouthwashes, and its antimicrobial abilities have also been harnessed to manage skin conditions such as acne and foot fungus. Some research suggests it may help with other dental hygiene issues, including reducing plaque formation, gingivitis, and cavities.

🌱 Growing

You don't need much time when growing thyme! This low-maintenance perennial enjoys tough conditions: It not only survives in poor soils, but has been known to thrive even in rocky conditions. (Good drainage is a must, however.) In the herb garden, thyme adds fragrance, flavour, and dainty flowers ranging from white to pink to purple. Trailing varieties of thyme can even be found flowing over the edges of mixed containers. Other varieties are used as ground cover, or even as a pathway plant growing between flagstones or patio stones, offering a sweet fragrance when stepped on.

Common Varieties: *Thymus vulgaris*, or common thyme, is most often used for cooking and medicinal purposes. Other useful garden species include lemon thyme (*T. citriodorus*) (right),

DIFFICULTY
Easy

HARDINESS
Perennial in zones 5 and above (depends on variety)

TIME TO PLANT
Spring or fall

TIME TO HARVEST
Summer through fall

LOCATION
Full sun

SOIL TYPE
Well-drained (tolerates poor soil)

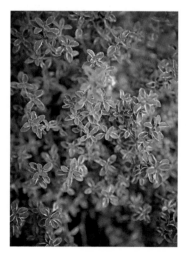

wild thyme (*T. serphyllum*), woolly thyme (*T. pseudolanuginosus*), and mother of thyme or creeping thyme (*T. praecox*).

PLANT

Some varieties of thyme can be propagated by seed or cuttings, but I recommend purchasing transplants. They're generally inexpensive and easy to find, and many are now grown organically. For die-hards, thyme can be sown directly in the garden in spring or fall, or started indoors 8 to 10 weeks before last frost date. The seeds require only a light covering. Remember to mark seeded areas: A common mistake is digging them up just before or after germinating, mistaking them for weeds!

Plant transplants in spring after the risk of frost, choosing a sunny location with well-drained soil. (Thyme can tolerate partial shade, but full sun is preferable.) Water deeply and infrequently until established, reducing the frequency of watering as the season progresses.

GROW

Thyme doesn't like to be overwatered or fertilized too often. In a container, overwatering is the number 1 reason for failure. Make sure drainage is good and sunshine is plentiful.

If thyme is struggling, it may be that you're treating it too well! I find thyme thrives more in the ornamental garden, where the soil conditions are not as rich as they are in the vegetable garden.

Thyme should be pruned vigorously twice during the season. Prune at least half the overall plant immediately after flowering and again a month prior to hard frost in fall. This "hard pruning" will improve the health of the plant.

Thyme is resistant to disease, insects, and rodents.

In areas with harsh winters, place boughs of evergreens over your crop before snowfall to add insulation.

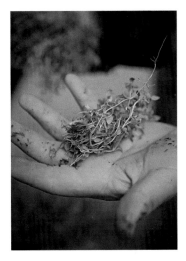

Thinking about planting a large area with thyme? Don't. Except for variegated cultivars (which are propagated by cutting), most thyme varieties produce a lot of seed and self-sow naturally every year, meaning they spread by themselves. In fact, you may need to tame the spread throughout the growing season to prevent it from migrating into unwanted locations.

HARVEST

Thyme can be harvested any time, but its flavour is most intense when the plant is just beginning to flower. Harvest mid-morning after the dew has dried using scissors, cutting a third to half the length of the stems.

STORE

Thyme can be used fresh or dried. To dry, tie the stems in small bundles, place in paper bags, and hang in a dark, dry place for about 2 weeks (see "Drying Herbs at Home" on page 365). You can also dry thyme in a dehydrator or on a baking sheet in an oven set to the lowest possible temperature. Bake for 1 hour, then turn the oven off but leave the thyme in overnight or at least until the oven has totally cooled. Once the herb is dried, carefully remove the leaves from stems, place in an airtight container, and store in a cool, dark place until needed.

Put It to Work

Upper respiratory infection? Thyme for honey!

Thyme honey is a popular product in Greece. The abundance of wild thyme in that country makes it the perfect source for bees that feast on the nectar and pollen of its tiny purple flowers. The essential oils of the thyme pass from the buds to the bees and end up in the honey. This process may or may not fortify the honey enough to give you a benefit during an upper respiratory infection. However, to up the concentration, you can further infuse the honey with dried thyme, which has antibacterial and cough suppressive effects.

Place ½ cup of dried thyme in a resealable glass jar (like a Mason jar) and pour in 1 cup of honey. (Be very careful that your thyme is fully dry to avoid any moisture getting into the honey and causing contamination.) Set aside for at least 1 week. If the herbs float to the top, turn the jar over a few times to keep them well coated.

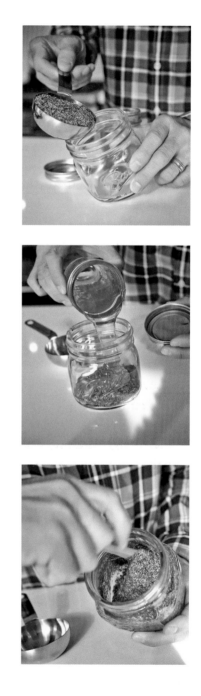

After a week, use a fine-mesh sieve to strain the infused honey into a sterile jar with a tight-fitting lid.

Whenever you have a cough, use 1 teaspoon of this honey 3 to 4 times daily as needed. Or boil a cup of water, squeeze half a lemon into it, add 1 tablespoon of thyme honey, and drink. The honey will keep indefinitely stored in a cool, dry place.

Bad acne? Tone with thyme!

Crush a handful of dried thyme and place in a resealable glass jar (like a Mason jar). Pour in enough witch hazel to cover it and fill the jar. Seal the jar, shake well, and set aside for 3 days in a cool, dark place (the witch hazel will look like a brown tea).

Cover the mouth of the jar with a coffee filter and strain the liquid into a sterile jar with a tight-fitting lid (discard solids).

Wash your face with soap and water. Using a cotton ball or swab, apply liberally to affected areas twice daily, in the morning and before bed. The toner will keep in a cool, dark place for up to 1 month.

Foot fungus? It's baththyme!

Fill a resealable glass jar (like a Mason jar) to the top with dried thyme leaves. Add enough vodka (at least 80 proof) to fill it to the brim. Place wax paper over the jar and then screw the lid on tightly to seal it. Shake vigorously. Set aside in a cool, dark place for at least 2 weeks, shaking the jar once daily.

To use, pour 4 to 5 cups of hot water into a large bowl or foot tub, add 4 ounces of the thyme alcohol tincture, and stir. Soak feet every night before bed for 1 month. The infusion will keep in a cool, dark place for at least a year.

» Fast Forward

Fast forward to the health food store to purchase Eclectic Institute's thyme tincture or equivalent. Follow the instructions on the label.

! Cautions

Do not ingest the essential oil of thyme—it can be toxic and may cause nausea and breathing problems.

Avoid thyme supplements if you have diabetes or low blood sugar, a bleeding disorder, blood pressure irregularity, or take drugs, herbs, or supplements for these conditions. Also avoid if you have a thyroid disorder, hormonal disorder, or are at risk for hormone imbalance. Use cautiously if you suffer from gastrointestinal irritation or peptic ulcer disease.

Avoid thyme supplements if you are pregnant or have a known allergy or hypersensitivity to members of the mint family (*Lamiaceae*) or to rosemary. Avoid topical use where the skin is broken.

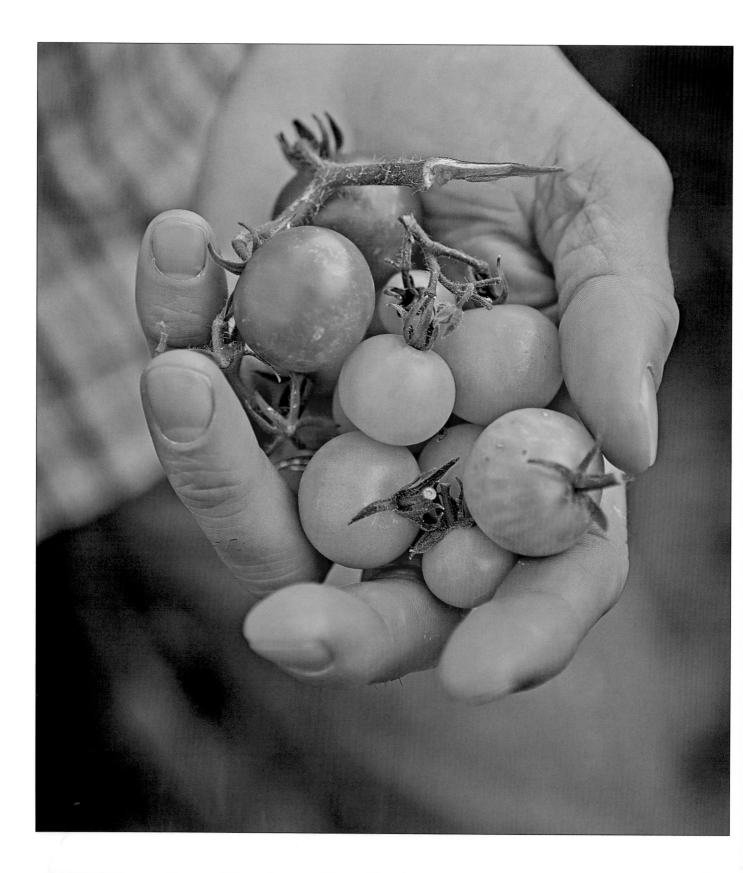

Tomato

Most of us grow up thinking tomatoes are vegetables because they show up in sauces, salads, and savoury dishes. Then one day someone who excels at Trivial Pursuit tells us that, because it grows above ground and contains seeds in its fleshy pulp, a tomato is actually a fruit. (More technically, it's a fruit because it develops from the ovary in the base of the flower and contains seeds.) However you want to classify it, the tomato is a superfood with incredible health benefits. So it may come as another surprise to learn that in the 17th century it was considered poisonous—or at least unfit to eat—in Britain. That wasn't an entirely crazy idea: Tomatoes are in fact a member of the nightshade family (*Solanaceae*), which does include some toxic species. But today there are thousands of tomato cultivars and it has become one of the most popular vegetables—make that fruits!—in the world.

⊕ Health Benefits

Lycopene is an antioxidant found in very high concentrations in tomatoes. It's a type of plant pigment called a carotenoid, and it's also present in carrots and red peppers. Lycopene enters your blood, liver, lungs, colon, and skin, protecting these tissues and organs from cancer. Studies have also correlated high levels of lycopene and carotenoids with lower incidence of heart disease and age-related macular degeneration, which affects your eyesight and can cause blindness.

Tomatoes are also great sources of vitamin C, folate, and potassium, all of which play an important role in human health.

Over the last decade or so, researchers have looked at the role tomatoes may have in the prevention of prostate cancer. Studies found a correlation between lower levels of lycopene in the blood or tissue and increased risk of prostate cancer. Scientists aren't yet convinced the link is causal, but lycopene certainly deserves a closer look.

Lycopene is better absorbed from tomato products (such as tomato paste or juice) than it is from fresh tomatoes. Tomato paste can double lycopene blood levels in healthy people. Although we still lack the hard evidence, researchers think that tomato products may even stimulate immunity.

🌱 Growing

Tomatoes are the superstars of the vegetable garden, and many feel they're the number 1 edible plant in the world. What says summer more than a freshly sliced tomato sandwich or caprese salad? Tomato talk dominates discussions at horticultural meetings and family gatherings (at least if you're Italian, like me!), and let's not forget the bragging rights given to whoever grows

DIFFICULTY
Easy

HARDINESS
Annual

TIME TO PLANT
Spring

TIME TO HARVEST
Summer through early fall

LOCATION
Full sun

SOIL TYPE
Rich, well-drained

the largest, juiciest beefsteak slicers. With good soil and a whole lot of sun, one tomato plant can yield enough for a family of four. From bush types (determinate) to vine types (indeterminate), the options in size, shape, colour, and flavour are endless, whether you're growing them in gardens or pots.

Common Varieties: There are more than 7,500 cultivars worldwide, including hybrid and heirloom varieties. My picks include 'Early Girl' (medium-size and quick to mature), 'Big Beef' (perfect for slicing), 'Brandywine' (an heirloom beefsteak variety), 'Roma' (plum-shaped, perfect for sauces and canning), 'Sugar Snack' (a cherry tomato), and 'Yellow Pear' (looks just like the name!).

PLANT

Sow seeds indoors 6 to 8 weeks before last frost date (don't start them too early!) or simply buy healthy transplants. Plant them outdoors only after all risk of frost has passed.

Are your tomatoes determinate or indeterminate? Determinate tomatoes grow as a bush and ripen all at one time (these are best suited for small spaces or pots); indeterminate tomatoes are produced on a vine that grows continually, producing fruit from late summer until frost. The latter require more staking, more support, and generally more space.

Also find out if the variety is resistant to disease. Unfortunately, heirloom tomatoes are not, but newer hybrids have resistance bred into them. On the tag or seed packet look for the letters VFN to indicate that your tomatoes will be resistant to verticillium wilt (V), fusarium wilt (F), and root-knot nematodes (N).

Tomatoes require at least 6 hours of direct sun—preferably in the afternoon—for optimum performance (8 hours or more is even better). If you lack adequate light, you're better to purchase locally grown tomatoes in season!

Plant in rich, organic, well-drained soil that's slightly acidic (pH 6 to 7). Remove the lower leaves from the plant, then slide

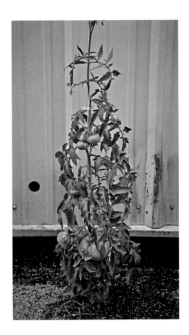

Staking tomatoes—especially vine types like these, also known as indeterminate tomatoes—increases yields by reducing disease and increasing pollination of tomato blooms.

it out of the container. Dig a hole and lay the root ball on its side in the hole so that the plant is lying sideways with its foliage hanging out over the side of the hole. Bury the bottom part of the stem where you removed the leaves, being careful to keep the top growth above soil level. Eventually the buried stem will send out roots.

When growing in a container, use potting soil and ensure there is adequate drainage. The larger the container, the better: I recommend a 40 cm (16 inch) diameter as a minimum.

Tomatoes and eggs make a great combo! Crumble some eggshells into the soil when you plant. The calcium will not only help the plants grow but also minimizes the risk of blossom end rot, which is the bruising that often appears on the underside of tomatoes just before harvest and is a result of a calcium deficiency in the soil and inconsistent watering.

Have you ever noticed some gardeners plant their tomatoes in tires? Why? Black absorbs heat, so planting tomatoes in tires—or even in black pots—will increase the temperature of the entire plant, including the roots. This encourages growth and can produce tomatoes up to 7 days earlier!

GROW

Tomato growers need to be strippers—of the stems! Suckers are clusters of leaves in the spot where the branch and the stem meet. These should always be removed (just pinch them with your fingers), as they don't bear fruit and take energy away from the plant. When your plant grows to a height of 65 to 90 cm (2 to 3 feet), remove the leaves from the bottom 25 cm (10 inches) of the stem, as they're the first to develop fungus.

In a vegetable garden, mulch tomato plants using clean straw. This helps to retain moisture while also reducing the amount of water and soil that splashes back onto the foliage or the tomatoes themselves. Back-splashes of water transfer soil-borne pathogens onto the plant, leading to disease.

Tomatoes can be heavy feeders, so for optimal production fertilize twice monthly with water-soluble fertilizer such as 15-15-30 or fish emulsion. If you're growing tomatoes in containers, this is essential!

Tomato plants need a lot of water. Water in the morning using a soaker hose rather than a sprinkler, as it's important to wet only the root zone and avoid the fruit or foliage. Thorough watering is essential on summer's brightest, windiest days.

Not all bugs are bad. You need to watch out for whiteflies, tomato hornworms, beetles, and slugs, but bees are a tomato's friend and help pollinate the plants. If you lack bees in your area, or are growing tomatoes on a high balcony, you can simply use a cotton swab to transfer pollen from bloom to bloom.

Monitor for disease, especially fusarium wilt! This fungal disease can be identified by the yellowing of bottom leaves and eventual

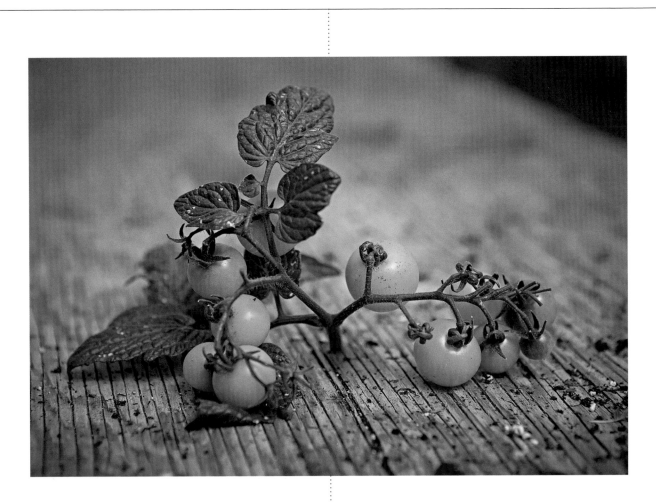

wilting of the entire plant. It may not kill your tomato plant, but it will destroy production. Fusarium wilt is a soil-borne disease, which is one reason why tomatoes should never be planted in the same location as previous years. Remove and destroy any infected plants to prevent spreading the disease.

HARVEST

Depending on the variety, your tomatoes will be ready 65 to 80 days from planting. Allow the fruit to fully ripen on the vine for the best, most flavourful results. A ripe tomato is firm and fully coloured. When harvesting, grasp the tomato firmly and twist off from the stem.

If you're stuck with green tomatoes at the end of the growing season, place one ripe fruit in a paper bag with a few green ones. The ripe tomato releases ethylene gas, helping to speed the green ones' ripening process.

STORE

Store your tomatoes on the counter, not in the refrigerator. Chilling a tomato does not increase its shelf life but does decrease its flavour. Keep your tomatoes indoors in a frost-free location out of direct light. Use fresh tomato purée in soups, preserve in jars, or make into sauce.

Put It to Work

Prostate problems? They'll be toast!
Whether it was in a pasta dish or pizza, you'd be hard pressed to remember a week when you didn't have tomato paste or sauce. It's not only delicious but also full of lycopene and other antioxidants that make it super-healthy.

Here's a delicious and healthier alternative to toast and jam that can be eaten any time of day. Slather a thick helping of the following spread on your favourite toast, drizzle with olive oil, and top with freshly ground black pepper and Parmesan cheese.

> *12 tomatoes*
> *1 red bell pepper*
> *1 tbsp pink Himalayan rock salt*
> *¼ tsp garlic powder*
> *Extra virgin olive oil*

In a blender, combine the tomatoes and bell pepper and purée. Pour into a large saucepan, bring to a boil, and boil for 5 minutes. Line a strainer with cheesecloth and place it over a pot. Pour the purée into the strainer and let it drain in the refrigerator overnight. Transfer

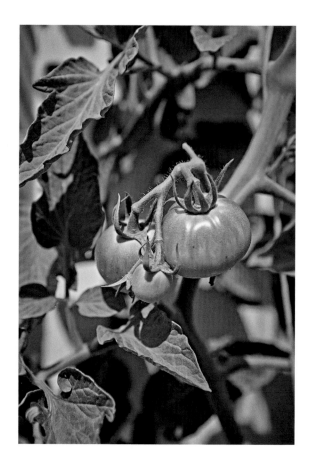

the now-drained purée to a glass baking dish (discard the strained liquid), stir in the salt and garlic powder, and spread evenly. Bake in a preheated 95°C (200°F) oven for 30 minutes. Transfer to resealable glass jars. Top with about 3 mm (⅛ inch) of olive oil to help preserve the paste. Store in an airtight container in the refrigerator for up to 2 weeks.

Tired of apples? Pack a tomato!
Apples are a delicious snack, but a perfectly ripe tomato is equally tasty and perhaps even

healthier. It may be a tiny bit messy, however, so bib up before diving in! To reduce the risk of prostate cancer, research suggests at least 4 servings of tomato products per week (equivalent to a lycopene intake of at least 6 milligrams daily). So swap a tomato for (or add to) your daily apple, orange, peach, or whatever other fruit accompanies you to work or school each day.

Want to prevent prostate cancer? Make the healthiest ketchup on the planet!
Ketchup is really simple to make, and it's a tasty (and kid-friendly) way to deliver lycopene and other antioxidants.

8 tomatoes, sliced
Red palm fruit oil
1 tbsp brown sugar
Sea salt and freshly ground black pepper
1 sweet onion, chopped
2 cloves garlic, crushed
½ tsp ground turmeric
2 tbsp balsamic vinegar
1 tsp apple cider vinegar

Arrange the tomatoes in a single layer on a baking sheet lined with parchment paper. Drizzle with oil. Sprinkle with the brown sugar and season with salt and pepper to taste. Bake in a preheated 200°C (400°F) oven for 30 minutes.

Meanwhile, in a skillet over medium heat, combine onions, garlic, and turmeric, and salt and pepper to taste. Sauté for 5 to 10 minutes, until soft. Pour in the vinegars and stir well.

Transfer the roasted tomatoes and the onion mixture to a blender and purée. Using a fine-mesh sieve, strain into the skillet (discard solids) and simmer over medium-low heat for 15 minutes, until thickened.

The ketchup will keep in an airtight container in the refrigerator for up to 4 weeks.

» Fast Forward

Fast forward to the health food store to purchase Natural Factors lycopene capsules or equivalent. Follow the instructions on the label.

! Cautions

Tomatoes are safe when eaten in normal amounts. Note that the leaves are potentially toxic to pets as well as humans.

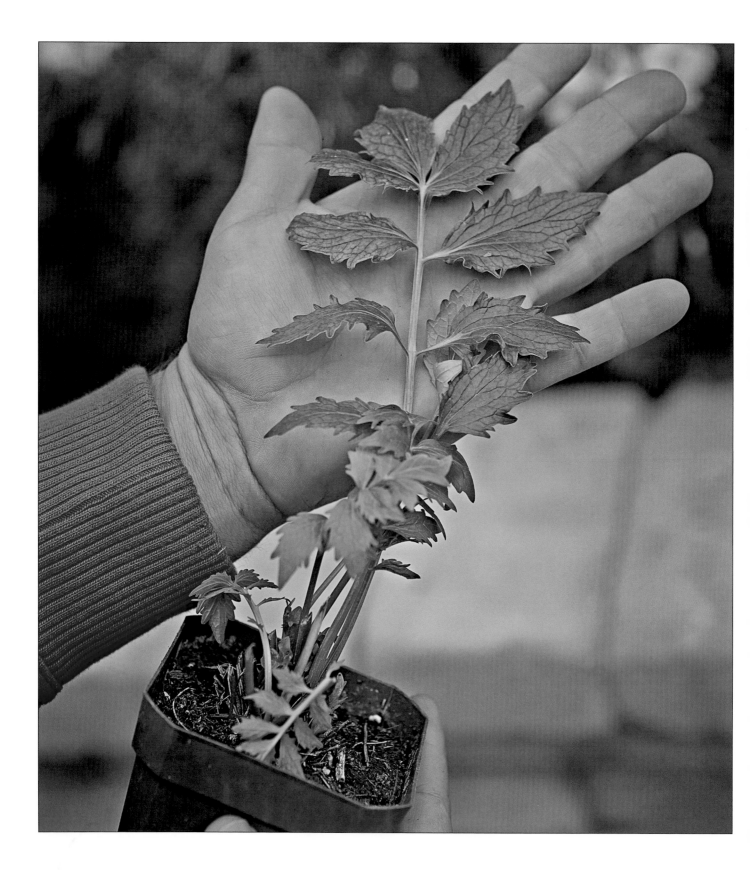

Valerian

Valerian is a flowering plant native to Europe and Asia and now widely grown in North America. It sends up stems about 60 cm (2 feet) high, with clusters of tiny white flowers. While it can be attractive to look at, valerian features a pungent, musky odour that some find offensive. It is primarily grown for its root, which has a long history of medicinal use in many cultures, primarily to treat anxiety and sleep disorders. Valerian root has been used since ancient times—both Hippocrates and Galen mentioned it in their writings. It's not surprising that it's still popular today: With stress affecting most of us, and with more than $21 billion spent annually on anti-anxiety benzodiazepine drugs, valerian is a natural alternative worthy of review.

Health Benefits

Valerian is primarily used as a relaxant and for managing anxiety. If you have problems sleeping because your mind is racing, valerian may be your saviour. Research shows it improves both quality and duration of sleep. However, it won't help much for the one-off disturbances you might endure when suffering from jet lag. Valerian works best if you have a more chronic sleep issue and you use it for 6 to 8 weeks to develop a good sleep schedule. The best time to dose up is about 2 hours before bedtime; this should help you fall asleep about 15 to 20 minutes faster.

If you have decided or been advised to stop taking a benzodiazepine drug (such as temazepam), valerian may help. In some studies, tapering benzodiazepine over 2 weeks and using valerian extract improved sleep quality. There is also new research suggesting that valerian can improve sleep in children with intellectual challenges who naturally have a higher incidence of sleep-related issues.

Best of all, valerian is much safer than pharmaceutical drugs. The German Commission E (a regulatory body for natural remedies) has approved the use of valerian as a mild sedative, and both the American Pharmaceutical Association and the Natural Health Products Directorate in Canada have given valerian a high rating for safety and efficacy.

Growing

Valerian (sometimes called garden heliotrope) is an attractive perennial. Unfortunately, while its flowers emit the sweet fragrance of vanilla, the plant itself stinks to high heaven! The smell is adored by cats, and if you have a feline friend you will

DIFFICULTY
Easy

HARDINESS
Perennial in zones 4 and above

TIME TO PLANT
Spring or early fall

TIME TO HARVEST
Fall or early spring

LOCATION
Full sun

SOIL TYPE
Rich, well-drained

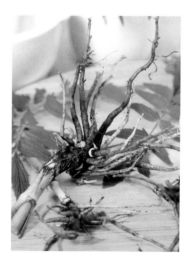

find it rolling and lying in your valerian. The blossoms of valerian are borne on tall stems and make an excellent cut flower (but note that cats love the smell of valerian and may knock over your vase). The plant itself is large and should be located to the rear of garden beds.

Common Varieties: There are many species of *Valeriana*, but only *V. officinalis* is used for medicinal purposes.

PLANT

Valerian can be propagated by seed or division. Divide the plant in spring or fall by lifting it out with a garden fork and removing sections using a sharp spade. Plant the divisions in fertile, well-drained soil in full sun.

You can also sow valerian seeds directly in the garden in spring: Press the seed into the soil but do not cover, as seeds require light to germinate. Plant 3 to 6 seeds per location, spacing locations 30 to 60 cm (1 to 2 feet) apart. Germination occurs within 7 to 14 days.

Valerian doesn't just attract cats; earthworms love it, too! This is primarily because of the phosphorous produced by its roots. That's good news, because earthworms are great for the garden.

GROW

Valerian needs very little maintenance beyond ensuring fertile, weed-free soil. The plant does enjoy nitrogen and will benefit if you amend the surrounding soil using coffee grounds or occasionally applying a high-nitrogen fertilizer like 30-12-12.

If you're growing valerian to harvest the roots for medicine, I recommend cutting the flower stalks as soon as they appear to improve the health and size of the roots. If you're growing it as an ornamental, just enjoy the white, fragrant flowers on spiky stalks.

Valerian is largely disease- and insect-resistant, though it may suffer from powdery mildew. This can be reduced if you increase air circulation in your garden by removing some existing plants.

Water deeply and infrequently, backing off during lengthy periods of rain and increasing during droughts.

HARVEST

Using a spade or garden fork, dig up roots in spring or fall when soil is moist. (Moist soil makes it easier to remove plants.) Remove the foliage and wash the roots.

STORE

Use valerian root fresh or dried. To dry, hang individual roots in a warm, dry place out of direct light, or arrange in a single layer on a baking sheet and bake in a preheated 120°C (250°F) oven until the roots are brittle. Store in an airtight container out of direct light. The dried root will keep indefinitely.

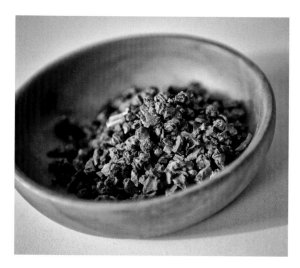
Chopped and dried valerian root.

⚙ Put It to Work

Sleepless? Let valerian root help!

While we tend to treat sleep as a luxury, plenty of research has revealed the negative health effects when we don't get enough of it. It's not necessarily the number of hours you sleep, but the quality of that sleep that counts. The real trick is to avoid waking up while you're in the deep stages of the sleep cycle, or the next day you won't feel rested. Controlled studies have shown valerian can help you enjoy deeper sleep, so you'll wake more refreshed.

The best way to use valerian is in tincture form. It is easy to prepare and convenient to have next to your bed.

Roughly chop ½ cup (4 ounces) of dried valerian root. Using a clean coffee or spice grinder, grind the root to a powder. Place in a large resealable glass jar (like a Mason jar). Pour vodka (at least 80 proof) into the jar until it covers the root by 6 mm (¼ inch). Place wax paper over the mouth of the jar and then screw the lid on tightly to seal it. Set aside for 12 hours. If the root powder has absorbed the alcohol, add enough vodka to re-establish the 6 mm (¼ inch) coverage. Set aside in a cool, dark place for at least 1 month, shaking the jar once daily.

After a month, cover the mouth of the jar with a coffee filter or cheesecloth and strain the liquid into a bowl. As much as you can, squeeze out all the liquid from the root powder without breaking the filter (discard solids). Transfer the tincture to sterile glass containers, ideally equipped with droppers.

Take several drops in warm water 3 times daily or before bed, and again at night if you wake up. The tincture will keep for up to 3 years in a cool, dark place.

Anxious? Valerian is the new Valium!

Getting through a busy day can be anxiety-provoking for many people. Most of the anti-anxiety drugs on the market are too strong for mild symptoms, and they may also be addictive. Here is how to make your own natural, milder, non-addictive treatment that you can keep in your purse or pocket.

3 ounces dried valerian root
3 cups boiling water
1 cup gum Arabic, crushed
2 cups icing sugar

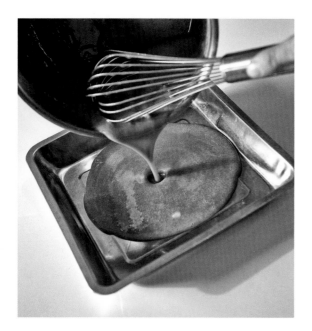

In a clean coffee or spice grinder, grind the dried valerian root to a powder. In a heatproof bowl, combine the valerian root powder with 2 cups of boiling water. Stir well and steep for 30 minutes.

In a saucepan over low heat, combine 1 cup of boiling water with the crushed gum Arabic; mix until it has a goopy consistency.

Strain the valerian solution through a fine-mesh strainer lined with cheesecloth into the gum Arabic. Stir in the icing sugar. Simmer over low heat, stirring frequently, for about 30 minutes. The preparation is done when it pulls away from the side of the pan and forms a thick ball in the centre.

Pour the mixture evenly onto a baking sheet lined with wax paper (optional). Let it set for about 15 minutes. When fully hard-ened, break it into bite-size pieces. Dust with icing sugar to prevent the pieces from sticking together (it will also help absorb any residual moisture). Store the lozenges in an airtight container.

Suck on one lozenge every 3 to 4 hours as needed for anxiety.

» Fast Forward

Fast forward to the health food store to purchase St. Francis valerian tincture or equivalent. Follow the instructions on the label.

! Cautions

Valerian may cause a slight "hangover" with symptoms of dizziness, foggy head, or headache. At regular doses it isn't considered a sedative and has little effect on reaction time, concentration, or coordination. Some studies report valerian may slow the processing of complex thoughts for a few hours after use.

Do not mix with alcohol, alprazolam (Xanax), benzodiazapines, or central nervous system suppressant medication.

Do not take if you are pregnant or nursing.

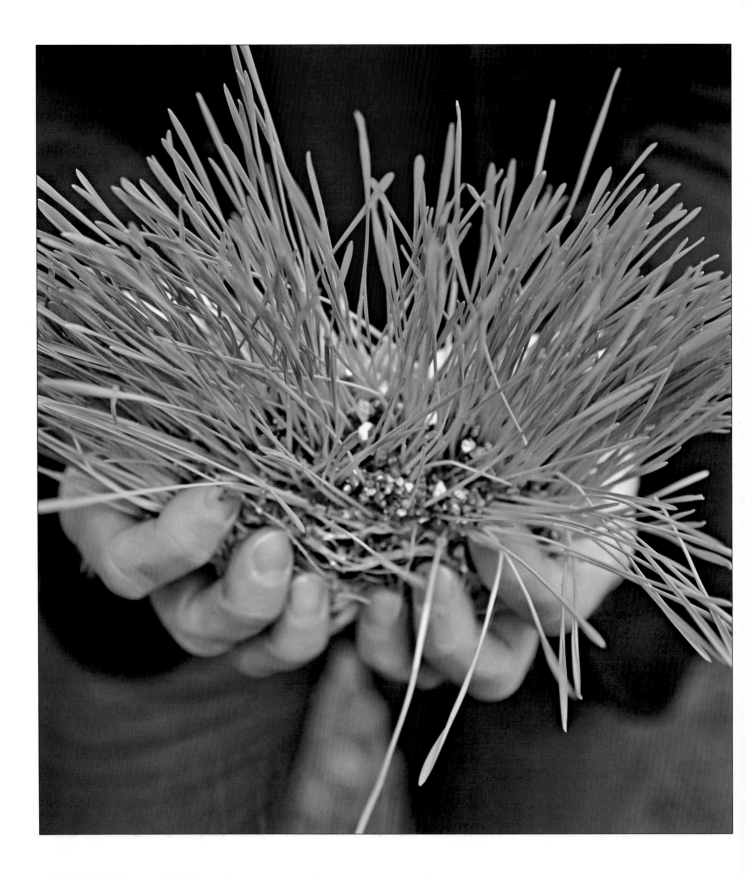

Wheatgrass

Even if you don't frequent health food stores, you've likely seen wheatgrass juice at the mall. It has become very popular in North America, where it's often added to vegetable juices as a "boost." Some people even shoot back an ounce of the juice on its own. That can be hard to do: Freshly cut grass, and that's essentially what it is, doesn't taste amazing unless you're a cow. Wheatgrass is simply the young green shoots of certain varieties of common wheat. Since it's not easily digested, it's pulverized to extract the juice, which is about 70% chlorophyll.

⊕ Health Benefits

Wheatgrass is like a package of sunshine. It is one of the best sources of dietary chlorophyll, and it can increase hemoglobin production in the blood, which in turn circulates more oxygen.

Wheatgrass can also improve blood sugar balance, and may reduce inflammation of the digestive tract. It has also been used to treat skin problems, including eczema or psoriasis. It may relieve constipation, since it contains a significant amount of magnesium. It has even been touted as a cancer remedy, although there is no evidence of its effectiveness for that.

A powerhouse of micronutrients, wheatgrass contains vitamins A, C, and E, calcium, iron, and selenium, as well antioxidants. Since it is harvested before the gluten develops, it's likely safe to consume if you are celiac or following a gluten-free diet.

🌱 Growing

Unless you happen to be a farmer, growing a crop of wheat is a bit of an ordeal. But if you enjoy the health benefits of wheatgrass, you can grow your own indoors year-round. Wheatgrass takes a little work and experience, and you need a lot of grass to extract a small amount of juice. Once you get the hang of it, however, you can produce a whole lawn's worth of this healthy herb!

Common Varieties: Look for varieties of *Triticum aestivum* suitable for using as wheatgrass, such as hard red winter wheat. Source the seeds (called "wheatberries") at health food stores or online, and ensure they have not been treated with chemicals or pesticides.

DIFFICULTY
Medium

HARDINESS
Annual

TIME TO PLANT
Can be grown indoors year-round

TIME TO HARVEST
14 to 20 days from seeding

LOCATION
Needs a window or full-spectrum light

SOIL TYPE
Rich, moist, well-drained

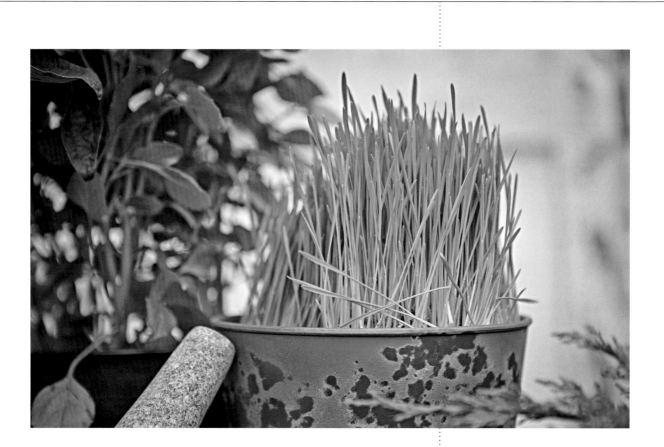

PLANT

To grow wheatgrass indoors, use 25 x 25 cm (10 x 10 inch) grow-ing trays, potting soil or seed-starting soil, and 8 ounces of wheat-grass seed per tray.

Soak the seeds in lukewarm water overnight. Fill the trays with soil and cover with seeds. Don't bury them; just cover lightly with soil. Gently water, and cover with clear plastic or plastic hoods (these can be purchased at garden centres).

Wheatgrass grown indoors requires indirect sunlight from a window or full-spectrum light bulbs (readily available at home improvement stores).

Once green blades are visible, remove the plastic cover and continue to keep moist . During the first few days of growth, gen-tly water every day, but don't soak!

GROW

Given enough water, and planted at the right depth, wheatgrass doesn't need a rocket scientist to grow. Common problems include overwatering, underwatering, and mould. If mould becomes a problem, reduce watering and increase air circulation by placing a fan in the room.

HARVEST

It's crucial to harvest wheatgrass at the right time! Wait for it to "split": This is when the shoots start to produce a second blade of grass. This typically occurs 7 to 12 days from the seed cracking, and when the blade measures 15 cm (6 inches). Use scissors to cut the wheatgrass just above the root. For fresh grass you'll need to plant new seed, so it might be helpful to keep a few trays growing.

STORE

Wheatgrass is best consumed immediately. Repeat the planting process every 10 to 15 days to ensure continual harvests through the year!

Put It to Work

Low iron? Down a green ice cube!

A craving for ice is often a symptom of iron deficiency. (Obviously, the best way to learn about your iron status is by having your doctor check your blood.) If you have low hemoglobin—and many women in their fertile years have slightly

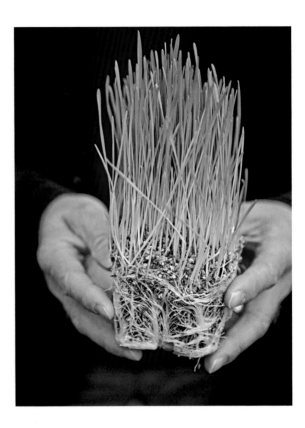

lower levels due to menstruation—supplementing the diet with wheatgrass is a good idea. And if you have a genetic iron deficiency known as thalassemia, iron supplementation won't help—but wheatgrass might!

Juicing wheatgrass requires a high-powered blender or juicer. Harvest as much wheatgrass as you can hold in one fist. Rinse well under cold running water. Chop into 2.5 cm (1 inch) pieces. Add to blender along with 1 cup of cold water and ½ cup of ice. Blend on high speed until smooth and there is a fibrous froth. Line a fine-mesh sieve with cheesecloth and slowly strain the mixture into a bowl.

Pour the juice evenly into a BPA-free ice-cube tray and freeze.

Blend 1 cube of frozen wheatgrass with ½ cup of your favourite citrus juice (this will limit the grassy flavour, and the vitamin C helps iron absorption), ½ cup of water, 1 tablespoon of isolated whey protein, and 1 can of sardines—OK, I'm kidding about the sardines, but now maybe the idea of just wheatgrass and juice doesn't sound so bad! Drink once a day to boost your iron levels.

Hung over? Bottoms up!

A hangover occurs when you have more toxins in your blood than your body can eliminate. Add that to the negative effects of dehydration and you're filled with regret about the night before! It's worth noting that different types of alcohol and the fermentation by-products (congeners) they contain can result in different hangover symptoms. The highest amounts of congeners are found in red wine and dark liquors such as bourbon, brandy, whisky, and tequila.

Consuming too much alcohol is never a good idea, but if you've awoken to a nasty hangover, this elixir should help. It tastes horrible, so plug your nose and kick it back!

4 cups water
Freshly squeezed juice of 1 lemon
1 99-mg potassium tablet, crushed
¼ tsp sea salt
1 tbsp blackstrap molasses
1 oz wheatgrass juice (fresh or frozen)

Combine all of the ingredients together in a bottle, mix vigorously, and force it all down!

» Fast Forward

Fast forward to the health food store to purchase NOW wheatgrass juice powder or equivalent. Follow the instructions on the label.

! Cautions

Because it is grown in soil or water that is potentially contaminated with bacteria, moulds, or other substances, avoid wheatgrass during pregnancy.

Avoid wheatgrass if you have any sensitivity or allergy to the plant. In a very few cases, there have been reports of nausea, headaches, hives, or swelling in the throat within minutes of drinking wheatgrass juice.

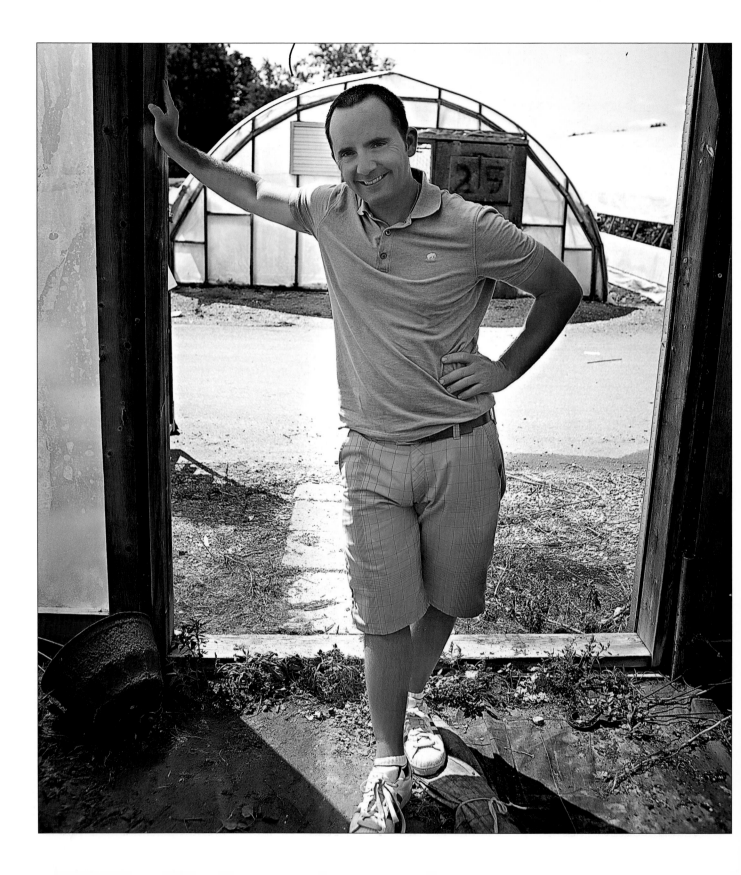

A Gardening Primer

If you're new to gardening, don't be intimidated. With the right guidance, the right location, and a willingness to learn, anyone can grow their own food and medicinal plants. From backyards to rooftops to terraces, if there's room for a plant or a pot, you can grow your own. The medicinal plants in this book can be grown in containers, formal vegetable gardens, formal herb gardens, or just mixed into your existing landscape.

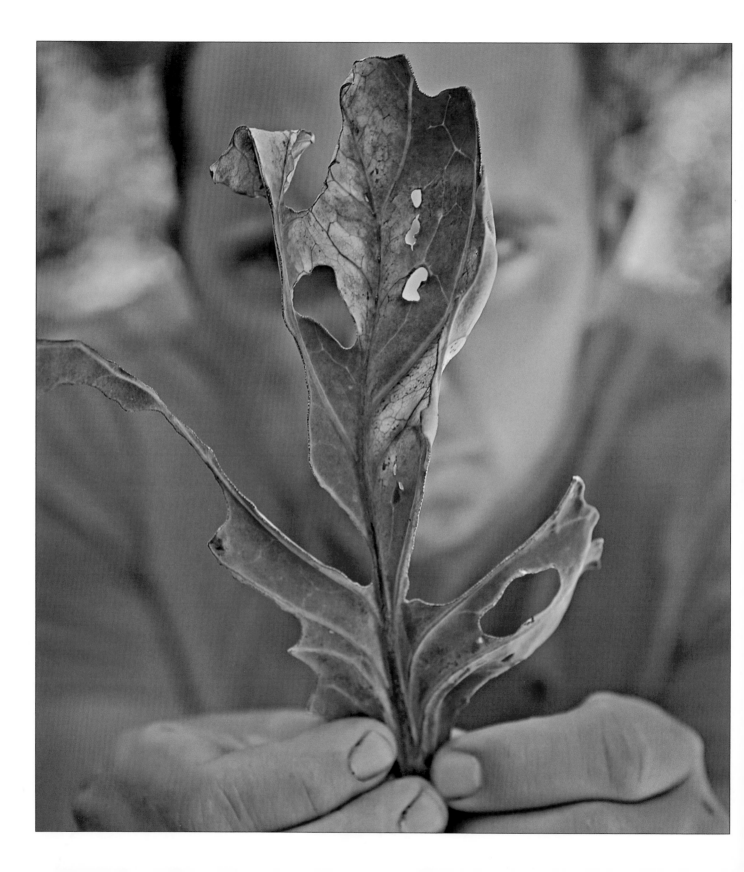

The first rule of gardening is to accept that some of your plants aren't going to make it. I've been working in gardens since I was two years old, and I have killed more than my share of plants—it happens to all of us. Just try to figure out what went wrong—was the plant getting enough light, was it in the right soil, did I remember to fertilize—and chalk it up to experience. The second rule is there's no such thing as a maintenance-free garden. Like all living things, plants have some basic requirements for survival. That largely comes down to finding the right location for each plant. Here are some important concepts you need to understand before you pick up your trowel.

Hardiness

When a plant survives for only one growing season and then dies during the winter, it's called an annual. A perennial is a plant that can survive the winter and come back again year after year. The catch is that a plant that is perennial in one area may be an annual in another; for example, plants in St. John's, Newfoundland, need to be a lot more winter-hardy than those in Victoria, B.C.

Before you even think about choosing plants, you need to know your hardiness zone. Every region of Canada has been assigned a zone number from 0 to 8, based on its climate. The lower the number, the lower the minimum temperature, and the fewer number of plants that will survive winter in that region. Your garden centre staff should be able to tell you what zone your community is in. If not, Agriculture and Agri-Food Canada has a complete plant hardiness zone map at http://atlas.agr.gc.ca/phz.

Whenever you buy a plant, the tag will tell you which zones it will survive in. Unfortunately, this can be a bit confusing. To begin with, many plant tags use the U.S. zone map, which is a bit different from the one used in Canada. For example, my hometown in southern Ontario is zone 5a according to the Canadian map, but it's zone 4b on the U.S. version. What's more, the U.S. scale goes up to zone 10, since many of the southern states are warmer than anywhere in Canada.

It's important not to take zone maps as gospel: Local conditions, such as winds and elevation, can create microclimates that can turn zone 6 into zone 4. If you're planting on a patio 10 storeys up, your zone will drop to a lower number.

Planting Time

Any time you grow plants outdoors you need to pay attention to the last frost date and the length of the growing season in your area. In Canada, the last frost date will be May or June (late April in some parts of B.C.). Do an internet search to find the last frost date in your area, or look to garden clubs, horticultural societies, garden centres, and agricultural agencies for advice.

The last frost date will help you determine when it's safe to sow seeds, when to plant frost-tender plants outdoors, and when tropical plants are safe to move outside. Just remember that historical averages don't mean you won't be surprised! Where I live, May 15 is my last frost date, but Jack Frost has shown his face many times later in the month. Newbies often feel the warmth of early spring air and they jump immediately into gardening, only to be surprised weeks later by a late snowfall or a "killing frost" that crushes their enthusiasm.

Remember, too, that not everything is planted in the spring; some bulbs, including garlic, require fall planting. Read plant tags carefully and ask questions at your garden centre.

The length of the growing season is the number of days between the last frost date in spring and the first frost date in fall. This will affect what types of fruits and vegetables you can grow in your area. For example, if your growing season is only 100 days and the hot peppers you desire take 120 days to maturity, you're out of luck! Dates to maturity can be found on plant tags and seed packs.

SOWING YOUR OWN SEEDS

A number of the plants in this book can be grown from seed. However, if you're a first-time gardener, I highly recommend against it. I want you to have the most positive experience possible, and growing from seed can be frustrating. It requires a lot of time, space, and knowledge—and that knowledge comes at the cost of a lot of failed experiments. Besides, do you really need that many plants? Remember, a single tomato plant, if properly maintained, can feed a family of four! That's why it's usually best to simply purchase healthy transplants from the garden centre.

However, if you are willing to put in the effort, there are some huge benefits to growing from seed. First, you know exactly how the plants were started, which is especially important if you're growing organic herbs. Second, you have access to great choices of plants, since many seed catalogues include items you'll never find at a garden centre. And finally, you'll save money!

To be successful growing from seed, you'll need the right soil, the right trays, the right location, and the time to take care of your young plants. But above all, you have to start them at the right time of year. The number 1 reason people fail is they start too early! Read the seed pack and follow the instructions closely. Most will tell you to sow seeds indoors 4 to 6 weeks before the last frost date.

While starting seeds outdoors may be challenging, some plants are best sown directly into the garden because they do not enjoy being transplanted. This includes most root vegetables like carrots, beets, and radishes, as well as some quick-germinating plants like squash, beans, spinach, and peas. When direct sowing into the garden, make sure you plant the seeds at the correct depth; instructions will be on the pack.

Light

About 90% of edible plants should be grown in full sunlight. But in the world of gardening (and in this book) you will encounter three types of light specifications:

Full sun means 6 or more hours of direct light: That's pretty much all afternoon in direct sunshine. West- or south-facing areas not shaded by buildings or large trees are typical full-sun gardens.

Part sun means 4 to 6 hours of morning sun or indirect light. Gardens facing north or east and gardens shaded by structures or trees are examples of part-sun locations.

Shade is considered 4 or fewer hours of sunlight. Gardens located directly under trees or blocked by structures are examples of shade gardens.

Water

Water is fundamental to all plants' survival. But many gardeners don't use water very efficiently. Be a soaker not a sprinkler! Water your plants deeply, ensuring the water penetrates the soil surface and gets down to the roots. Shallow sprinkling forces plants to send roots close to the surface to absorb water.

Using a soaker hose reduces the risk of water sitting on the plants' foliage for lengthy periods, which can lead to disease. It's also best to water in the morning so the afternoon sun will dry the foliage. Never put your gardens to bed wet!

Some containers need to be watered twice: If you water a pot and notice the water has drained immediately, you need to water it again. Containers typically use soilless mixes that are like sponges: When they are very dry, they can't absorb moisture. So after watering once to open up the soil, give them another drink about 5 minutes later.

Air

During photosynthesis—the process by which plants turn sunlight into sugars—plants remove carbon dioxide from the air and release oxygen. Air circulation is important in the garden; giving plants the space they need will aid photosynthesis and reduce the risk of diseases (such as powdery mildew) by allowing foliage to dry quickly.

With any type of gardening, spacing plants is critical for success. Planting too close together is one of the most common mistakes made by novice gardeners: Those transplants look so small, and it's hard to imagine they can grow several feet tall and wide in a single season! Refer to seed packs and plant tags to learn each plant's space requirements, and follow the instructions closely.

Soil

Your plants are only as good as the soil you grow them in! Most properties have poor soil—it's rare to find one where the soil is well drained and rich in organic matter, especially in new residential areas. Your planned garden may even be sitting on top of "builder's fill," a mix of bad soil, rocks, and random pieces of junk.

There are three basic types of soil. Sand is made up of coarse particles, so it drains well but is lacking in nutrients. Silt contains finer particles than sand and often contains some organic material. It can become very hard and compacted when it dries. Clay is made up of very fine particles of minerals. It retains a lot of moisture, is usually acidic, and doesn't allow good drainage.

The ideal garden soil is called loam, a mix of about two parts sand, two parts silt, and one part clay. If your soil has too much sand or silt, your goal is to improve moisture retention and add nutrients. You can do this by adding equal amounts of topsoil and peat moss, or use triple mix (a blend of topsoil, peat moss, and composted manure). If the soil has too much clay, you'll need to improve the drainage. To be honest, this is not easy to do. The only long-term solutions are to dig it out and replace it with better soil, or to build on top of it. I recommend building a raised bed edged with stone or pressure-treated lumber. Dig out as much clay as you can, put down a layer of coarse stone for drainage, and then add your new soil on top.

How much soil should you add? An investment in soil is well worth it, though replacing the soil in a large garden can be costly. At a minimum I recommend 20 cm (8 inches) of rich organic matter, but my preference is 40 to 45 cm (16 to 18 inches) for new gardens.

You've heard the saying "you get what you give"—it holds true for soil, too. You should always give back to your soil by improving and amending it every year. Many people like to add rich new soil to the garden (called "topdressing") in spring, but the best time is actually the fall. The freezing and thawing that occurs in winter will help work it into the soil naturally. My favourite amendment for herb and vegetable gardens is sheep manure: It's a natural nutrient booster that minimizes the need to use fertilizer.

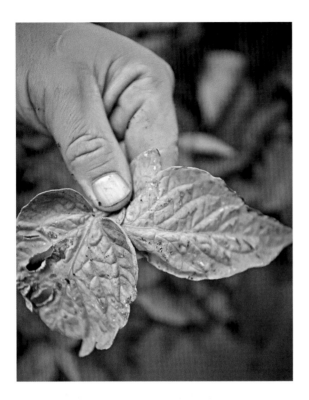

Yellowing foliage on any plant is an indicator of plant stress, which can be caused by a multitude of factors, including too much or too little water, a lack of iron, disease, and insect damage.

Fertilizer

Many plants need to be fertilized during the growing season. Fertilizers come in many different shapes and sizes: water-soluble, liquid, spikes, slow-release granular. They can be organic (fish emulsion, composted manure) or synthetic.

You may have noticed that fertilizer labels have three numbers, such as 20-20-20. The numbers indicate the relative amounts of nitrogen, phosphorus, and potassium (NPK) in the product. These are the primary nutrients plants need to grow, though there are many others, including calcium, magnesium, sulphur, copper, and iron.

Plants typically obtain nutrients by absorbing them through the soil, but the rate of absorption and the amount of nutrients available vary widely with location. For example, rich loamy soil has more nutrients than sandy or clay soil. Soilless mixes and potting soils, used for growing plants in containers, may have no nutrients at all, making fertilizing essential.

The appropriate type of fertilizer, and the right time to apply it, depends on the plant variety and soil. These are outlined in the plant descriptions throughout the book. But as a general rule, the best time to apply water-soluble fertilizer is when gardens are wet, as the fertilizer will be taken up by the roots much more easily.

Location

When choosing an appropriate location for your plant, light, soil, and air aren't the only factors to consider. What good is growing your own plants if you don't use them? Edible plants located far away from the kitchen or porch will never see the mouths they're intended for! When possible, locate your edibles close to areas where they will be consumed.

My favourite herbs are in pots on my back deck, close to my kitchen door and beside my barbecue. They get used often and, because they're so visible, they receive all the watering and fertilizer they deserve.

When growing edible plants, I tend to prefer raised beds. They're easier to maintain—you don't have to bend down too far to weed or harvest—and when you raise a garden you can determine the type of soil your plants will grow in. Raised gardens also warm faster in early spring and generally produce yields more quickly, though they can require extra watering.

For this book, I grew the bulk of the plants in water troughs generally used for horses and cattle. They're portable, they're cheaper than purchasing cedar to build planter boxes, and they come with a drain to ensure the plants will not drown. Besides, I think they look cool—a little rural chic that would fit a funky urban setting! You can easily find these water troughs at farm supply stores, antique stores, online, or even at the occasional rural garage sale or auction.

Unfortunately, once you find a good location, it may not be suitable every year. Crop rotation is the process of making sure you never plant the same types of plants in the same space year after year. By rotating green crops (like spinach or Swiss chard) with root crops (like beets), you will minimize the risk of disease and improve overall garden health, as the soil will have time to replenish nutrients.

Some plants make great partners, while others don't! For example, I've learned that planting marigolds near tomatoes can help deter insects. Nasturtiums play the same role if you plant them near squash. I've suggested a number of other companion ideas in the plant profiles in this book.

Weeding

Weeding is the most loathed task in the garden, but where there is soil there will eventually be weeds. Some offer health benefits (such as dandelion and plantain), but many just interfere with the plants you desire. Weeds are bullies that choke out gardens by reducing light and taking moisture and nutrients away from your plants. So get in there and weed often.

The best time to weed is when gardens are wet, such as immediately after a rain. The weeds will come out much more easily. Always try to pull out weeds before they flower and set seed, and do your best to remove the entire root. Be careful when discarding weeds: Place them immediately into a bag or container to capture any seeds and reduce their broadcast into other areas.

Mulch

Mulch is garden gold! Dry straw, shredded cedar, pine chips, and even used newspapers are all examples of mulch. A good layer of mulch around your plants can reduce weeds by up to 90%, retains moisture, keeps roots cool, and improves soil health by naturally decomposing and adding organic material to the soil underneath. (I prefer organic mulches like those mentioned above, though there are inorganic mulches available, too, such as shredded rubber and stone.)

The recommended depth for most mulches is 6.5 to 10 cm (2.5 to 4 inches). This can be expensive, but it's well worth the investment since mulch helps prevent plant loss from disease. It reduces the splashing of soil during watering and rain, which keeps the soil off the foliage of plants and reduces the spread of pathogens.

Cleaning

Cleanliness is godliness in the garden. After harvesting your plants, make sure leaves, stems, and other unwanted plant material are removed and placed into the composter. If you allow those greens to sit in the garden and rot, you're encouraging a breeding ground for insects and disease.

One of the most important chores is deadheading, or removing flowers after the blooms are spent. To deadhead, simply remove the spent flower and the stem that it's located on.

If you're not harvesting the seeds, you should deadhead your flowering plants often.

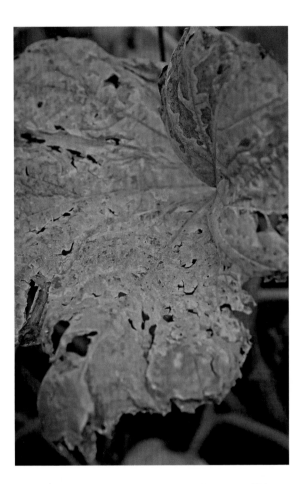

Powdery mildew is a common disease for many edible plants, including beans, cucumbers, and squash. To control, immediately remove and discard infected leaves. For severe cases, removal of the entire plant may be necessary.

This ensures more energy goes to support other parts of the plant rather than the flowers that have just finished. By deadheading you'll increase yields and also see more flowers produced.

Bugs

Cutworms (caterpillars), aphids, slugs, and whiteflies are just some of the insects that may visit your garden during the growing season. If caught early they can usually be managed easily, but if left alone they will destroy your garden. Just about every plant has an insect that enjoys eating it, and every insect requires a different type of control. Cutworms may be stopped by making collars from empty soup cans with the ends cut out and placing them around seedlings. Other insects can be controlled by a sprinkle of crushed eggshells.

Inspect your gardens often for insects: Look for them at night, as many insects are nocturnal. Try to identify the insect and then research the proper treatment. When in doubt, pick and squish! You may also be able to use a high-pressure nozzle to wash bugs away—just be careful not to damage your plants.

An effective and non-toxic control is insecticidal soap. It's available at garden centres, or you can make your own. Just use 2½ tablespoons of liquid dish soap (free of degreasers) and 2½ tablespoons of vegetable oil per gallon of distilled warm water. Mix together and apply with a spray bottle when necessary. Never spray during the hottest part of the day or when temperatures are over 32°C (90°F). It may cause leaf burn.

Disease

Rain, heat, humidity, reduced air circulation, and weak plants are the perfect ingredients for a disease-ridden garden. Plant diseases are often fungal infections, such as powdery mildew, black spot, and fusarium wilt. Many of these can be controlled by applications of a fungicide, but some are not treatable. When a tomato plant is infected with fusarium wilt, for example, your best bet is to carefully remove it before it infects other plants.

One of the best ways to reduce disease is to increase air circulation in the garden by proper plant spacing, clearing away fallen leaves, and immediately removing any diseased foliage. You can also limit the spread by washing your hands, discarding old gloves, and sterilizing pruners when dealing with plants with disease.

When to Give Up

Don't try too hard to rescue a plant that's plagued by disease or infested with bugs. You're probably better off removing it and starting over. Remember, you're trying to grow for health, so get rid of those plants before they harm the health of others!

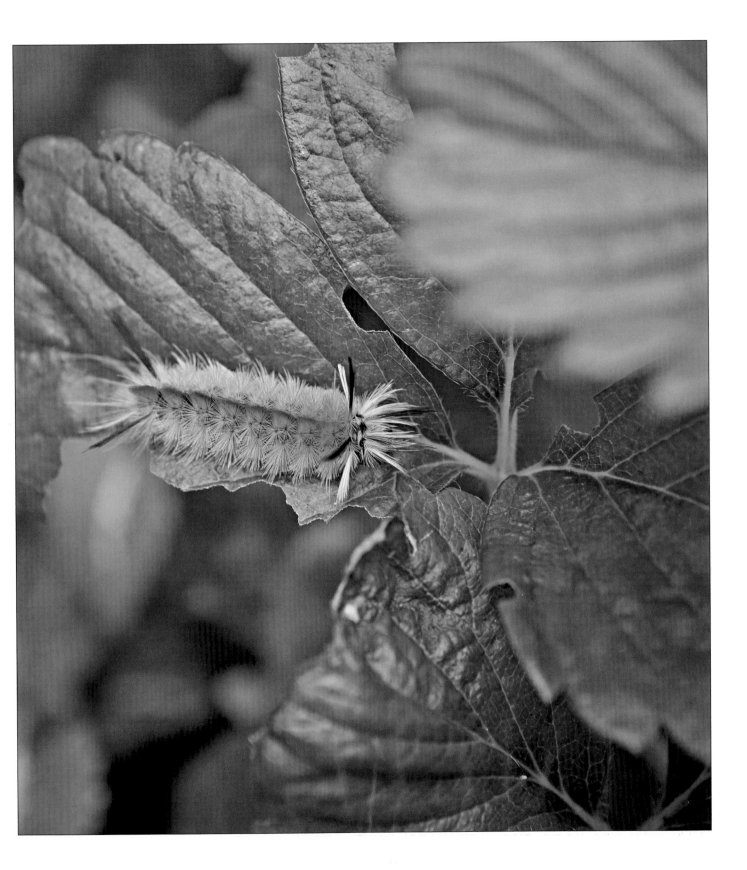

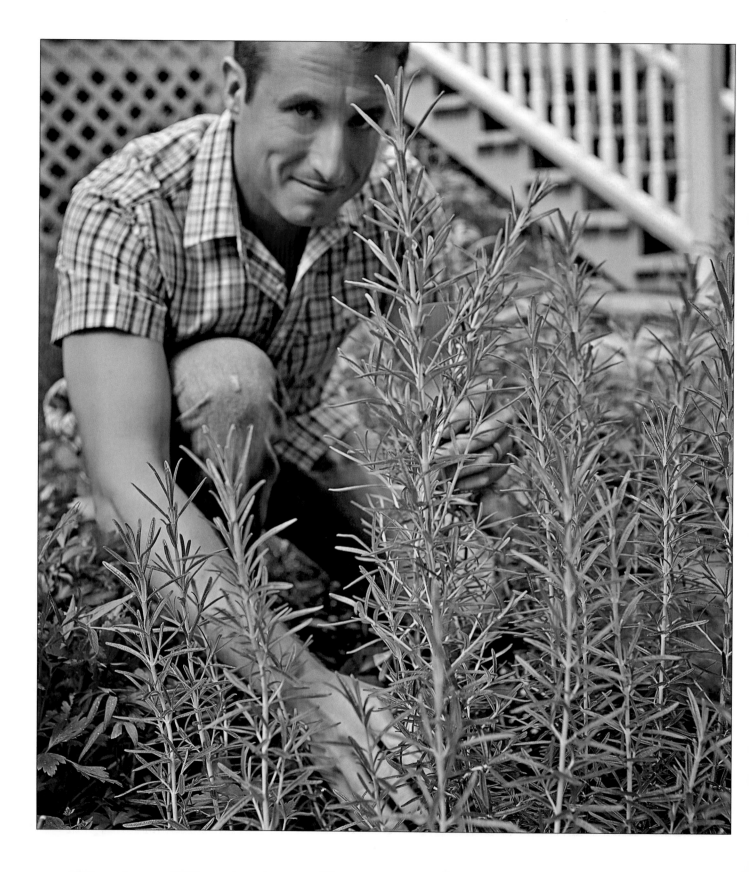

Drying Herbs at Home

Many of the preparations in this book are made with dried herbs, so if you're growing your own, you'll need to get comfortable with the drying process. For the most part this is quite easy—sage and parsley are a snap—but others such as basil and mint can be more challenging.

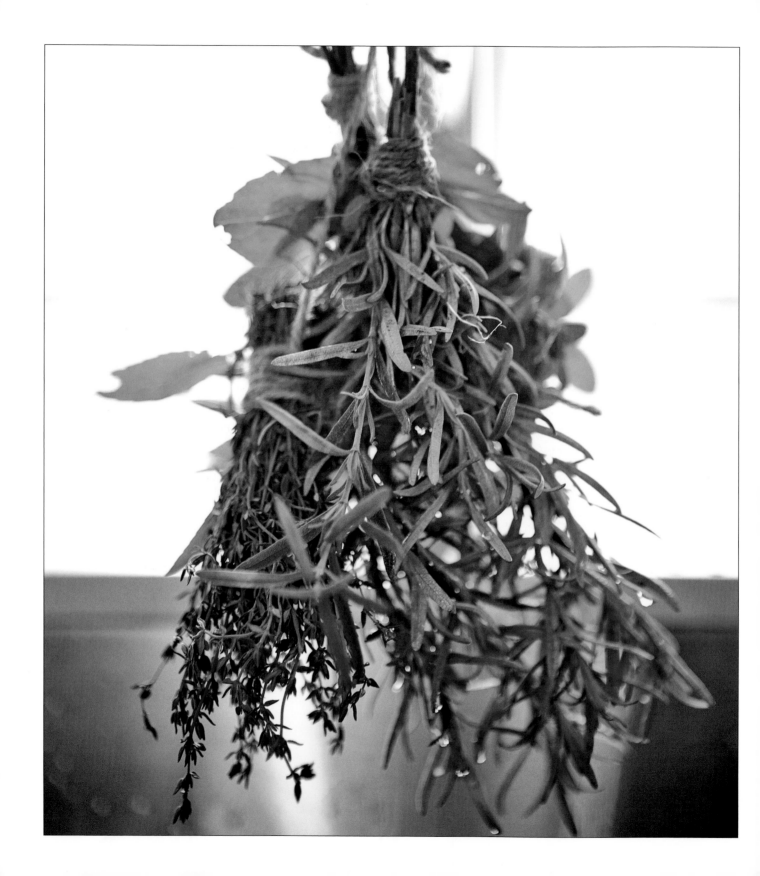

Start by harvesting herbs in late morning, after the dew has evaporated. Remove any dead or damaged leaves. If the foliage is dirty you can give your herb harvest a rinse under cold running water. Shake off the excess water and spread the herb on a paper towel or cloth and leave until all the moisture has evaporated. Then follow one of these three drying methods:

To Air-Dry

Make small bundles by tying the stems with string or twine. The bundles shouldn't be too large, and you should keep them loose to allow for greater airflow. Hang the bundles out of direct light. UV rays from the sun will discolour and reduce the potency of many herbs. You can also place them loosely in paper bags before hanging. This will help shade them and keep them dry and dust-free. Hang them in a closet, attic, garage, or any room that is dry, remains above freezing, and is usually dark.

Another option is to use drying trays (best described as window screens). The holes in the screen help increase airflow. Arrange herbs in a single layer (do not crowd them) on the trays and place in a dry, warm location out of direct light until the herbs are thoroughly dry and brittle (usually 2 to 4 weeks).

To Oven-Dry

Arrange the herbs in a single layer on a baking sheet lined with parchment paper. Spread them out evenly, ensuring they're not crowded. Bake in the oven at the lowest temperature setting for 1 hour. Then turn off the heat and leave the herbs in the oven overnight.

To Dry in the Microwave

Arrange a single layer of herbs between two paper towels and place in a microwave set on high for 1 to 2 minutes (you may need more or less time depending on the herb you are drying), until completely dried and brittle. If the herbs are not brittle, heat for another 30 to 40 seconds. Repeat as needed.

How Do You Know When Herbs Are Dried?

That depends on the method you used and the thickness of the leaf: Each herb dries differently. As a general rule, you know an herb is dried when it is brittle and crumbles when touched.

Dried herbs should always be stored out of direct light, moisture, and extreme heat. Some can be stored for up to a year in the right conditions. See the recommendations listed under each plant in this book.

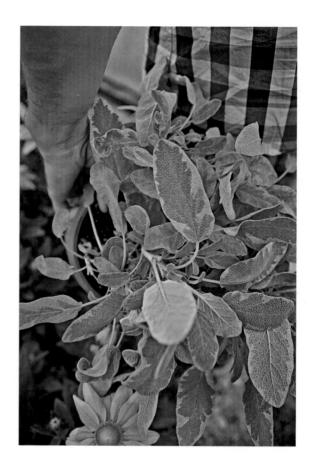

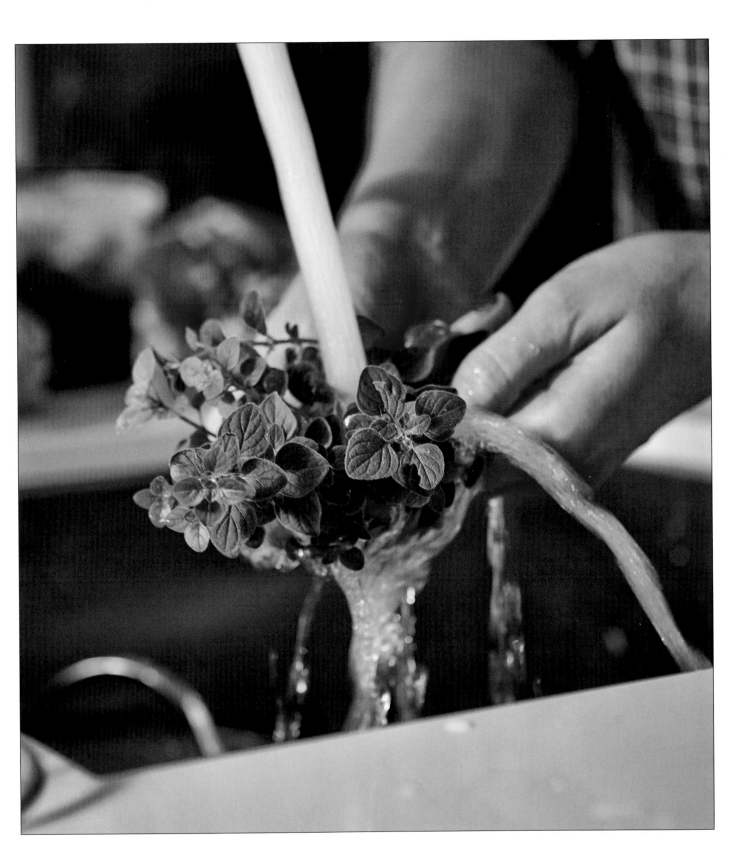

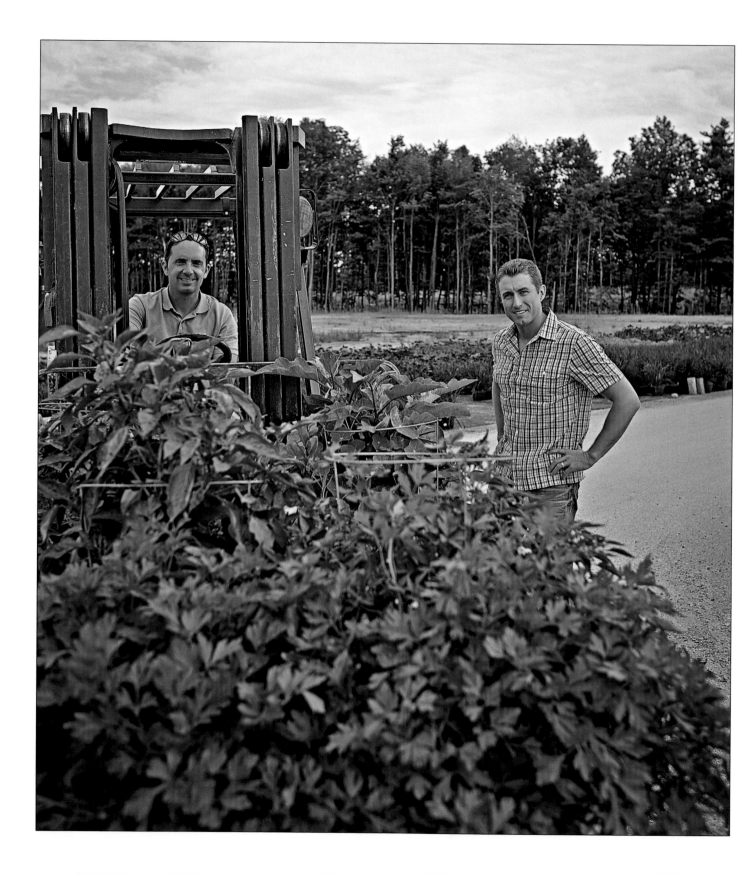

Acknowledge-
ments

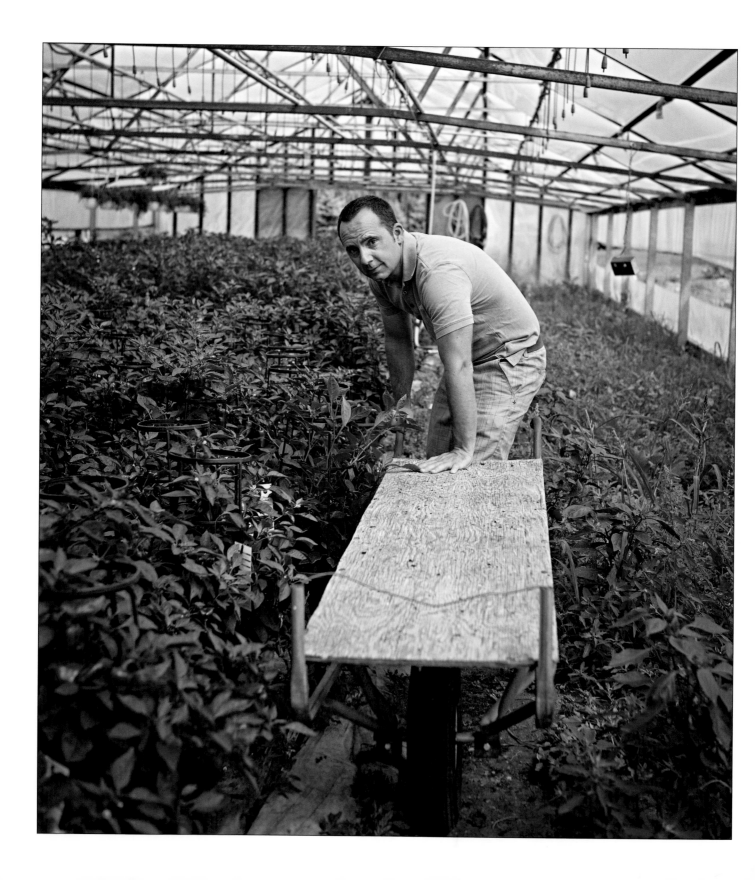

My co-author, Bryce Wylde, has travelled the world seeking the truth about how individuals can improve their quality of life through natural elements, especially plants. I've always known how to grow plants, but Bryce has taught me to put them to use in ways that have already been rewarding, and hopefully will make me live longer!

I've always had an interest in using plants medicinally. It began in my childhood with my Nonna's belief that generous portions of dandelion make the heart stronger. I learned more from my friend Rylan Vallee's father, Dr. Brian Vallee, who was a naturopathic doctor in Abbotsford, B.C. He taught me about the healing powers of plants that have been known for thousands of years.

A project like this requires countless hours of research, writing, planting, watering, and photography. That workload requires the support of my immediate family. My wife, Laurie, is always patient and supportive of any project I take on, and I love her for that. My boys, Gavin and Matheson, came together to help me tend many of the plants featured in this book. My family business, Bradford Greenhouses, cultivated my knowledge from childhood to present day. I thank my mother, Alyce; my father, Tony; my sister, Chiara; my uncles, Sam, Peter, Mickey, and Len; my aunts, Mary, Eileen, Jen, Lucy, and Rosalba; and my many cousins for their support and love.

The horticultural industry in Canada has always been a source of inspiration: It includes many of the hardest-working and most passionate people I know. Freeman Herbs provided me with a host of plants for this book, and I want to acknowledge the exceptional quality of plants they produce, many of which are grown organically. To my cousins at Riga Farms, who work from sunrise to sunset growing some of Ontario's best Swiss chard, beets, and kale: Thank you for providing this book with some great plants, and also for the food you put on Canadian tables throughout the growing season.

In life it takes a team to build a home, a business, a car. A book is no different, so I would like to acknowledge the team of talented people who helped create *Power Plants*: from the exceptional photography of Shannon J. Ross to the vision and guidance (and downright pestering!) of HarperCollins senior editor Kate Cassaday—you're amazing! Dan Bortolotti has to be recognized, too—before his editing, some of this book looked more like notes on a sketch pad. To my publicists, Julia Barrett and Carolyn Ovell, thank you for helping keep me on track and in the public eye. I consider you both a part of my extended family.

We hope the work of our team will help you grow a healthy life!

—Frankie

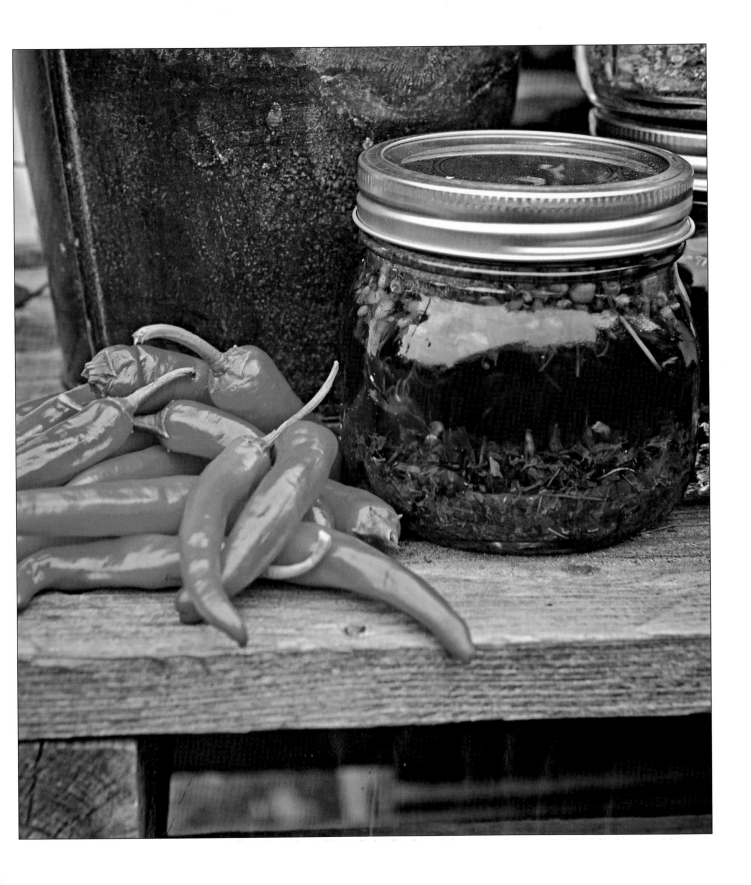

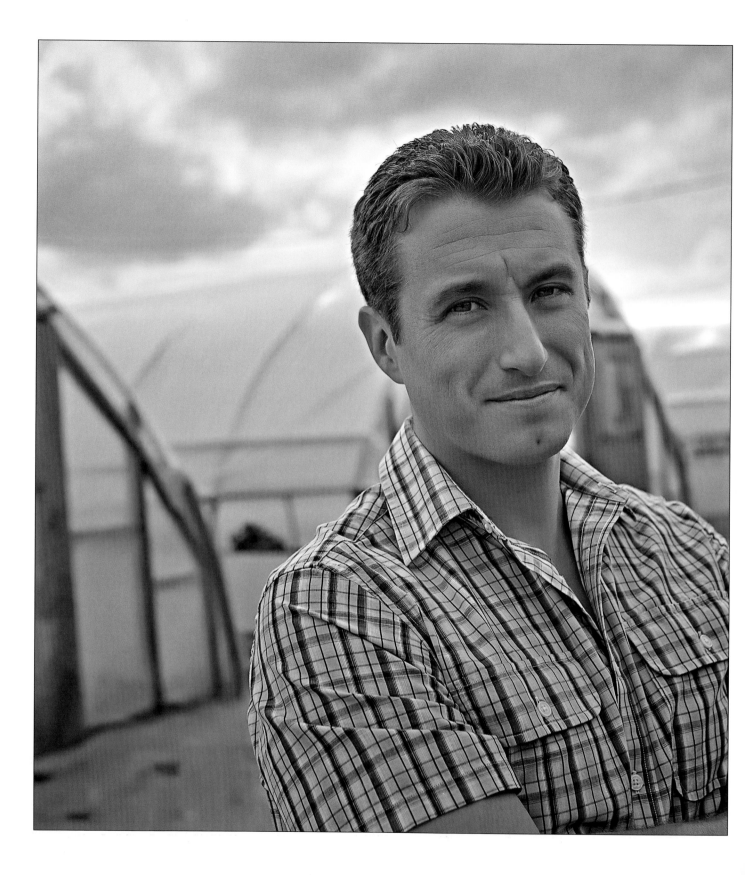

This book wouldn't have been possible if it wasn't for Frank's idea, many years ago, that we collaborate on a project that could benefit the general public. So I'd like to deeply thank Frank for his ingenuity, and for bringing me even closer to nature through this initiative. His passion for growing plants is contagious!

I came into this project "green" in more ways than one. Natural medicine is my life, but I only ever had a basic understanding when it came to growing plants. In this day and age, people need to remember the wisdom their grandparents and elders once held with respect to the miracles of nature. Until I met Frankie Flowers, I too was stuck in the mentality that "natural" and "complementary alternative" meant herbs or nutrients encapsulated and bottled to look like a medicine. That's fine in most cases, but there is something special about getting back to nature and growing a medicine yourself.

My mother was an avid gardener. She insisted my two sisters and I share in the responsibility of watering and fertilizing the annual Wylde family bounty. We used an all-natural approach, of course. Among other now widely accepted practices, my mother raised us to compost before it was a household term and a municipal requirement. For all of this, I thank you, Momsie!

I'd also like to share my deepest gratitude to HarperCollins Canada, and in particular our editor, Kate Cassaday. I've met few others with such incredible vision, positive motivation, and strong determination to see the project come alive to its full potential.

The amount of time and energy spent by Dan Bortolotti focusing our prose so the book was ready for publishing was also impressive. Thank you!

It's one thing to grow and bottle nature's beauty, but capturing the process with such a keen eye and under significant time constraints required the genius work of Shannon J. Ross, for whom I'm very grateful.

I want to acknowledge a very important person without whom this project couldn't have happened. My literary agent, Chris Casuccio, of Westwood Creative Artists once again stepped up and went way above and beyond the call of duty to support me. Thanks also to John Pearce at Westwood Creative Artists.

To my team at Argyle Communications—you guys know what you do and there aren't enough pages here anyway. My sincere gratitude to Nick Williams, Caroline DeSilva, Anna Campbell, and especially Rob McEwan.

To my "mushy" manager, Sharon Feldstein, thank you for all your constant efforts and belief in me.

To Dr. Mehmet Oz and Dr. Andy Weil, we are very grateful for all the time it took to review this work.

I also want to thank my many patients for being so, well, patient with me during my time away from the clinic.

A very special appreciation goes to my wonderful wife and family. "Thank you" doesn't begin to express how deeply I am grateful for their support during this project. Seeing my daughter, Zaya, picking and eating fresh basil and tomatoes from our garden, and my son, Devin, collecting the strawberries we grow out back of our house warms my heart and speaks to the success of this project.

—Bryce

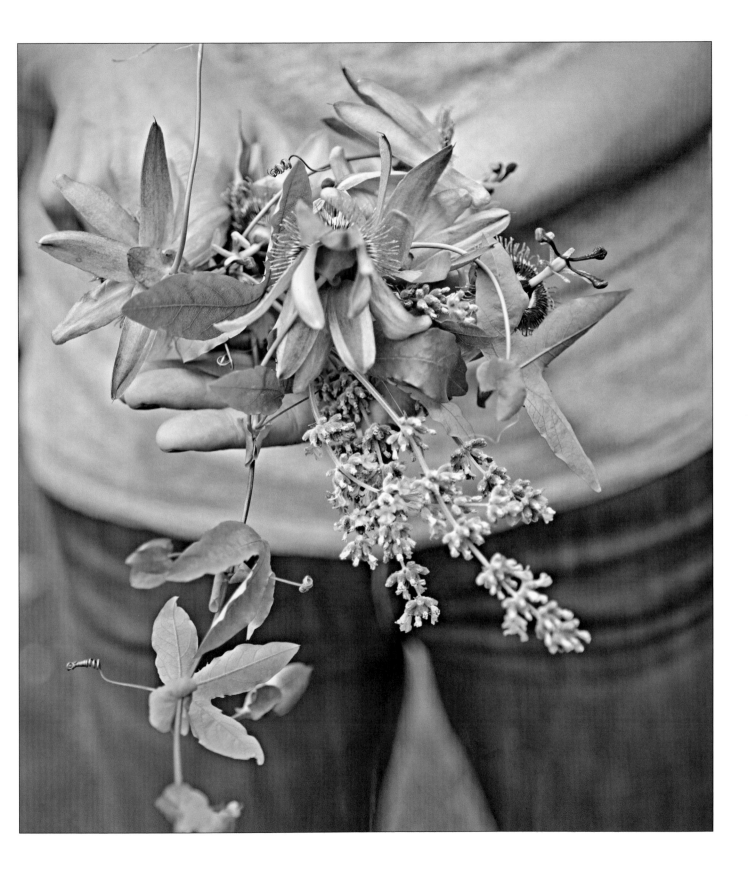

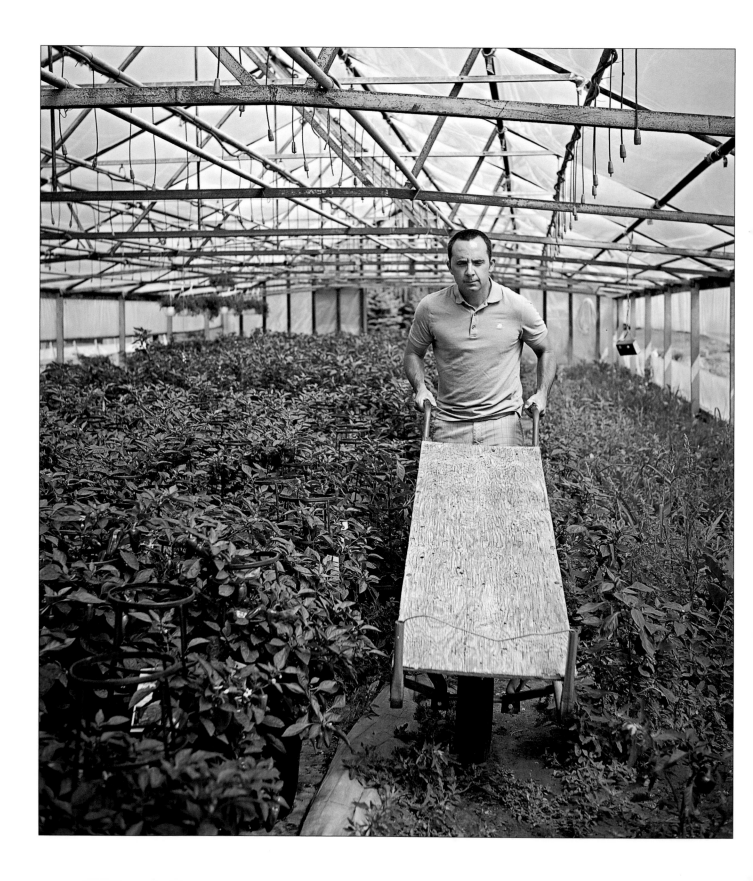

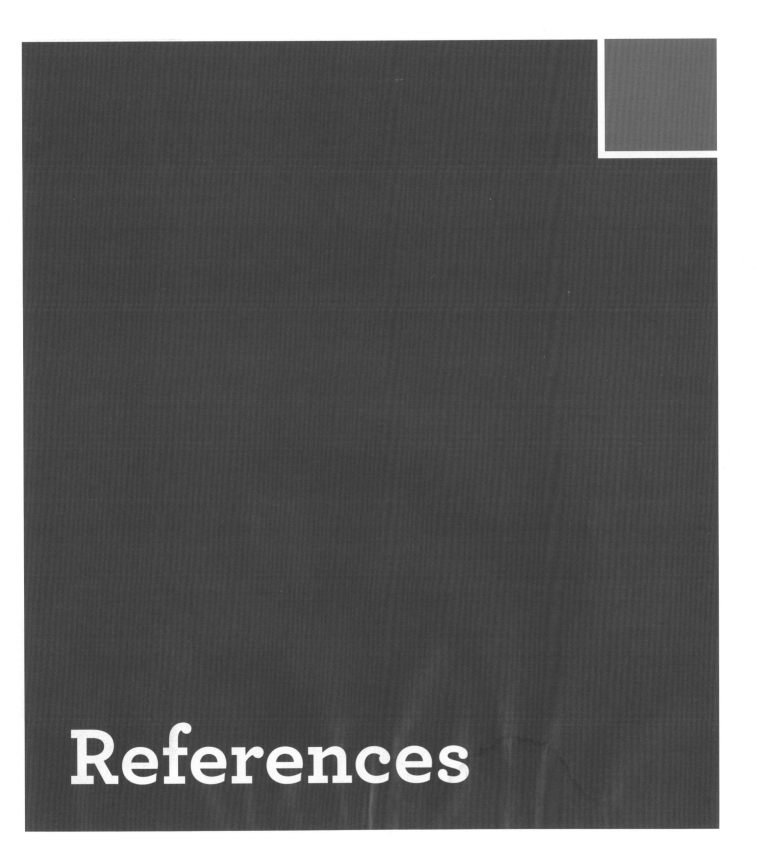

References

ALFALFA

Basch, E., et al. Alfalfa (*Medicago sativa L.*): a clinical decision support tool. *J Herb Pharm* 2003;3(2):69–90.

Boue, S.M., et al. Evaluation of the estrogenic effects of legume extracts containing phytoestrogens. *J Agric Food Chem* 4-9-2003;51(8): 2193–99.

Briggs, C. Alfalfa. *Canadian Pharm J* 1994;Mar:84–5, 115.

De Leo, V., et al. Treatment of neurovegetative menopausal symptoms with a phytotherapeutic agent. *Minerva Ginecol* 1998 May;50(5):207–11.

Foster, S. *Herbs for Your Health*. Loveland, CO: Interweave Press, 1996, 2–3.

Gray, A.M., & Flatt, P.R. Pancreatic and extra-pancreatic effects of the traditional anti-diabetic plant, *Medicago sativa* (lucerne). *Br J Nutr* 1997;78(2):325–34.

Malinow, M.R., McLaughlin, P., & Stafford, C. Alfalfa seeds: Effects on cholesterol metabolism. *Experientia* 5-15-1980;36(5):562–64.

Mölgaard, J., et al. Alfalfa seeds lower low-density lipoprotein cholesterol and apolipoprotein B concentrations in patients with type II hyperlipoproteinemia. *Atherosclerosis* 1987 May;65(1–2):173–79.

Story, J.A. Alfalfa saponins and cholesterol interactions. *Am J Clin Nutr* 1984;39:917–29.

Swanston-Flatt, S.K., et al. Traditional plant treatments for diabetes: Studies in normal and streptozotocin-diabetic mice. *Diabetologia* 1990;33(8): 462–64.

ALOE VERA

Blumenthal, M., et al. (eds.). *The Complete Commission E Monographs: Therapeutic Guide to Herbal Medicines*. Boston, MA: Integrative Medicine Communications, 1998, 80–81.

Chevrel, B. A comparative crossover study on the treatment of heartburn and epigastric pain: Liquid Gaviscon and a magnesium-aluminum antacid gel. *J Int Med Res* 1980;8:300–03.

Davis, R.H., Leitner, M.G., Russo, J.M., & Byrne, M.E. Wound healing: Oral and topical activity of aloe vera. *J Am Podiatr Med Assoc* 1989;79:559–62.

Syed, T.A., et al. Management of psoriasis with aloe vera extract in a hydrophilic cream: A placebo-controlled, double-blind study. *Tropical Med Inter Health* 1996;1:505–09.

Vardy, D.A., et al. A double-blind, placebo-controlled trial of an aloe vera (*A. barbadensis*) emulsion in the treatment of seborrheic dermatitis. *J Dermatol Treat* 1999;10:7–11.

Visuthikosol, V., et al. Effect of aloe vera gel to healing of burn wound: A clinical and histologic study. *J Med Assoc Thai* 1995;78:403–09.

Williams, M.S., et al. Phase III double-blind evaluation of an aloe vera gel as a prophylactic agent for radiation-induced skin toxicity. *Int J Rad Oncol Biol Phys* 1996;36:345–49.

BASIL

Brinker, F. *Herb Contraindications and Drug Interactions*, 2nd ed. Sandy, OR: Eclectic Medical Publications, 1998.

Farnsworth, N.R., & Bunyapraphatsara, N. (eds.). *Thai Medicinal Plants*. Bangkok: Medicinal Plant Information Center, 1992, 180–82.

Grieve, M. *A Modern Herbal*, Vol. 1. New York: Hafner, 1967, 86.

Nadkarni, A.K., & Nadkarni, K.M. *Indian Materia Medica*, Vol. 1. Bombay: Popular Prakashan, 1976, 861–67.

BEET

Lansley, K.E., et al. Acute dietary nitrate supplementation improves cycling time trial perfomance. *Med Sci Sports Exerc* 2011;43(6):1125–31.

Lundberg, J.O., Larsen, F.J., & Weitzberg, E. Supplementation with nitrate and nitrite salts in exercise: A word of caution. *J Appl Physiol* 2011;111:616–17.

Presley, T.D., et al. Acute effect of a high nitrate diet on brain perfusion in older adults. *Nitric Oxide* 2011 Jan 1;24(1):34–42. doi: 10.1016/j.niox.2010.10.002. Epub 2010 Oct 15.

Wylie, L.J., et al. Beetroot juice and exercise: Pharmacodynamic and dose-response relationships. *J Appl Physiol* (1985). 2013 Aug 1; 115(3):325–36.

BERGAMOT

Duke, J.A. *The Green Pharmacy*. Boston: St. Martin's Press, 1997, 35, 78, 152, 431.

Gruenwald, J., et al. *PDR for Herbal Medicines*, 1st ed. Montvale, NJ: Medical Economics Company, Inc., 1998.

McGuffin, M., et al. *American Herbal Products Association's Botanical Safety Handbook*. Boca Raton, FL: CRC Press, LLC, 1997.

BLACKBERRY

Blomhoff, R. Antioxidants and oxidative stress. *Tidsskr. Nor Laegeforen* 6-17-2004;124(12):1643–45.

Pellegrini, N., et al. Total antioxidant capacity of plant foods, beverages, and oils consumed in Italy assessed by three different in vitro assays. *J Nutr* 2003;133(9):2812–19.

Serraino, I., et al. Protective effects of cyanidin-3-O-glucoside from blackberry extract against peroxynitrite-induced endothelial dysfunction and vascular failure. *Life Sci* 7-18-2003;73(9):1097–1114.

BLUEBERRY

Abidov, M., et al. Effect of Blueberin on fasting glucose, C-reactive protein, and plasma aminotransferases, in female volunteers with diabetes type 2: Double-blind, placebo-controlled clinical study. *Georgian Med News* 2006;(141):66–72.

Kay, C.D., & Holub, B.J. The effect of wild blueberry (*Vaccinium angustifolium*) consumption on postprandial serum antioxidant status in human subjects. *Br J Nutr* 2002;88(4):389–98.

Melzig, M.F., & Funke, I. Inhibitors of alpha-amylase from plants: A possibility to treat diabetes mellitus type II by phytotherapy? *Wien Med Wochenschr* 2007; 157(13-14):320–24.

Nemes-Nagy, E., et al. Effect of a dietary supplement containing blueberry and sea buckthorn concentrate on antioxidant capacity in type 1 diabetic children. *Acta Physiol Hung* 2008;95(4):383–93.

Prior, R.L., et al. Plasma antioxidant capacity changes following a meal as a measure of the ability of a food to alter in vivo antioxidant status. *J Am Coll Nutr* 2007;26(2):170–81.

Wedick, N.W., et al. Dietary flavonoid intakes and risk of type 2 diabetes in US men and women. *Am J Clin Nutr* 2012 Apr;95(4):925–33.

Wilms, L.C., et al. Impact of multiple genetic polymorphisms on effects of a 4-week blueberry juice intervention on ex vivo induced lymphocytic DNA damage in human volunteers. *Carcinogenesis* 2007;28(8):1800–06.

BURDOCK

Cicero, A.F., Derosa, G., & Gaddi, A. What do herbalists suggest to diabetic patients in order to improve glycemic control? Evaluation of scientific evidence and potential risks. *Acta Diabetol* 2004;41(3):91–98.

Iwakami, S., Wu, J.B., Ebizuka, Y., & Sankawa, U. Platelet activating factor (PAF) antagonists contained in medicinal plants: Lignans and sesquiterpenes. *Chem Pharm Bull* (Tokyo) 1992;40:1196–98.

Zick, S.M., et al. Trial of Essiac to ascertain its effect in women with breast cancer (TEA-BC). *J Altern Complement Med* 2006;12(10):971–80.

CALENDULA

Amirghofran, Z., Azadbakht, M., & Karimi, M.H. Evaluation of the immunomodulatory effects of five herbal plants. *J Ethnopharmacol* 2000;72(1–2):167–72.

Basch, E., et al. (*Calendula officinalis* L.): An evidence-based systematic review by the Natural Standard Research Collaboration. *J Herb Pharmacother* 2006; 6(3-4):135–59.

Bogdanova, N.S., et al. Study of antiviral properties of *Calendula officinalis*. *Farmskolto Ksikol* 1970;33:349–55 [in Russian].

Weiss, R.F. *Herbal Medicine.* Gothenburg, Sweden: Ab Arcanum, 1988, 344.

Yoshikawa, M., et al. Medicinal flowers. III. Marigold. (1): Hypoglycemic, gastric emptying inhibitory, and gas-troprotective principles and new oleanane-type triterpene oligoglycosides, calendasaponins A, B, C, and D, from Egyptian *Calendula officinalis*. *Chem Pharm Bull* (Tokyo) 2001;49(7):863–70.

CAMELLIA

Chantre, P., & Lairon, D. Recent findings of green tea extract AR25 (Exolise) and its activity for the treatment of obesity. *Phytomedicine* 2002;9(1):3–8.

Coimbra, S., et al. The effect of green tea in oxidative stress. *Clin Nutr* 2006;25(5):790–96.

Cooper, M.J., Cockell, K.A., & L'Abbé, M.R. The iron status of Canadian adolescents and adults: Current knowledge and practical implications. *Can J Diet Pract Res* 2006;67(3):130–38.

Green, R.J., et al. Common tea formulations modulate in vitro digestive recovery of green tea catechins. Department of Food Science, Purdue University, West Lafayette, IN 47907, USA. *Mol Nutr Food Res* 2007;51(9):1152–62.

Stensvold, I., et al. Tea consumption: Relationship to cholesterol, blood pressure, and coronary and total mortality. *Prev Med* 1992;21:546–53.

CAPISCUM

Bortolotti, M., Coccia, G., & Grossi, G. Red pepper and functional dyspepsia. *N Engl J Med* 2002;346:947–48.

Chrubasik, S., Weiser, W., & Beime, B. Effectiveness and safety of topical capsaicin cream in the treatment of chronic soft tissue pain. *Phytother Res* 2010;24:1877–85.

Mason, L., et al. Systematic review of topical capsaicin for the treatment of chronic pain. *BMJ* 2004;328:991.

Whiting, S., et al. Capsaicinoids and capsinoids: A potential role for weight management? A systematic review of the evidence. *Appetite* 2012 Oct;59(2):341–48.

Yoshioka, M., et al. Effects of red pepper on appetite and energy intake. *Br J Nutr* 1999;82:115–23.

Yoshioka, M., St-Pierre, S., Suzuki, M., & Tremblay, A. Effects of red pepper added to high-fat and high-carbohydrate meals on energy metabolism and substrate utilization in Japanese women. *Br J Nutr* 1998;80:503–10.

CHAMOMILE

Avallone, R., et al. Benzodiazepine-like compounds and GABA in flower heads of *Matricaria chamomilla*. *Phyto Res* 1996;10:S177–S179.

Glowania, H. J., Raulin, C., & Swoboda, M. Effect of chamomile on wound healing: A clinical double-blind study. *Z.Hautkr.* 9-1-1987;62(17):1262, 1267–71.

Hormann, H., & Korting, H. Evidence for the efficacy and safety of topical herbal drugs in dermatology: Part 1: Anti-inflammatory agents. *Phytomed* 1994;1(2):161–71.

Jakolev, V., & Schlichtegroll, A. Anti-inflammatory activity of (-)-alpha-bisabolol: An essential component of chamomile oil. *Arzneimittelforschung* 1969;19(4):615–16.

Tubaro, A., Zilli, C., Redaelli, C., & Della, Loggia R. Evaluation of anti-inflammatory activity of a chamomile extract topical application. *Planta Med* 1984;50(4):359.

Viola, H., et al. Apigenin, a component of *Matricaria recutita* flowers, is a central benzodiazepine receptors-ligand with anxiolytic effects. *Planta Med* 1995;61:213–16.

COMFREY

D'Anchise, R., et al. Comfrey extract ointment in comparison to diclofenac gel in the treatment of acute unilateral ankle sprains (distortions). *Arzneimittelforschung* 2007; 57(11):712–16.

Duke, J.A. *Handbook of Phytochemical Constituents of GRAS Herbs and Other Economic Plants.* Boca Raton, FL: CRC Press, 1992.

Koll, R., et al. Efficacy and tolerance of a comfrey root extract (*Extr. Rad. Symphyti*) in the treatment of ankle distortions: Results of a multicenter, randomized, placebo-controlled, double-blind study. *Phytomed* 2004;11(6):470–77.

Kucera, M., Kalal, J., & Polesna, Z. Effects of Symphytum ointment on muscular symptoms and functional locomotor disturbances. *Adv Ther* 2000;17(4):204–10.

Mills, S.Y. *Out of the Earth: The Essential Book of Herbal Medicine.* New York: Viking Arkana, 1991, 544–47.

Predel, H.G., et al. Efficacy of a comfrey root extract ointment in comparison to a diclofenac gel in the treatment of ankle distortions: Results of an observer-blind, randomized, multicenter study. *Phytomed* 2005;12:707–14.

DANDELION

Baba, K., Abe, S., & Mizuno, D. [Anti-tumor activity of hot water extract of dandelion, *Taraxacum officinale*: Correlation between antitumor activity and timing of administration (Author's transl.)]. *Yakugaku Zasshi* 1981;101(6):538–43.

Blumenthal, M., et al. (eds.). *The Complete German Commission E Monographs: Therapeutic Guide to Herbal Medicines.* Austin: American Botanical Council and Boston: Integrative Medicine Communications, 1998, 425–26.

Kuusi, T., Pyylaso, H., & Autio, K. The bitterness properties of dandelion. II. Chemical investigations. *Lebensm-Wiss Technol* 1985;18:347–49.

Racz-Kotilla, E., Racz, G., & Solomon, A. The action of *Taraxacum officinale* extracts on body weight and diuresis of laboratory animals. *Planta Med* 1974:26:212–17.

Schulz, V., Hänsel, R., & Tyler, V.E. *Rational Phytotherapy: A Physician's Guide to Herbal Medicine,* 3rd ed. Berlin: Springer, 1998, 168–73.

ECHINACEA

Braunig, B., Dorn, M., & Knick, E. *Echinacea purpurea* root for strengthening the immune response to flu-like infections. *Z Phyto* 1992;13:7–13.

Brikenborn, R.M., Shah, D.V., & Degenring, F.H. Echinaforce° and other echinacea fresh plant preparations in the treatment of the common cold: A randomized, placebo-controlled, double-blind clinical trial. *Phytomed* 1999;6:1–5.

Di Pierro, F., et al. Use of a standardized extract from *Echinacea angustifolia* (Polinacea°) for the prevention of respiratory tract infections. *Alterna Med Rev* Mar 2012;17(1):36–41.

Dorn, M., Knick, E., & Lewith, G. Placebo-controlled, double-blind study of *Echinacea pallida redix* in upper respiratory tract infections. *Comp Ther Med* 1997;5:40–42.

Hoheisel, O., et al. Echinagard treatment shortens the course of the common cold: A double-blind, placebo-controlled clinical trial. *Eur J Clin Res* 1997;9:261–68.

Jawad, M., et al. Safety and efficacy profile of *Echinacea purpurea* to prevent common cold episodes: A randomized, double-blind, placebo-controlled trial. *Evid Based Comp Alternat Med.* 2012:841315. Epub 2012 Sep 16.

Lakier Smith, L. Overtraining, excessive exercise, and altered immunity: Is this a T helper-1 versus T helper-2 lymphocyte response? *Sports Med* 2003;33(5):347–64.

Melchart, D., et al. Immunomodulation with echinacea: A systematic review of controlled clinical trials. *Phytomed* 1994;1:245–54.

Schoop, R., Klein, P., Suter, A., & Johnston, S.L. Echinacea in the prevention of induced rhinovirus colds: A meta-analysis. *Clin The* Feb 2006;28(2):174–83.

See, D.M., Broumand, N., Sahl, L., & Tilles, J.G. In vitro effects of echinacea and ginseng on natural killer and antibody-dependent cell cytotoxicity in healthy subjects and chronic fatigue syndrome or acquired immunodeficiency syndrome patients. *Immunopharmacology* 1997;35:229–35.

ELDERBERRY

Kong, F. Pilot clinical study on a proprietary elderberry extract: Efficacy in addressing influenza symptoms. *OJP* 2009;5:32–43.

Newall, C.A., Anderson, L.A., & Phillipson, J.D. *Herbal Medicines: A Guide for Health-Care Professionals.* London: The Pharmaceutical Press, 1996, 104–05.

Roschek, B., et al. Elderberry flavonoids bind to and prevent H1N1 infection in vitro. *Phytochemistry* 2009;70:1255–61.

Serkedjieva, J., et al. Antiviral activity of the infusion (SHS-174) from flowers of *Sambucus nigra L.*, aerial parts of *Hypericum perforatum L.*, and roots of *Saponaria officinalis L.* against influenza and herpes simplex viruses. *Phytother Res* 1990;4:97–100.

Uncini Manganelli, R.E., Zaccaro, L., & Tomei, P.E. Antiviral activity in vitro of *Urtica dioica L., Parietaria diffusa M. et K.* and *Sambucus nigra L. J Ethnopharmacol* 2005 Apr 26;98(3):323–27.

Vlachojannis, J.E., Cameron, M., & Chrubasik, S. A systematic review on the sambuci fructus effect and efficacy profiles. *Phytother Res* 2010 Jan;24(1):1–8. Review.

Youdim, K.A., Martin, A., & Joseph, J.A. Incorporation of the elderberry anthocyanins by endothelial cells increases protection against oxidative stress. *Free Radical Biol Med* 2000;29:51–60.

Zakay-Rones, Z., et al. Inhibition of several strains of influenza virus in vitro and reduction of symptoms by an elderberry extract (*Sambucus nigra L*) during an outbreak of influenza B Panama. *J Altern Complement Med* 1995;1:361–69.

FEVERFEW

Diener, H.C., et al. Efficacy and safety of 6.25 mg t.i.d. feverfew CO_2-extract (MIG-99) in migraine prevention: A randomized, double-blind, multicentre, placebo-controlled study. *Cephalalgia* 2005;25:1031–41.

Green, J. *The Herbal Medicine Maker's Handbook: A Home Manual.* Darlinghurst, AU: Crossing Press, 2000.

Johnson, E.S., Kadam, N.P., Hylands, D.M., & Hylands, P.J. Efficacy of feverfew as prophylactic treatment of migraine. *Br Med J* (Clin Res Ed) 1985;291:569–73.

Murphy, J.J., Hepinstall, S., & Mitchell, J.R. Randomized double-blind placebo-controlled trial of feverfew in migraine prevention. *Lancet* 1988;2:189–92.

Palevitch, D., Earon, G., & Carasso, R. Feverfew (*Tanacetum parthenium*) as a prophylactic treatment for migraine: A double-blind, placebo-controlled study. *Phytother Res* 1997;11:508–11.

FRENCH BEANS

Azinge, N.O. Use of beans diet for control of diabetes. *Trop Doct* 1985;15(3):139.

Barrett, M.L., & Udani, J.K. A proprietary alpha-amylase inhibitor from white bean (*Phaseolus vulgaris*): A review of clinical studies on weight loss and glycemic control. *Nutr J* 2011;10:24.

Birketvedt, G.S., Travis, A., Langbakk, B., & Florholmen, J.R. Dietary supplementation with bean extract improves lipid profile in overweight and obese subjects. *Nutrition* 2002;18(9):729–33.

Bo-Linn, G.W., Santa Ana, C.A., Morawski, S.G., & Fordtran, J.S. Starch blockers: Their effect on calorie absorption from a high-starch meal. *N Engl J Med* 12-2-1982;307(23):1413–16.

Celleno, L., Tolaini, M.V., D'Amore, A., Perricone, N.V., and Preuss, H.G. A dietary supplement containing standardized *Phaseolus vulgaris* extract influences body composition of overweight men and women. *Int J Med Sci* 2007;4(1):45–52.

Layer, P., Carlson, G.L., & DiMagno, E.P. Partially purified white bean amylase inhibitor reduces starch digestion in vitro and inactivates intraduodenal amylase in humans. *Gastroenterology* 1985;88(6):1895–1902.

Preuss, H.G. Bean amylase inhibitor and other carbohydrate absorption blockers: Effects on diabesity and general health. *J Am Coll Nutr* 2009;28(3):266–76.

GARLIC

Berthold, H.K., Sudhop, T., & von Bergmann, K. Effect of a garlic oil preparation on serum lipoproteins and cholesterol metabolism. *JAMA* 1998;279:1900–02.

Isaacsohn, J.L., et al. Garlic powder and plasma lipids and lipoproteins. *Arch Intern Med* 1998;158:1189–94.

Kleijnen, J., Knipschild, P., & Ter Riet, G. Garlic, onion, and cardiovascular risk factors: A review of the evidence from human experiments with emphasis on commercially available preparations. *Br J Clin Pharmacol* 1989;28:535–44.

Koscielny, J., et al. The antiatherosclerotic effect of *Allium sativum*. *Atherosclerosis* 1999;144:237–49.

Legnani, C., et al. Effects of a dried garlic preparation on fibrinolysis and platelet aggregation in healthy subjects. *Arzneim-Forsch Drug Res* 1993;43:119–22.

McCrindle, B.W., Helden, E., & Conner, W.T. Garlic extract therapy in children with hypercholesterolemia. *Arch Pediatr Adolesc Med* 1998;152:1089–94.

Neil, H.A., et al. Garlic powder in the treatment of moderate hyperlipidaemia: A controlled trial and a meta-analysis. *J R Coll Phys Lond* 1996;30:329–34.

Silagy, C, & Neil, A. Garlic as a lipid-lowering agent: A meta-analysis. *J R Coll Phys Lond* 1994;28:39–45.

Silagy, C., & Neil, A meta-analysis of the effect of garlic on blood pressure. *J Hyperten* 1994;12:463–68.

Warshafsky, S., Kamer, R., & Sivak, S. Effect of garlic on total serum cholesterol: A meta-analysis. *Ann Int Med* 1993;119:599–605.

Zeng, T., et al. A meta-analysis of randomized, double-blind, placebo-controlled trials for the effects of garlic on serum lipid profiles. *J Sci Food Agric* 2012;92(9):1892–1902. doi:10.1002/jsfa.5557.

GINKGO

Clostre, F. From the body to the cell membranes: The different levels of pharmacological action of *Ginkgo biloba* extract. In: *Rokan (Ginkgo biloba): Recent Results in Pharmacology and Clinic*. Fünfgeld, EW, ed. Berlin: Springer-Verlag, 1988, 180–98.

Drieu, K. Preparation and definition of *Ginkgo biloba* extract. In: *Rokan (Ginkgo biloba): Recent Results in Pharmacology and Clinic*. Fünfgeld EW, ed. Berlin: Springer-Verlag, 32–36.

Ferrandini, C., Droy-Lefaix, M.T., & Christen, Y. (eds.). *Ginkgo biloba extract (EGb 761) as a free radical scavenger*. Paris: Elsevier, 1993.

Jung, F., Mrowietz, C., Kiesewetter, H., & Wenzel, E. Effect of *Ginkgo biloba* on fluidity of blood and peripheral microcirculation in volunteers. *Arzneimittelforschung* 1990;40:589–93.

Krieglstein, J. Neuroprotective properties of Ginkgo biloba: Constituents. *Zeitschrift Phytother* 1994;15:92–96.

Lanthony, P., & Cosson, J.P. Evolution of color vision in diabetic retinopathy treated by extract of *Ginkgo biloba*. *J Fr Ophthalmol* 1988;11:671–74 [in French].

Lebuisson, D.A., Leroy, L., & Rigal, G. Treatment of senile macular degeneration with *Ginkgo biloba* extract:

A preliminary double-blind, drug versus placebo study. *Presse Med* 1986;15:1556–58 [in French].

Matthews, M.K., Jr. Association of *Ginkgo biloba* with intracerebral hemorrhage. *Neurology* 1998;50:1933–34 [letter].

Mix, J.A., & Crews, W.D. An examination of the efficacy of *Ginkgo biloba* extract EGb761 on the neuropsychologic functioning of cognitively intact older adults. *J Altern Complement* Med 2000;6:219–29.

Rosenblatt, M., & Mindel, J. Spontaneous hyphema associated with ingestion of *Ginkgo biloba* extract. *N Engl J Med* 1997;336:1108 [letter].

HASKAP

Bhooshan Pandey, K. & Rizvi, S.I. Plant polyphenols as dietary antioxidants in human health and disease. *Oxid Med Cell Longev* 2009 Nov–Dec;2(5):270–78.

Jurikova, T., et al. Phenolic profile of edible honeysuckle berries (genus lonicera) and their biological effects. *Molecules* 2011 Dec 22;17(1):61–79.

Vasantha Rupasinghe, H.P., Yu, L.J., Bhullar, K.S., & Bors, B. Short Communication: Haskap (*Lonicera caerulea*): A new berry crop with high antioxidant capacity. Department of Environmental Sciences, Faculty of Agriculture, Dalhousie University, Truro, Nova Scotia.

HAWTHORN

Degenring, F.H., et al. A randomized double-blind placebo-controlled clinical trial of a standardized extract of fresh Crataegus berries (*Crataegisan*) in the treatment of patients with congestive heart failure NYHA II. *Phytomedicine* 2003;10(5):363–69.

Holubarsch, C.J., et al. Survival and prognosis: Investigation of Crataegus extract WS 1442 in congestive heart failure (SPICE): Rationale, study design and study protocol. *Eur J Heart Fail* 2000;2(4):431–37.

Iwamoto, M., Sato, T., & Ishizaki, T. The clinical effect of Crataegus in heart disease of ischemic or hypertensive origin: A multicenter double-blind study. *Planta Med* 1981;42(1):1–16.

Koller, M., et al. Crataegus special extract WS 1442 in the treatment of early stages of CHD-associated heart failure. *MMW Fortschr Med* 2006;148(6):42.

Leuchtgens, H. Crataegus Special Extract WS 1442 in NYHA II heart failure: A placebo-controlled randomized double-blind study. *Fortschr Med* 1993;111(20–21):352–54.

Pittler, M.H., Schmidt, K., & Ernst, E. Hawthorn extract for treating chronic heart failure: meta-analysis of randomized trials. *Am J Med* 2003 Jun 1;114(8):665–74.

HOPS

Abourashed, E.A., Koetter, U., & Brattstrom, A. In vitro binding experiments with a Valerian, hops and their fixed combination extract to selected central nervous system receptors. *Phytomedicine* 2004;11(7-8):633–38.

Blumenthal, M., et al. (eds.). *The Complete German Commission E Monographs: Therapeutic Guide to Herbal Medicines.* Austin: American Botanical Council and Boston: Integrative Medicine Communications, 1998, 147, 160–61.

Koetter, U., Schrader, E., Käufeler, R., & Brattström, A. A randomized, double-blind, placebo-controlled, prospective clinical study to demonstrate clinical efficacy of a fixed valerian

hops extract combination (Ze 91019) in patients suffering from non-organic sleep disorder. *Phytother Res* 2007;21:847–51.

Lee, K.M., et al. Effects of *Humulus lupulus* extract on the central nervous system in mice. *Planta Med* 1993;59(Suppl):A691.

Nikolic, D., et al. Metabolism of 8-prenyl-naringenin, a potent phytoestrogen from hops (Humulus lupulus), by human liver microsomes. *Drug Metab Dispos* 2004;32(2):272–79.

Oerter, K.K., Janfaza, M., Wong, J.A., & Chang, R.J. Estrogen bioactivity in fo-ti and other herbs used for their estrogen-like effects as determined by a recombinant cell bioassay. *J Clin Endocrinol Metab* 2003;88(9):4077–79.

Shellie, R.A., et al. Varietal characterization of hop (*Humulus lupulus L.*) by GC-MS analysis of hop cone extracts. *J Sep Sci* 2009;32(21):3720–25.

JUNIPER

Leung, A.Y., & Foster, S. *Encyclopedia of Common Natural Ingredients Used in Food, Drugs and Cosmetics*, 2nd ed. New York, NY: John Wiley & Sons, 1996.

Newall, C.A., Anderson, L.A., & Philpson, J.D. *Herbal Medicine: A Guide for Healthcare Professionals.* London, UK: The Pharmaceutical Press, 1996.

Robbers, J.E., & Tyler, V.E. *Tyler's Herbs of Choice: The Therapeutic Use of Phytomedicinals.* New York, NY: The Haworth Herbal Press, 1999.

Sanchez de Medina, F., et al. Hypoglycemic activity of juniper "berries." *Planta Med* 1994;60:197–200.

Swanston-Flatt, S.K., Day, C., Bailey, C.J., & Flatt, P.R. Traditional plant treat-

ments for diabetes: Studies in normal and streptozotocin-diabetic mice. *Diabetologia* 1990;33:462–64.

KALE

Asbell, R. Kale. *Vegetarian Times* 2011 Jan–Feb;(382):78–81.

Bolton-Smith, C., et al. Compilation of a provisional UK database for the phylloquinone (vitamin K1) content of foods. *Br J Nutr* 2000;83:389–99.

Sikora, E. Composition and antioxidant activity of kale (*Brassica oleracea L.* var. *acephala*) raw and cooked. *Technologia Alimentaria* 2012 Jul–Sep;11(3):239–48.

Tufts University. Try kale for vitamin K and cancer protection. *Tufts University Health & Nutrition Letter*, 2013 Jul;31(5):6.

LAVENDER

Basch, E., et al. Lavender (*Lavandula angustifolia Miller*). *J Herb Pharmacother* 2004;4(2):63–78.

Denner, S.S. *Lavandula angustifolia Miller*: English lavender. *Holist Nurs Pract* 2009;23(1):57–64.

Gabbrielli, G., et al. Activity of lavandino essential oil against non-tubercular opportunistic rapid grown mycobacteria. *Pharmacol Res Commun* 1988;20 Suppl 5:37–40.

Kane, F.M., et al. The analgesic effect of odour and music upon dressing change. *Br J Nurs* 10-28-2004;13(19):S4–12.

Lewith, G.T., Godfrey, A.D., & Prescott, P. A single-blinded, randomized pilot study evaluating the aroma of Lavandula augustifolia as a treatment for mild insomnia. *J Altern Complement Med* 2005 Aug;11(4):631–37.

Snow, L.A., Hovanec, L., & Brandt, J. A controlled trial of aromatherapy for agitation in nursing home patients with dementia. *J Altern Complement Med* 2004;10(3):431–37.

Soden, K., et al. A randomized controlled trial of aromatherapy massage in a hospice setting. *Palliat Med* 2004;18 (2):87–92.

LEMON BALM

Consumer Reports. Lemon balm. (2011). Retrieved from http://consumerreports.adam.com/content.aspx?productId=107&pid=33&gid=000261.

Herb Society of America. *Lemon Balm: An Herb Society of America Guide.* (2007). Retrieved from http://www.herbsociety.org/factsheets/Lemon%20Balm%20Guide.pdf.

Hncianu, M., et al. Chemical composition and in vitro antimicrobial activity of essential oil *Melissa officinalis L.* from Romania. *Rev Med Chir Soc Med Nat Iasi* 2008;112(3):843–47.

Kennedy, D.O., et al. Modulation of mood and cognitive performance following acute administration of *Melissa officinalis* (Lemon balm). *Pharmacol Biochem Behav* 2002 Jul;72(4):953–64.

Kennedy, D.O., et al. Modulation of mood and cognitive performance following acute administration of single doses of *Melissa officinalis* (Lemon balm) with human CNS nicotinic and muscarinic receptor-binding properties. *Neuropsychopharmacology* 2003 Oct;28(10):1871–81.

Mrlianova, M., et al. Comparison of the quality of *Melissa officialis L.* cultivar Citra with *Mellissas* of Europian origin. *Pharmacopsychiatry* 2001;34:27–36.

Muller, S.F., & Klement, S. A combination of valerian and lemon balm is effective in the treatment of restlessness and dyssomnia in children. *Phytomedicine* 2006;13(6):383–87.

University of Maryland Medical Center. Lemon balm. (2011). Retrieved from http://www.umm.edu/altmed/articles/lemon-balm-000261.htm.

MILK THISTLE

Agarwal, R., et al. Anticancer potential of silymarin: From bench to bed side. *Anticancer Res.* 2006 Nov–Dec;26(6B):4457–98. Review.

Andrade, R.J., et al. Effects of silymarin on the oxidative stress in patients with alcoholic liver cirrhosis. Results from a controlled, double-blind, randomized pilot clinical trial. *Hepatology* 1998;28(4):629.

Angulo, P., et al. Silymarin in the treatment of patients with primary biliary cirrhosis with a suboptimal response to ursodeoxycholic acid. *Hepatology* 2000;32(5):897–900.

Feher, J. & Lengyel, G. Silymarin in the treatment of chronic liver diseases: Past and future. *Orv Hetil* 12-21-2008;149(51):2413–18.

Lahiri-Chatterjee, M., Katiyar, S.K., Mohan, R.R., & Agarwal, R. A flavonoid antioxidant, silymarin, affords exceptionally high protection against tumor promotion in the SENCAR mouse skin tumorigenesis model. *Cancer Res* 2-1-1999;59(3):622–32.

Luper, S. A review of plants used in the treatment of liver disease: Part 1. *Altern Med Rev* 1998;3(6):410–21.

Pares, A., et al. Effects of silymarin in alcoholic patients with cirrhosis of the liver: Results of a controlled, double-blind, randomized and multicenter trial. *J Hepatol* 1998;28(4):615–21.

Saller, R., Brignoli, R., Melzer, J., & Meier, R. An updated systematic review with meta-analysis for the clinical evidence of silymarin. *Forsch Komplementmed* 2008 Feb;15(1):9–20. Review.

Zi, X., Feyes, D.K., & Agarwal, R. Anticarcinogenic effect of a flavonoid antioxidant, silymarin, in human breast cancer cells MDA-MB 468: Induction of G1 arrest through an increase in Cip1/p21 concomitant with a decrease in kinase activity of cyclin-dependent kinases and associated cyclins. *Clin Cancer Res* 1998;4(4):1055–64.

Zi, X., Grasso, A.W., Kung, H.J., & Agarwal, R. A flavonoid antioxidant, silymarin, inhibits activation of erbB1 signaling and induces cyclin-dependent kinase inhibitors, G1 arrest, and anticarcinogenic effects in human prostate carcinoma DU145 cells. *Cancer Res* 5-1-1998;58(9):1920–29.

Zou, C.G., Agar, N.S., & Jones, G.L. Oxidative insult to human red blood cells induced by free radical initiator AAPH and its inhibition by a commercial antioxidant mixture. *Life Sci* 5-25-2001;69(1):75–86.

NETTLE

Bombardelli, E., & Morazzoni, P. *Urtica dioica L. Fitoterapia* 1997;68(5):387–402.

Dantas, S.M. Menopausal symptoms and alternative medicine. *Prim Care Update Ob/Gyns* 1999; 6:212–20.

Koch, E., & Biber, A. Pharmacological effects of sabal and *Urtica* extracts as a basis for a rational medication of benign prostatic hyperplasia. *Urologe* 1994;334:90–95.

Metzker, H., Kieser, M., & Hölscher, U. Efficacy of a combined Sabal-Urtica preparation in the treatment of benign prostatic hyperplasia (BPH). *Urologe B* 1996;36:292–300.

Mittman, P. Randomized, double-blind study of freeze-dried Urtica dioica in the treatment of allergic rhinitis. Planta Med 1990;56:44–47.

Patten, G. Medicinal plant review: Urtica. *Aust J Med Herbalism* 1993;5(1):5–13.

Randall, C., Meethan, K., Randall, H., & Dobbs, F. Nettle sting of Urtica dioica for joint pain: An exploratory study of this complementary therapy. *Compl Ther Med* 1999;7:126–31.

Safarinejad, M.R. *Urtica dioica* for treatment of benign prostatic hyperplasia: A prospective, randomized, double-blind, placebo-controlled, crossover study. *J Herb Pharmacother* 2005;5:1–11.

Tahri, A., et al. Acute diuretic, natriuretic and hypotensive effects of a continuous perfusion of aqueous extract of *Urtica dioica* in the rat. *J Ethnopharmacol* 2000;73(1-2):95–100.

OREGANO

Burt, S.A., & Reinders, R.D. Antibacterial activity of selected plant essential oils against *Escherichia coli* O157:H7. *Lett Appl Microbiol* 2003;36(3):162–67.

Chami, F., et al. Oregano and clove essential oils induce surface alteration of *Saccharomyces cerevisiae*. *Phytother Res* 2005;19(5):405–08.

Chorianopoulos, N., et al. Essential oils of *Satureja, Origanum,* and *Thymus* species: Chemical composition and antibacterial activities against foodborne pathogens. *J Agric Food Chem* 2004;52(26):8261–67.

Dorman, H.J., & Deans, S.G. Antimicrobial agents from plants: Antibacterial activity of plant volatile oils. *J Appl Microbiol* 2000;88(2):308–16.

Exarchou, V., et al. Antioxidant activities and phenolic composition of extracts from Greek oregano, Greek sage, and summer savory. *J Agric Food Chem* 2002;50(19):5294–5299.

Force, M. Inhibition of enteric parasites by emulsified oil of oregano in vivo. *Phytotherapy Research* May 1, 2000;14(3):213–4.

Force, M., Sparks, W.S., Ronzio, R.A. Inhibition of enteric parasites by emulsified oil of oregano in vivo. *Phytother Res* 2000;14(3):213–214.

Jarmuda S., et al. Potential role of Demodex mites and bacteria in the induction of rosacea. *J Med Microbiol* 2012 Nov;61(Pt 11):1504–10.

Lambert, R.J., et al. A study of the minimum inhibitory concentration and mode of action of oregano essential oil, thymol, and carvacrol. *J Appl Microbiol* 2001;91(3):453–462.

Stensvold, C.R., et al. Blastocystis: Unravelling potential risk factors and clinical significance of a common but neglected parasite. *Epidemiol Infect* 2009 Nov.;137(11):1655–63.

PARSLEY

Heck, A.M., DeWitt, B.A., & Lukes, A.L. Potential interactions between alternative therapies and warfarin. *Am J Health Syst Pharm* 7-1-2000;57(13):1221–27.

Meyer, H., et al. Bioavailability of apigenin from apiin-rich parsley in humans. *Ann Nutr Metab* 2006;50(3):167–72.

Nielsen, S.E., et al. Effect of parsley (*Petroselinum crispum*) intake on urinary apigenin excretion, blood antioxidant enzymes, and biomarkers for oxidative stress in human subjects. *Br J Nutr* 1999;81(6):447–55.

PASSIONFLOWER

Akhondzadeh, S., et al. Passionflower in the treatment of generalized anxiety: A pilot double-blind randomized controlled trial with oxazepam. *J Clin Pharm Ther* 2001;26(5):363–67.

Aoyagi, N., Kimura, R., & Murata, T. Studies on *Passiflora incarnata* dry extract. I. Isolation of maltol and pharmacological action of maltol and ethyl maltol. *Chem Pharm Bull* (Tokyo) 1974;22(5):1008–13.

Brown, E., Hurd, N.S., McCall, S., & Ceremuga, T.E. Evaluation of the anxiolytic effects of chrysin, a *Passiflora incarnata* extract, in the laboratory rat. *AANA J* 2007;75(5):333–37.

Dhawan, K., Kumar, S., & Sharma, A. Comparative biological activity study on *Passiflora incarnata* and *P. edulis*. *Fitoterapia* 2001;72(6):698–702.

Speroni, E., & Minghetti, A. Neuropharmacological activity of extracts from *Passiflora incarnata*. *Planta Med* 1988;54(6):488–91.

Wolfman, C., Viola, H., Paladini, A., Dajas, F., & Medina, J.H. Possible anxiolytic effects of chrysin, a central benzodiazepine receptor ligand isolated from *Passiflora coerulea*. *Pharmacol Biochem Behav* 1994;47(1):1–4.

PEPPERMINT

Alam, M.S., et al. Efficacy of peppermint oil in diarrhea predominant IBS: A double-blind randomized placebo-controlled study. *Mymensingh Med J* 2013 Jan;22(1):27–30.

Cappello, G., et al. Peppermint oil (Mintoil) in the treatment of irritable

389

bowel syndrome: A prospective double-blind placebo-controlled randomized trial. *Dig Liver Dis* 2007 Jun;39(6):530–36.

Ford, A.C., et al. Effect of fibre, antispasmodics, and peppermint oil in the treatment of irritable bowel syndrome: Systematic review and meta-analysis. *BMJ* (International Edition), 2008 Dec 13;337(7683):1388–92.

Göbel, H., et al. Effectiveness of *Oleum menthae piperitae* and paracetamol in therapy of headache of the tension type. *Nervenarzt* 1996 Aug;67(8): 672–81.

Grigoleit, H.G., & Grigoleit, P. Pharmacology and preclinical pharmacokinetics of peppermint oil. *Phytomedicine* 2005 Aug;12(8):612–16.

Kligler, B., & Chaudhary, S. Peppermint oil. *Am Fam Physician* 2007 Apr 1;75(7):1027–30.

Lech, Y., et al. Treatment of irritable bowel syndrome with peppermint oil: A double-blind study with a placebo. *Ugeskr Laeger* 1988; 150(40):2388–89.

Liu, J.H., et al. Enteric-coated peppermint oil capsules in the treatment of irritable bowel syndrome: A prospective, randomized trial. *J Gastroenterol* 1997 Dec.;32(6):765–68.

PLANTAIN

Blumenthal, M. (ed.). *Herbal Medicine: Expanded Commission E Monographs.* Newton, MA: Integrative Medicine Communications, 2000, 307–10.

Chiang, L.C., Chiang, W., Chang, M.Y., & Lin, C.C. In vitro cytotoxic, antiviral, and immunomodulatory effects of *Plantago major* and *Plantago asiatica*. *Am J Chin Med* 2003;31(2):225–34.

Koichev A. Complex evaluation of the therapeutic effect of a preparation from *Plantago major* in chronic bronchitis. *Probl Vatr Med* 1983;11:61–69.

Matev, M., et al. Clinical trial of *Plantago major* preparation in the treatment of chronic bronchitis. *Vutr Boles* 1982;21:133–37.

McGuffin, M., Hobbs, C., Upton, R., Goldberg, A. (eds.). *American Herbal Products Association's Botanical Safety Handbook.* Boca Raton, FL: CRC Press, LLC, 1997.

Wegener, T., & Kraft, K. [Plantain (*Plantago lanceolata L.*): Anti-inflammatory action in upper respiratory tract infections]. *Wien Med Wochenschr* 1999;149(8–10): 211–16.

Wichtl, M., & Bisset, N.G. (eds.). *Herbal Drugs and Phytopharmaceuticals.* Stuttgart: Medpharm Scientific Publishers, 1994.

RASPBERRY

Patel, A.V., Rojas-Vera, J., & Dacke, C.G. Therapeutic constituents and actions of *Rubus* species. *Curr Med Chem* 2004;11(11):1501–12.

Rojas-Vera, J., Patel, A.V., & Dacke, C.G. Relaxant activity of raspberry (*Rubus idaeus*) leaf extract in guinea-pig ileum in vitro. *Phytother Res* 2002;16(7):665–68.

Ryan, T., Wilkinson, J.M., & Cavanagh, H.M. Antibacterial activity of raspberry cordial in vitro. *Res Vet Sci* 2001;71(3):155–59.

Simpson, M., Parsons, M., Greenwood, J., & Wade, K. Raspberry leaf in pregnancy: Its safety and efficacy in labor. *J Midwifery Womens Health* 2001;46(2):51–59.

RED CLOVER

Atkinson, C., et al. The effects of phytoestrogen isoflavones on bone density in women: A double-blind, randomized, placebo-controlled trial. *Amer J Clin Nutr* 2004;79(2):326–33.

Bown, D. *The Herb Society of America New Encyclopedia of Herbs and Their Uses.* London: Dorling Kindersley Ltd., 2001.

Howes, J., et al. Effects of dietary supplementation with isoflavones from red clover on ambulatory blood pressure and endothelial function in postmenopausal type 2 diabetes. *Diabetes Obes Metab* 2003;(5):325–32.

Huntley, A.L., & Ernst, E. A systematic review of herbal medicinal products for the treatment of menopausal symptoms. *Menopause* 2003 Sep–Oct;10(5):465–76.

Kelly, G., Husband, A., & Waring, M. *Standardized red clover extract clinical monograph.* Natural Products Research Consultants 1998. Seattle, WA 1998, Herb Clip, 080590 (Trifolium pratense; isoflavones).

Mannella, P., et al. Effects of red clover extracts on breast cancer cell migration and invasion. *Gynecol endocrinol* 2012;28(1):29–33.

Mueller, M., & Jungbauer, A. Red clover extract: A putative source for simultaneous treatment of menopausal disorders and the metabolic syndrome. *Menopause* 2008 Nov–Dec;15(6): 1120–31.

Nachtigall, L.E. Isoflavones in the management of menopause. *J Brit Meno Soc* 2001;Supplement S1:8–12.

Nestel, P.J., et al. Isoflavones from red clover improve systemic arterial compliance but not plasma lipids in menopausal women. *J Clin Endocrinol Metab* 1999;84(3):895–98.

Smith, R. Red Clover in the "Twenty-First" Century. 2000. Retrieved from: http://www.uwex.edu/ces/forage/wfc/proceedings2000/smith/htm. Accessed March 4, 2005.

Van de Weijer, P., & Barentsen, R. Isoflavones from red clover (*Promensil*) significantly reduce menopausal hot flush symptoms compared with placebo. *Maturitas* 2002;42;187–93.

RHUBARB

Albrecht, U.W. [The efficacy and tolerability of Pyralvex solution and Pyralvex gel in the treatment of gingivitis: Results of double-blind, randomized, controlled clinical trials]. *Der Freie Zahnarzt* 1997;9:76–80.

Borgia, M., et al. Pharmacological activity of a herbs extract: A controlled clinical study. *Curr Ther Res Clin Exp* 1981;29(3):525–36.

Renggli, H. [Gingivitis- and plaque-inhibiting action of Pyralvex Berna and its components]. *SSO Schweiz Monatsschr Zahnheilkd* 1980;90(8):718–24.

Xin, S.F., et al. [Clinical observation on patients with constipation using Rhubarb and Mangxiao]. *Chin J Nurs* 1995;7(30):420–22.

Zhou, L., Hao, R., & Jiang, L. [Clinical study on retarding aging effect of tongbu recipe to traditional Chinese medicine]. *Zhongguo Zhong Xi Yi Jie He Za Zhi* 1999;19(4):218–20.

ROSEMARY

Aqel, M.B. Relaxant effect of the volatile oil of *Rosmarinus officinalis* on tracheal smooth muscle. *J Ethnopharmacol* 1991;33:57–62.

Burnett, K.M., Solterbeck, L.A., & Strapp, C.M. Scent and mood state following an anxiety-provoking task. *Psychol Rep* 2004;95(2):707–22.

Hay, I.C., Jamieson, M., & Ormerod, A.D. Randomized trial of aromatherapy: Successful treatment for alopecia areata. *Arch Dermatol* 1998;134(11):1349–52.

Huhtanen, C. Inhibition of *Clostridium botulinum* by spice extract and aliphatic alcohols. *J Food Protect* 1980;43:195–96.

Leung, A.Y., & Foster, S. *Encyclopedia of Common Natural Ingredients Used in Foods, Drugs, and Cosmetics,* 2nd ed. New York: John Wiley & Sons, 1996, 446–48.

Martinez, A.L., et al. Antinociceptive effect and GC/MS analysis of *Rosmarinus officinalis* L. essential oil from its aerial parts. *Planta Med* 2009;75(5):508–11.

McCaffrey, R., Thomas, D.J., & Kinzelman, A.O. The effects of lavender and rosemary essential oils on test-taking anxiety among graduate nursing students. *Holist Nurs Pract* 2009;23(2):88–93.

Minich, D.M., et al. Clinical safety and efficacy of NG440: A novel combination of rho iso-alpha acids from hops, rosemary, and oleanolic acid for inflammatory conditions. *Can J Physiol Pharmacol* 2007;85(9):872–83.

Moss, M., et al. Aromas of rosemary and lavender essential oils differentially affect cognition and mood in healthy adults. *Int J Neurosci* 2003;113(1):15–38.

Park, M.K., & Lee, E.S. [The effect of aroma inhalation method on stress responses of nursing students.]. *Taehan Kanho Hakhoe Chi* 2004;34(2):344–51.

Peng, Y., Yuan, J., Liu, F., & Ye, J. Determination of active components in rosemary by capillary electrophoresis with electrochemical detection. *J Pharm Biomed Anal* 9-15-2005;39(3–4):431–37.

Sayorwan, W., et al. Effects of inhaled rosemary oil on subjective feelings and activities of the nervous system. *Scientia Pharmaceutica* 2013 Jun;81(2):531–42.

Singletary, K., MacDonald, C., & Wallig, M. Inhibition by rosemary and carnosol of 7,12-dimethyl-benz[a]anthracene (DMBA)-induced rat mammary tumorigenesis and in vivo DMBA-DNA adduct formation. *Cancer Lett* 1996;104:43–48.

SAGE

Abascal, K., & Yarnell, E. A botanical approach to Alzheimer's disease. *Nat Pharm* 2004;8(5):1–17.

Abascal, K., & Yarnell, E. Alzheimer's disease—Part 2—A botanical treatment plan. *Alter Comp Ther* 2004;10:67–72.

Adams, M., Gmunder, F., & Hamburger, M. Plants traditionally used in age-related brain disorders: A survey of ethnobotanical literature. *J Ethnopharmacol* 9-25-2007;113(3):363–81.

Blumenthal, M., et al. (eds.). *The Complete German Commission E Monographs: Therapeutic Guide to Herbal Medicines*. Austin: American Botanical Council and Boston: Integrative Medicine Communications, 1998, 198.

De Leo, V., Lanzetta, D., Cazzavacca, R., Morgante, G. [Treatment of neurovegetative menopausal symptoms with a phytotherapeutic agent] [Article in Italian]. *Minerva Ginecol* 1998;50:207–11.

Duke, J.A. *CRC Handbook of Medicinal Herbs*. Boca Raton, FL: CRC Press, 1985, 420–21.

Weiss, R.F. *Herbal Medicine*. Gothenburg, Sweden: Ab Arcanum and Beaconsfield, UK: Beaconsfield Publishers Ltd., 1988, 229–30.

SLIPPERY ELM

Blumenthal, M., et al. (eds.). *The Complete German Commission E Monographs: Therapeutic Guide to Herbal Medicines*. Austin: American Botanical Council and Boston: Integrative Medicine Communications, 1998, 167.

Duke, J.A. *CRC Handbook of Medicinal Herbs*. Boca Raton, FL: CRC Press, 1985, 495–96.

Kaegi, E. Unconventional therapies for cancer: 1. Essiac. The Task Force on Alternative Therapies of the Canadian Breast Cancer Research Initiative. *CMAJ* 4-7-1998;158(7):897–902.

Langmead, L., Dawson, C., Hawkins, C., Banna, N., Loo, S., & Rampton, D.S. Antioxidant effects of herbal therapies used by patients with inflammatory bowel disease: An in vitro study. *Aliment Pharmacol Ther* 2002;16(2):197–205.

Pizzorno, J.E., & Murray, M.T. *Textbook of Natural Medicine*. London: Churchill Livingstone, 1999, 1335–49.

Rakel, D. *Rakel: Integrative Medicine*, 2nd ed. Philadelphia, PA: Saunders Elsevier Inc., 2007, 43.

Rotblatt, M., & Ziment, I. *Evidence-based Herbal Medicine*. Philadelphia, Penn: Hanley & Belfus, Inc., 2002, 337–38.

Wong, C.K., Leung, K.N., Fung, K.P., & Choy, Y.M. Immunomodulatory and anti-tumour polysaccharides from medicinal plants. *J Int Med Res* 1994;22(6):299–312.

Wren, R.C., Williamson, E.M., & Evans, F.J. *Potter's New Cyclopedia of Botanical Drugs and Preparations*. Essex, UK: CW Daniel Company, 1988, 252.

SPINACH

Asai, A., Terasaki, M., & Nagao, A. An epoxide-furanoid rearrangement of spinach neoxanthin occurs in the gastrointestinal tract of mice and in vitro: Formation and cytostatic activity of neochrome stereoisomers. *J Nutr* 2004 Sep;134(9):2237–43. 2004. PMID:15333710.

Asai, A., Yonekura, L., & Nagao, A. Low bioavailability of dietary epoxyxanthophylls in humans. *Br J Nutr* 2008 Aug;100(2):273–77.

Chung, H.Y., Rasmussen, H.M., & Johnson, E.J. Lutein bioavailability is higher from lutein-enriched eggs than from supplements and spinach in men. *J Nutr* 2004 Aug;134(8):1887–93. 2004. PMID:15284371.

Edenharder, R., Keller, G., Platt, K.L., & Unger, K.K. Isolation and characterization of structurally novel antimutagenic flavonoids from spinach (*Spinacia oleracea*). *J Agric Food Chem* 2001 Jun;49(6):2767–73. 2001. PMID:12950.

Gates, M.A., et al. A prospective study of dietary flavonoid intake and incidence of epithelial ovarian cancer. *Int J Cancer* 2007 Apr 30; [Epub ahead of print]. 2007. PMID:17471564.

Genannt Bonsmann, S.S., et al. Oxalic acid does not influence nonhaem iron absorption in humans: A comparison of kale and spinach meals. *Eur J Clin Nutr* 2008 Mar;62(3):336–41. Epub 2007 Apr 18.

Longnecker, M.P., et al. Intake of carrots, spinach, and supplements containing vitamin A in relation to risk of breast cancer. *Cancer Epidemiol Biomarkers Prev* 1997 Nov;6(11):887–92. 1997. PMID:12980.

Lucarini, M., et al. Intake of vitamin A and carotenoids from the Italian population: Results of an Italian total diet study. *Int J Vitam Nutr Res* 2006 May;76(3):103–09.

Makiko, I., Mutsuko, T., & Takashi, N. Influence of the amount of boiling water on the sensory evaluation, oxalic acid and potassium content of boiled spinach. *Journal of Cookery Science of Japan* 2005;38(4):343–49.

Manach, C., et al. Polyphenols: Food sources and bioavailability. *Am J Clin Nutr* 2004 May;79(5):727–47. 2004. PMID:15113710.

Morris, M.C., et al. Associations of vegetable and fruit consumption with age-related cognitive change. *Neurology* 2006 Oct 24;67(8):1370–76. 2006. PMID:17060562.

Okazaki, K., et al. Differences in the metabolite profiles of spinach (*Spinacia oleracea* L.) leaf in different concentrations of nitrate in the culture solution. *Plant Cell Physio* 2008 Feb;49(2):170–77. Epub 2007 Dec 17.

Song, W., et al. Cellular antioxidant activity of common vegetables. *J Agric Food Chem* 2010 Jun 9; 58(11):6621–29.

Tang, G., et al. Spinach or carrots can supply significant amounts of vitamin A as assessed by feeding with intrinsically deuterated vegetables. *Am J Clin Nutr* 2005 Oct;82(4):821–28.

Wang, Y., et al. Dietary supplmentation with blueberries, spinach, or spirulina reduces ischemic brain damage. *Exp Neurol* 2005 May;193(1):75–84. 2005. PMID:15817266.

Yang, Y., et al. Isolation and antihypertensive effect of angiotensin I-converting enzyme (ACE) inhibitory peptides from spinach. *Rubisco*. *J Agric Food Chem* 2003 Aug 13;51(17):4897–02.

SQUASH

Albanes, D., et al. Alpha-tocopherol and beta-carotene supplements and lung cancer incidence in the Alpha-Tocopherol, Beta-Carotene Cancer Prevention Study: Effects of base-line characteristics and study compliance. *J Natl Cancer Inst* 1996;88:1560–70.

The Alpha-Tocopherol, Beta Carotene Cancer Prevention Study Group. The effect of vitamin E and beta carotene on the incidence of lung cancer and other cancers in male smokers. *N Engl J Med* 1994;330:1029–35.

Bone, R.A., & Landrum, J.T. Distribution of macular pigment components, zeaxanthin and lutein, in human retina. *Methods Enzymol* 1992:213:360–66.

Greenburg, E.R., et al. Mortality associated with low plasma concentration of beta carotene and the effect of oral supplementation. *JAMA* 1996;275: 699–703.

Hennekens, C.H., et al. Lack of effect of long-term supplementation with beta carotene on the incidence of malignant neoplasms and cardiovascular disease. *N Engl J Med* 1996;334:1145–49.

Probstfield, J.L., Lin, T., Peters, J., & Hunninghake, D.B. Carotenoids and vitamin A: The effect of hypocholesterolemic agents on serum levels. *Metabolism* 1985;34:88–91.

Seddon, J.M., et al. Dietary carotenoids, vitamins A, C, and E, and advanced age-related macular degeneration. *JAMA* 1994;272:1413–20.

ST JOHN'S WORT

Kasper, S., et al. Continuation and long-term maintenance treatment with Hypericum extract WS 5570 after recovery from an acute episode of moderate depression: A double-blind, randomized, placebo-controlled long-term trial. *Eur Neuropsychopharmacol* 2008;18(11):803–13.

Linde, K., Berner, M.M., & Kriston, L. St John's wort for major depression. *Cochrane Database Syst Rev* 2008;(4):CD000448.

Muller, T., et al. Treatment of somatoform disorders with St. John's wort: A randomized, double-blind and placebo-controlled trial. *Psychosom Med* 2004;66(4):538–47.

Randlov, C., et al. The efficacy of St. John's Wort in patients with minor depressive symptoms or dysthymia: A double-blind placebo-controlled study. *Phytomedicine* 2006 Mar;13(4):215–21.

Saarto, T., & Wiffen, P.J. Antidepressants for neuropathic pain. *Cochrane Database Syst Rev* 2007 Oct 17; (4):CD005454.

Schulz, V. Safety of St. John's wort extract compared to synthetic antidepressants. *Phytomedicine* 2006 Feb;13(3):199–204.

Shelton, R.C., et al. Effectiveness of St John's wort in major depression: A randomized controlled trial. *JAMA* 4-18-2001;285(15):1978–86.

STRAWBERRY

Ballot, D., et al. The effects of fruit juices and fruits on the absorption of iron from a rice meal. *Br J Nutr* 1987;57(3):331–43.

Cheel, J., et al. E-cinnamic acid derivatives and phenolics from Chilean strawberry fruits, *Fragaria chiloensis* ssp. *chiloensis*. *J Agric Food Chem* 11-2-2005;53(22):8512–18.

Hannum, S.M. Potential impact of strawberries on human health: A review of the science. *Crit Rev Food Sci Nutr* 2004;44(1):1–17.

Joseph, J.A., et al. Long-term dietary strawberry, spinach, or vitamin E supplementation retards the onset of age-related neuronal signal-transduction and cognitive behavioral deficits. *J Neurosci* 1998;18:8047–55.

Joseph, J.A., et al. Reversals of age-related declines in neuronal signal transduction, cognitive, and motor behavioral deficits with blueberry, spinach, or strawberry dietary supplementation. *J Neurosci* 1999;19:8114–21.

Lukasik, J., et al. Reduction of poliovirus 1, bacteriophages, *Salmonella montevideo,* and *Escherichia coli* O157:H7 on strawberries by physical and disinfectant washes. *J Food Prot* 2003;66(2):188–93.

Meyers, K.J., Watkins, C.B., Pritts, M.P., & Liu, R.H. Antioxidant and antiproliferative activities of strawberries. *J Agric Food Chem*.11-5 2003;51(23):6887–92.

Puupponen-Pimia, R., Nohynek, L., Alakomi, H.L., & Oksman-Caldentey, K.M. The action of berry phenolics against human intestinal pathogens. *Biofactors* 2005;23(4):243–51.

Ramos, S., Alia, M., Bravo, L., & Goya, L. Comparative effects of food-derived polyphenols on the viability and apoptosis of a human hepatoma cell line (HepG2). *J Agric Food Chem* 2005;53:1271–80.

Wang, S.Y., et al. Inhibitory effect on activator protein-1, nuclear factor-kappaB, and cell transformation by extracts of strawberries (*Fragaria x ananassa Duch.*). *J Agric Food Chem* 2005;53:4187–93.

SWISS CHARD

Bolkent, S., et al. Effects of chard (*Beta vulgaris* L. var. *Cicla*) extract on pancreatic B cells in streptozotocin-diabetic rats: A morphological and biochemical study. *J Ethnopharmacol.* 2000 Nov;73(1–2):251–59.

Calderón-Montaño, J.M., et al. A review on the dietary flavonoid kaempferol. *Mini Rev Med Chem* 2011 Apr;11(4):298–344.

Kugler, F., Stintzing, F.C., & Carle, R. Identification of betalains from petioles of differently colored Swiss chard (*Beta vulgaris* L. ssp. *Cicla* [L.] Alef. Cv. Bright Lights) by High-Performance Liquid Chromatography-Electrospray Ion. *J Agric Food Chem* 2004;52(10):2975–81.

Ozsoy-Sacan, O., et al. Effects of chard (*Beta vulgaris* L. var *Cicla*) on the liver of the diabetic rats: A morphological and biochemical study. *Bioscience, Biotechnology, and Biochemistry* 2004;68(8):1640–48.

Pyoa, Y.H., et al. Antioxidant activity and phenolic compounds of Swiss chard (*Beta vulgaris* ssp. *Cycla*) extracts. *Food Chem* 2004 March;85(1):19–26.

Song, W., et al. Cellular antioxidant activity of common vegetables. *J Agric Food Chem* 2010 Jun 9; 58(11):6621–29.

Yanardag, R., et al. The effects of chard (*Beta vulgaris* L. var. *Cicla*) extract on the kidney tissue, serum urea and creatinine levels of diabetic rats. *Phytother Res* 2002 Dec;16(8):758–61.

THYME

Alissandrakis, E., Tarantilis, P.A., Harizanis, P.C., & Polissiou, M. Comparison of the volatile composition in thyme honeys from several origins in Greece.

J Agric Food Chem 10-3-2007; 55(20):8152–57.

Blumenthal, M., et al. (eds.). *The Complete German Commission E Monographs: Therapeutic Guide to Herbal Medicines.* Austin: American Botanical Council and Boston: Integrative Medicine Communications, 1998, 425–26.

Charles, C.H., et al. Comparative efficacy of an antiseptic mouthrinse and an antiplaque/antigingivitis dentifrice: A six-month clinical trial. *J Am Dent Assoc* 2001;132(5):670–75.

Cosentino, S., et al. In vitro antimicrobial activity and chemical composition of Sardinian *Thymus* essential oils. *Lett Appl Microbiol* 1999;29:130–35.

Dapkevicius, A., et al. Isolation and structure elucidation of radical scavengers from *Thymus vulgaris* leaves. *J Nat Prod* 2002;65(6):892–96.

Forster, H.B., Niklas, H., & Lutz, S. Antispasmodic effects of some medicinal plants. *Planta Med* 1980;40:303–19.

Haukali, G., & Poulsen, S. Effect of a varnish containing chlorhexidine and thymol (Cervitec) on approximal caries in 13- to 16-year-old schoolchildren in a low caries area. *Caries Res* 2003;37(3):185–89.

Kato, T., et al. Antibacterial effects of Listerine on oral bacteria. *Bull Tokyo Dent Coll* 1990;31:301–07.

Miura, K., Kikuzaki, H., & Nakatani, N. Antioxidant activity of chemical components from sage (*Salvia officinalis L.*) and thyme (*Thymus vulgaris L.*) measured by the oil stability index method. *J Agric Food Chem* 2002;50(7):1845–51.

Nozal Nalda, M.J., Bernal Yague, J.L., Diego Calva, J.C., & Martin Gomez, M.T. Classifying honeys from the

Soria Province of Spain via multivariate analysis. *Anal Bioanal Chem* 2005;382(2):311–19.

Youdim, K.A., & Deans, S.G. Effect of thyme oil and thymol dietary supplementation on the antioxidant status and fatty acid composition of the aging rat brain. *Br J Nutr* 2000;83(1):87–93.

TOMATO

Clinton, S.K., et al. Cis-trans lycopene isomers, carotenoids, and retinol in the human prostate. *Cancer Epidemiol Biomarkers Prev* 1996;5:823–33.

Gann, P.H., et al. Lower prostate cancer risk in men with elevated plasma lycopene levels: Results of a prospective analysis. *Cancer Res* 1999;59:1225–30.

Giovannucci, E. Tomatoes, tomato-based products, lycopene, and cancer: Review of the epidemiologic literature. *J Natl Cancer Inst* 1999;91:317–31.

Giovannucci, E., et al. Intake of carotenoids and retinol in relation to risk of prostate cancer. *J Natl Cancer Inst* 1995;87:1767–76.

Kristal, A., et al. Serum lycopene concentration and prostate cancer risk: Results from the Prostate Cancer Prevention Trial. *Cancer Epidemiol Biomarkers Prev* 2011;20(4):638–46.

Magbanua, M.J., et al. Gene expression and biological pathways in tissue of men with prostate cancer in a randomized clinical trial of lycopene and fish oil supplementation. *PLoS One* 2011;6(9):e24004.

McClean, C.M., et al. The impact of acute moderate intensity exercise on arterial regional stiffness, lipid peroxidation, and antioxidant status in healthy males. *Res Sports Med* 2011;19(1):1–13.

Miyazawa, T., et al. Plasma carotenoid concentrations before and after supplementation with astaxanthin in middle-aged and senior subjects. *Biosci Biotechnol Biochem* 2011;75(9):1856–58.

VALERIAN

Bent, S., et al. Valerian for sleep: A systematic review and meta-analysis. *Am J Med* 2006;119:1005–12.

Bent, S., Patterson, M., & Garvin, D. Valerian for sleep: A systematic review and meta-analysis. *Alt Ther* 2001;7:S4.

Donath, F., et al. Critical evaluation of the effect of valerian extract on sleep structure and sleep quality. *Pharmacopsychiatry* 2000;33:47–53.

Francis, A.J., & Dempster, R.J. Effect of valerian, *Valeriana edulis,* on sleep difficulties in children with intellectual deficits: Randomized trial. *Phytomedicine* 2002;9:273–79.

Gadsby, J.E. *Addiction by Prescription: One Woman's Triumph and Fight for Change.* Toronto, ON: Key Porter Books, 2000.

Glass, J.R., et al. Acute pharmacological effects of temazepam, diphenhydramine, and valerian in healthy elderly subjects. *J Clin Psychopharmacol* 2003;23:260–68.

Leathwood, P.D., & Chauffard, F. Aqueous extract of valerian reduces latency to fall asleep in man. *Planta Med* 1985;2:144–48.

Leathwood, P.D., Chauffard, F., Heck, E., & Munoz-Box, R. Aqueous extract of valerian root (*Valeriana officinalis L.*) improves sleep quality in man. *Pharmacol Biochem Behav* 1982;17:65–71.

Plushner, S.L. Valerian: *Valerian officinalis. Am J Health Syst Pharm* 2000;57:328, 333, 335.

Poyares, D.R., Guilleminault, C., Ohayon, M.M., & Tufik, S. Can valerian improve the sleep of insomniacs after benzodiazepine withdrawal? *Prog Neuropsychopharmacol Biol Psychiatry* 2002;26:539–45.

Wheatley, D. Stress-induced insomnia treated with kava and valerian: Singly and in combination. *Hum Psychopharmacol* 2001;16:353–56.

WHEATGRASS

Ben Arye, E., et al. Wheatgrass juice in the treatment of active distal ulcerative colitis: A randomized double-blind placebo-controlled trial. *Scand J Gastroenterol* 2002;37(4):444–49.

Duke, J. Wheat. Dr. Duke's Phytochemical and Ethnobotanical Databases. (2013.) Retrieved from http://sun.ars-grin.gov:8080/npgspub/xsql/duke/plantdisp.xsql?taxon=1025.

Forgionne, G.A. Bovine cartilage, coenzyme Q10, and wheatgrass therapy for primary peritoneal cancer. *J Altern Complement Med* 2005;11(1):161–65.

Marawaha, R.K., Bansal, D., Kaur, S., & Trehan, A. Wheatgrass juice reduces transfusion requirement in patients with thalassemia major: A pilot study. *Indian Pediatr* 2004;41(7):716–20.

Rauma, A.L., Nenonen, M., Helve, T., & Hanninen, O. Effect of a strict vegan diet on energy and nutrient intakes by Finnish rheumatoid patients. *Eur J Clin Nutr* 1993;47(10):747–49.

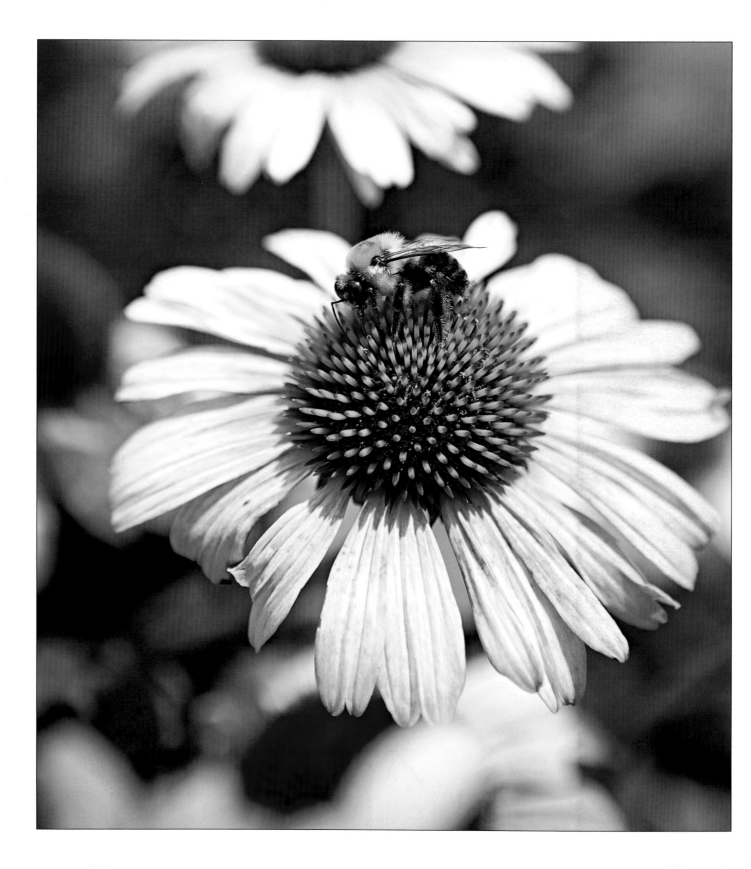

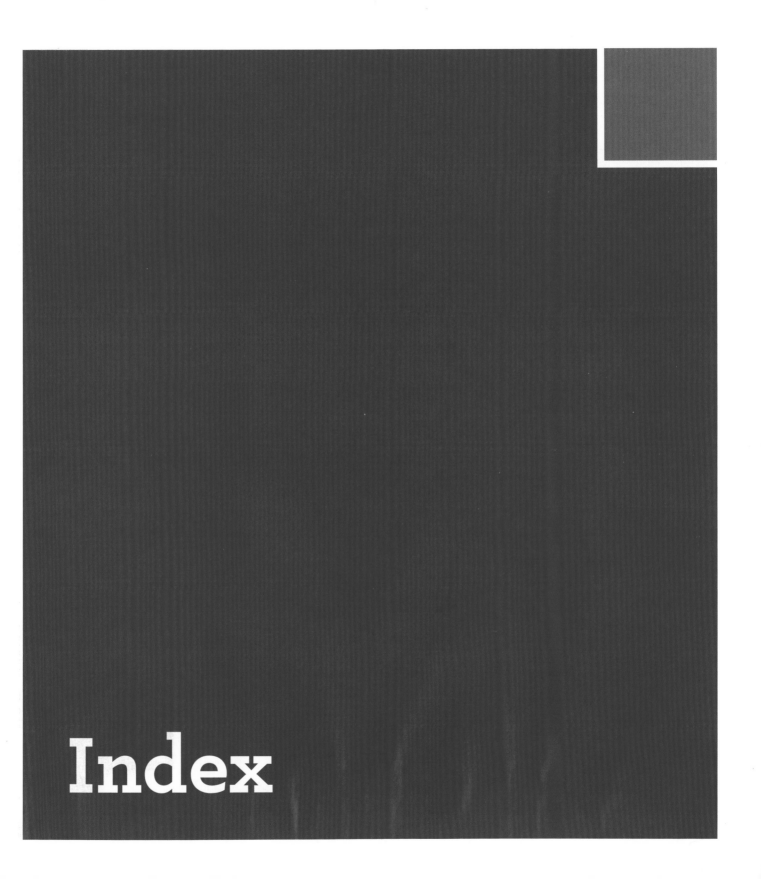

Index

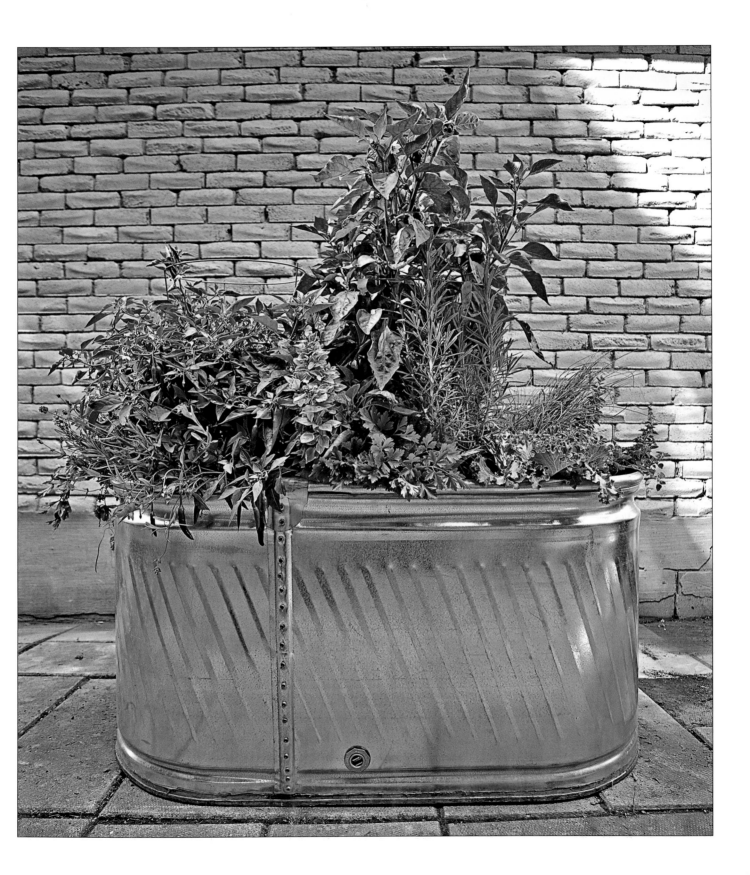

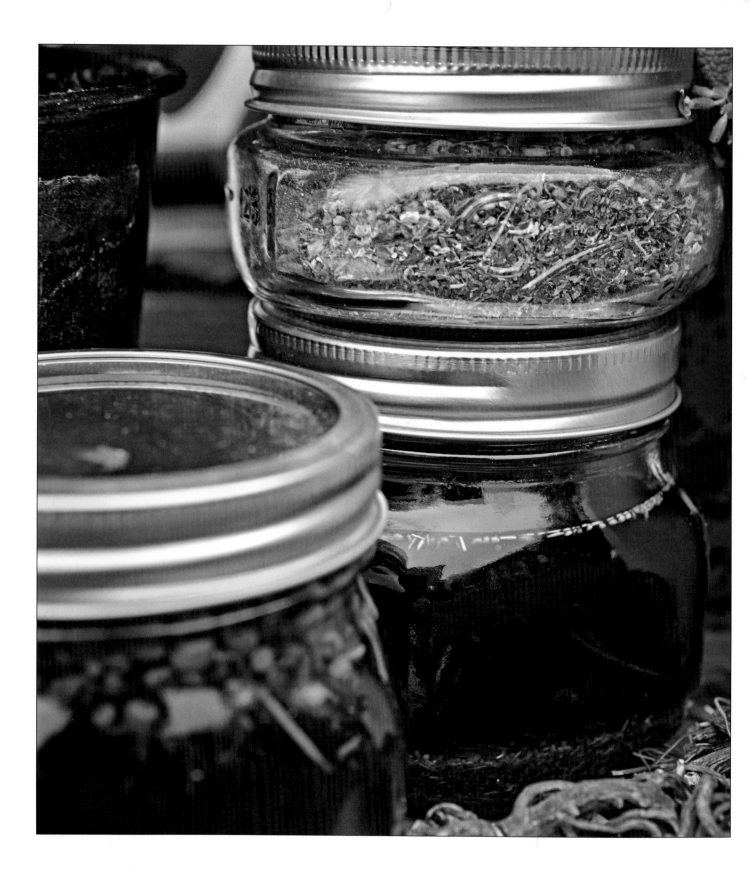

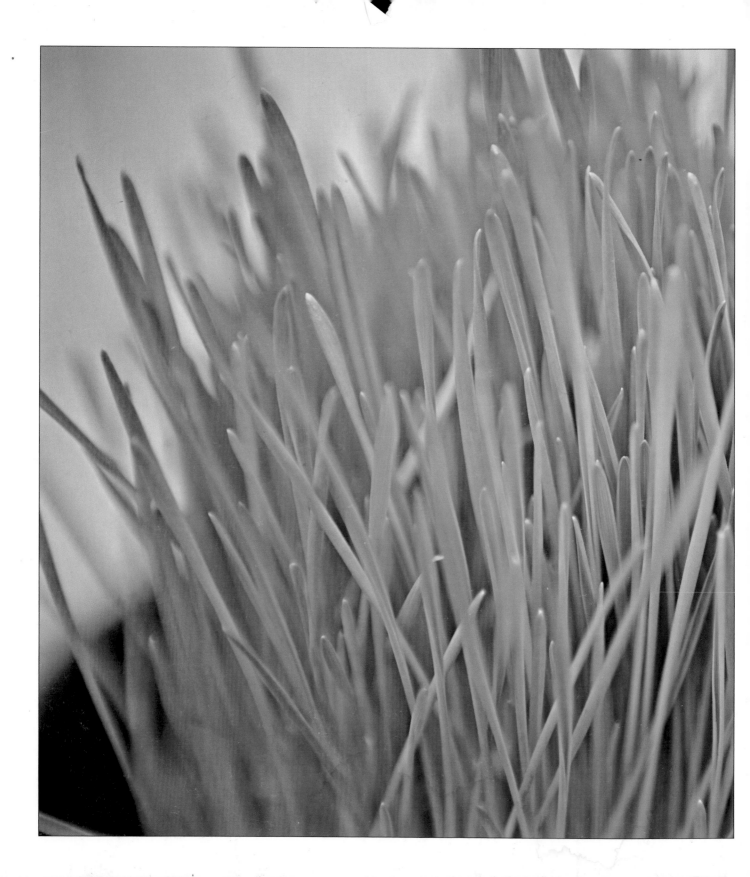